Lecture Notes in Computer Science   11045

Commenced Publication in 1973
Founding and Former Series Editors:
Gerhard Goos, Juris Hartmanis, and Jan van Leeuwen

More information about this series at http://www.springer.com/series/7412

Danail Stoyanov · Zeike Taylor
Gustavo Carneiro · Tanveer Syeda-Mahmood et al. (Eds.)

Deep Learning in Medical Image Analysis
and Multimodal Learning
for Clinical Decision Support

4th International Workshop, DLMIA 2018
and 8th International Workshop, ML-CDS 2018
Held in Conjunction with MICCAI 2018
Granada, Spain, September 20, 2018
Proceedings

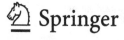 Springer

Editors
Danail Stoyanov
University College London
London
UK

Zeike Taylor
University of Leeds
Leeds
UK

Gustavo Carneiro (iD)
University of Adelaide
Adelaide, SA
Australia

Tanveer Syeda-Mahmood
IBM Research – Almaden
San Jose, CA
USA

Additional Workshop Editors *see next page*

ISSN 0302-9743   ISSN 1611-3349   (electronic)
Lecture Notes in Computer Science
ISBN 978-3-030-00888-8   ISBN 978-3-030-00889-5   (eBook)
https://doi.org/10.1007/978-3-030-00889-5

Library of Congress Control Number: 2018955639

LNCS Sublibrary: SL6 – Image Processing, Computer Vision, Pattern Recognition, and Graphics

This Springer imprint is published by the registered company Springer Nature Switzerland AG
The registered company address is: Gewerbestrasse 11, 6330 Cham, Switzerland

Additional Workshop Editors

Tutorial and Educational Chair

Anne Martel
University of Toronto
Toronto, ON
Canada

Workshop and Challenge Co-chair

Lena Maier-Hein
German Cancer Research Center (DKFZ)
Heidelberg
Germany

4th International Workshop on Deep Learning in Medical Image Analysis, DLMIA 2018

João Manuel R. S. Tavares (iD)
Universidade do Porto
Porto
Portugal

Andrew Bradley (iD)
Queensland University of Technology
Brisbane, QLD
Australia

João Paulo Papa (iD)
São Paulo State University
São Paulo
Brazil

Vasileios Belagiannis (iD)
OSRAM GmbH
Munich
Germany

Jacinto C. Nascimento (iD)
Instituto Superior Técnico
Lisboa
Portugal

Zhi Lu
ReFUEL4
Singapore
Singapore

Sailesh Conjeti
German Center for Neurodegenerative
    Diseases (DZNE)
Munich
Germany

8th International Workshop on Multimodal Learning for Clinical Decision Support, ML-CDS 2018

Mehdi Moradi
IBM Research – Almaden
San Jose, CA
USA

Hayit Greenspan
Tel Aviv University
Tel Aviv
Israel

Anant Madabhushi
Case Western Reserve University
Cleveland, OH
USA

DLMIA 2018 Preface

Welcome to the fourth edition of the MICCAI Workshop on Deep Learning in Medical Image Analysis (DLMIA). DLMIA has become one of the most successful MICCAI satellite events, with hundreds of attendees and more than 80 paper submissions in 2018. The fourth edition of DLMIA was dedicated to the presentation of papers focused on the design and use of deep learning methods in medical image analysis applications. We believe that this workshop is setting the trends and identifying the challenges of the deep learning methods in medical image analysis. Another important objective of the workshop is to continue and increase the connection between software developers, researchers, and end users from diverse fields related to medical image and signal processing, which are the main scopes of MICCAI. For the keynote talks, we invited Prof. Hayit Greenspan from Tel Aviv University, Prof. Alison Noble from the University of Oxford, and Mr. Christopher Semturs from Google Research – they represent three prominent researchers in the field of deep learning in medical image analysis. The first call of papers for the fourth DLMIA was released March 20, 2018, and the last call on June 7, 2018, with the paper deadline set to June 15, 2018. The submission site of DLMIA received 85 paper registrations, from which 77 papers turned into full paper submissions, where each submission was reviewed by between two and four reviewers. The chairs decided to select 39 out of the 77 submissions, based on the scores and comments made by the reviewers and meta-reviewers (i.e., a 50% acceptance rate). We would like to acknowledge the financial support provided by Nvidia, Hyperfine, Imsight, and Maxwell MRI for the realization of the workshop. Finally, we would like to acknowledge the support from the Australian Research Council for the realization of this workshop (discovery project DP180103232). We would also like to thank the program chair and Program Committee members of DLMIA.

September 2018

Gustavo Carneiro
João Manuel R. S. Tavares
Andrew Bradley
João Paulo Papa
Vasileios Belagiannis
Jacinto C. Nascimento
Zhi Lu
Sailesh Conjeti

ML-CDS 2018 Preface

On behalf of the organizing committee, we welcome you to the 8th Workshop on Multimodal Learning for Clinical Decision Support (ML-CDS 2018). The goal of this series of workshops is to bring together researchers in medical imaging, medical image retrieval, data mining, text retrieval, and machine learning/AI communities to discuss new techniques of multimodal mining/retrieval, and their use in clinical decision support. Although the title of the workshop has been changing slightly over the years, the common theme preserved is the notion of clinical decision support and the need for multimodal analysis. The previous seven workshops on this topic were well-received at MICCAI, specifically Quebec City (2017), Athens (2016), Munich (2015), Nagoya (2013), Nice (2012), Toronto (2011), and London (2009).

Continuing on the momentum built by these workshops, our focus remains on multimodal learning. As has been the norm with these workshops, the papers were submitted in eight-page double-blind format, and were accepted after the review. As in previous years, the program featured an invited lecture by a practicing radiologist to form a bridge between medical image interpretation and clinical informatics. This year we brought a neurologist to tell us about problems facing decision support for neurology where the modalities expand beyond diagnostic imaging to camera-grabbed imaging (monitoring epileptic patients) and electroencephalograms (EEGs). The workshop retained an oral format for all the presentations. The day ended with a lively panel composed of more doctors, medical imaging researchers, and industry experts.

With less than 5% of medical image analysis techniques translating to clinical practice, workshops on this topic have helped raise the awareness of our field to clinical practitioners. The approach taken in the workshop is to scale it to large collections of patient data exposing interesting issues of multimodal learning and its specific use in clinical decision support by practicing physicians. With the introduction of intelligent browsing and summarization methods, we hope to also address the ease-of-use in conveying derived information to clinicians to aid their adoption. Finally, the ultimate impact of these methods can be judged when they begin to affect treatment planning in clinical practice.

We hope you will enjoy the proceedings we have assembled in this volume.

September 2018

Tanveer Syeda-Mahmood
Hayit Greenspan
Anant Madabhushi
Mehdi Moradi

Organization

DLMIA 2018 Organizing Committee

Gustavo Carneiro   University of Adelaide, Australia
João Manuel R. S. Tavares   Universidade do Porto, Portugal
Andrew Bradley   Queensland University of Technology, Australia
João Paulo Papa   Universidade Estadual Paulista, Brazil
Vasileios Belagiannis   Osram, Germany
Jacinto C. Nascimento   Instituto Superior Tecnico, Portugal
Zhi Lu   Guangdong University of Technology, China

ML-CDS 2018 Program Committee

Amir Amini   University of Louisville, USA
Sameer Antani   National Library of Medicine, USA
Rivka Colen   MD Andersen Research Center, USA
Keyvan Farahani   National Cancer Institute, USA
Alejandro Franji   University of Sheffield, UK
Guido Gerig   University of Utah, USA
David Gutman   Emory University, USA
Allan Halpern   Memorial Sloan-Kettering Research Center, USA
Ghassan Hamarneh   Simon Fraser University, Canada
Jayshree Kalpathy-Kramer   Mass General Hospital, USA
Ron Kikinis   Harvard University, USA
Georg Lands   Medical University of Vienna, Austria
Robert Lundstrom   Kaiser Permanente, USA
B. Manjunath   University of California, Santa Barbara, USA
Dimitris Metaxas   Rutgers University, USA
Nikos Paragios   Ecole Centrale de Paris, France
Daniel Racoceanu   National University of Singapore, Singapore
Eduardo Romero   Universidad Nationale Colombia, Colombia
Daniel Rubin   Stanford University, USA
Russ Taylor   Johns Hopkins University, USA
Agma Traina   São Paulo University, Brazil
Max Viergewer   Utrecht University, The Netherlands
Sean Zhou   Siemens Corporate Research, USA

Contents

**8th International Workshop on Multimodal Learning
for Clinical Decision Support, ML-CDS 2018**

4th International Workshop on Deep Learning in Medical Image Analysis, DLMIA 2018

UNet++: A Nested U-Net Architecture for Medical Image Segmentation

Zongwei Zhou, Md Mahfuzur Rahman Siddiquee, Nima Tajbakhsh, and Jianming Liang[✉]

Arizona State University, Tempe, USA
{zongweiz,mrahmans,ntajbakh,jianming.liang}@asu.edu

Abstract. In this paper, we present UNet++, a new, more powerful architecture for medical image segmentation. Our architecture is essentially a deeply-supervised encoder-decoder network where the encoder and decoder sub-networks are connected through a series of nested, dense skip pathways. The re-designed skip pathways aim at reducing the semantic gap between the feature maps of the encoder and decoder sub-networks. We argue that the optimizer would deal with an easier learning task when the feature maps from the decoder and encoder networks are semantically similar. We have evaluated UNet++ in comparison with U-Net and wide U-Net architectures across multiple medical image segmentation tasks: nodule segmentation in the low-dose CT scans of chest, nuclei segmentation in the microscopy images, liver segmentation in abdominal CT scans, and polyp segmentation in colonoscopy videos. Our experiments demonstrate that UNet++ with deep supervision achieves an average IoU gain of 3.9 and 3.4 points over U-Net and wide U-Net, respectively.

1 Introduction

The state-of-the-art models for image segmentation are variants of the encoder-decoder architecture like U-Net [9] and fully convolutional network (FCN) [8]. These encoder-decoder networks used for segmentation share a key similarity: skip connections, which combine deep, semantic, coarse-grained feature maps from the decoder sub-network with shallow, low-level, fine-grained feature maps from the encoder sub-network. The skip connections have proved effective in recovering fine-grained details of the target objects; generating segmentation masks with fine details even on complex background. Skip connections is also fundamental to the success of instance-level segmentation models such as Mask-RCNN, which enables the segmentation of occluded objects. Arguably, image segmentation in natural images has reached a satisfactory level of performance, but do these models meet the strict segmentation requirements of medical images?

Segmenting lesions or abnormalities in medical images demands a higher level of accuracy than what is desired in natural images. While a precise segmentation

© Springer Nature Switzerland AG 2018
D. Stoyanov et al. (Eds.): DLMIA 2018/ML-CDS 2018, LNCS 11045, pp. 3–11, 2018.
https://doi.org/10.1007/978-3-030-00889-5_1

mask may not be critical in natural images, even marginal segmentation errors in medical images can lead to poor user experience in clinical settings. For instance, the subtle spiculation patterns around a nodule may indicate nodule malignancy; and therefore, their exclusion from the segmentation masks would lower the credibility of the model from the clinical perspective. Furthermore, inaccurate segmentation may also lead to a major change in the subsequent computer-generated diagnosis. For example, an erroneous measurement of nodule growth in longitudinal studies can result in the assignment of an incorrect Lung-RADS category to a screening patient. It is therefore desired to devise more effective image segmentation architectures that can effectively recover the fine details of the target objects in medical images.

To address the need for more accurate segmentation in medical images, we present UNet++, a new segmentation architecture based on nested and dense skip connections. The underlying hypothesis behind our architecture is that the model can more effectively capture fine-grained details of the foreground objects when high-resolution feature maps from the encoder network are gradually enriched prior to fusion with the corresponding semantically rich feature maps from the decoder network. We argue that the network would deal with an easier learning task when the feature maps from the decoder and encoder networks are semantically similar. This is in contrast to the plain skip connections commonly used in U-Net, which directly fast-forward high-resolution feature maps from the encoder to the decoder network, resulting in the fusion of semantically dissimilar feature maps. According to our experiments, the suggested architecture is effective, yielding significant performance gain over U-Net and wide U-Net.

2   Related Work

Long et al. [8] first introduced fully convolutional networks (FCN), while U-Net was introduced by Ronneberger et al. [9]. They both share a key idea: skip connections. In FCN, up-sampled feature maps are summed with feature maps skipped from the encoder, while U-Net concatenates them and add convolutions and non-linearities between each up-sampling step. The skip connections have shown to help recover the full spatial resolution at the network output, making fully convolutional methods suitable for semantic segmentation. Inspired by DenseNet architecture [5], Li et al. [7] proposed H-denseunet for liver and liver tumor segmentation. In the same spirit, Drozdzal et al. [2] systematically investigated the importance of skip connections, and introduced short skip connections within the encoder. Despite the minor differences between the above architectures, they all tend to fuse semantically dissimilar feature maps from the encoder and decoder sub-networks, which, according to our experiments, can degrade segmentation performance.

The other two recent related works are GridNet [3] and Mask-RCNN [4]. GridNet is an encoder-decoder architecture wherein the feature maps are wired in a grid fashion, generalizing several classical segmentation architectures. GridNet, however, lacks up-sampling layers between skip connections; and thus, it does not represent UNet++. Mask-RCNN is perhaps the most important meta framework for object detection, classification and segmentation. We would like to note that UNet++ can be readily deployed as the backbone architecture in Mask-RCNN by simply replacing the plain skip connections with the suggested nested dense skip pathways. Due to limited space, we were not able to include results of Mask RCNN with UNet++ as the backbone architecture; however, the interested readers can refer to the supplementary material for further details.

3   Proposed Network Architecture: UNet++

Figure 1a shows a high-level overview of the suggested architecture. As seen, UNet++ starts with an encoder sub-network or backbone followed by a decoder sub-network. What distinguishes UNet++ from U-Net (the black components in Fig. 1(a) is the re-designed skip pathways (shown in green and blue) that connect the two sub-networks and the use of deep supervision (shown red).

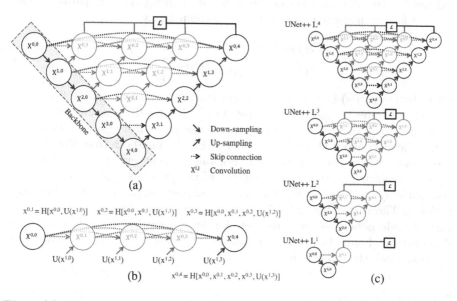

Fig. 1. (a) UNet++ consists of an encoder and decoder that are connected through a series of nested dense convolutional blocks. The main idea behind UNet++ is to bridge the semantic gap between the feature maps of the encoder and decoder prior to fusion. For example, the semantic gap between $(X^{0,0}, X^{1,3})$ is bridged using a dense convolution block with three convolution layers. In the graphical abstract, black indicates the original U-Net, green and blue show dense convolution blocks on the skip pathways, and red indicates deep supervision. Red, green, and blue components distinguish UNet++ from U-Net. (b) Detailed analysis of the first skip pathway of UNet++. (c) UNet++ can be pruned at inference time, if trained with deep supervision. (Color figure online)

3.1   Re-designed Skip Pathways

Re-designed skip pathways transform the connectivity of the encoder and decoder sub-networks. In U-Net, the feature maps of the encoder are directly received in the decoder; however, in UNet++, they undergo a dense convolution block whose number of convolution layers depends on the pyramid level. For example, the skip pathway between nodes $X^{0,0}$ and $X^{1,3}$ consists of a dense convolution block with three convolution layers where each convolution layer is preceded by a concatenation layer that fuses the output from the previous convolution layer of the same dense block with the corresponding up-sampled output of the lower dense block. Essentially, the dense convolution block brings the semantic level of the encoder feature maps closer to that of the feature maps awaiting in the decoder. The hypothesis is that the optimizer would face an easier optimization problem when the received encoder feature maps and the corresponding decoder feature maps are semantically similar.

Formally, we formulate the skip pathway as follows: let $x^{i,j}$ denote the output of node $X^{i,j}$ where i indexes the down-sampling layer along the encoder and j indexes the convolution layer of the dense block along the skip pathway. The stack of feature maps represented by $x^{i,j}$ is computed as

$$x^{i,j} = \begin{cases} \mathcal{H}\left(x^{i-1,j}\right), & j = 0 \\ \mathcal{H}\left(\left[\left[x^{i,k}\right]_{k=0}^{j-1}, \mathcal{U}(x^{i+1,j-1})\right]\right), & j > 0 \end{cases} \tag{1}$$

where function $\mathcal{H}(\cdot)$ is a convolution operation followed by an activation function, $\mathcal{U}(\cdot)$ denotes an up-sampling layer, and $[\,]$ denotes the concatenation layer. Basically, nodes at level $j = 0$ receive only one input from the previous layer of the encoder; nodes at level $j = 1$ receive two inputs, both from the encoder sub-network but at two consecutive levels; and nodes at level $j > 1$ receive $j + 1$ inputs, of which j inputs are the outputs of the previous j nodes in the same skip pathway and the last input is the up-sampled output from the lower skip pathway. The reason that all prior feature maps accumulate and arrive at the current node is because we make use of a dense convolution block along each skip pathway. Figure 1b further clarifies Eq. 1 by showing how the feature maps travel through the top skip pathway of UNet++.

3.2   Deep Supervision

We propose to use deep supervision [6] in UNet++, enabling the model to operate in two modes: (1) accurate mode wherein the outputs from all segmentation branches are averaged; (2) fast mode wherein the final segmentation map is selected from only one of the segmentation branches, the choice of which determines the extent of model pruning and speed gain. Figure 1c shows how the choice of segmentation branch in fast mode results in architectures of varying complexity.

Owing to the nested skip pathways, UNet++ generates full resolution feature maps at multiple semantic levels, $\{x^{0,j}, j \in \{1, 2, 3, 4\}\}$, which are amenable to deep supervision. We have added a combination of binary cross-entropy and dice coefficient as the loss function to each of the above four semantic levels, which is described as:

$$\mathcal{L}(Y, \hat{Y}) = -\frac{1}{N} \sum_{b=1}^{N} \left(\frac{1}{2} \cdot Y_b \cdot \log \hat{Y}_b + \frac{2 \cdot Y_b \cdot \hat{Y}_b}{Y_b + \hat{Y}_b} \right) \tag{2}$$

where $\hat{Y}_b$ and Y_b denote the flatten predicted probabilities and the flatten ground truths of bth image respectively, and N indicates the batch size.

In summary, as depicted in Fig. 1a, UNet++ differs from the original U-Net in three ways: (1) having convolution layers on skip pathways (shown in green), which bridges the semantic gap between encoder and decoder feature maps; (2) having dense skip connections on skip pathways (shown in blue), which improves gradient flow; and (3) having deep supervision (shown in red), which as will be shown in Sect. 4 enables model pruning and improves or in the worst case achieves comparable performance to using only one loss layer.

4 Experiments

Datasets: As shown in Table 1, we use four medical imaging datasets for model evaluation, covering lesions/organs from different medical imaging modalities. For further details about datasets and the corresponding data pre-processing, we refer the readers to the supplementary material.

Table 1. The image segmentation datasets used in our experiments.

Dataset	Images	Input Size	Modality	Provider
Cell nuclei	670	96×96	microscopy	Data Science Bowl 2018
Colon polyp	7,379	224×224	RGB video	ASU-Mayo [10, 11]
Liver	331	512×512	CT	MICCAI 2018 LiTS Challenge
Lung nodule	1,012	$64 \times 64 \times 64$	CT	LIDC-IDRI [1]

Baseline Models: For comparison, we used the original U-Net and a customized wide U-Net architecture. We chose U-Net because it is a common performance baseline for image segmentation. We also designed a wide U-Net with similar number of parameters as our suggested architecture. This was to ensure that the performance gain yielded by our architecture is not simply due to increased number of parameters. Table 2 details the U-Net and wide U-Net architecture.

Implementation Details: We monitored the Dice coefficient and Intersection over Union (IoU), and used *early-stop* mechanism on the validation set. We also used Adam optimizer with a learning rate of 3e−4. Architecture details for U-Net and wide U-Net are shown in Table 2. UNet++ is constructed from the

Table 2. Number of convolutional kernels in U-Net and wide U-Net.

Encoder/decoder	$X^{0,0}/X^{0,4}$	$X^{1,0}/X^{1,3}$	$X^{2,0}/X^{2,2}$	$X^{3,0}/X^{3,1}$	$X^{4,0}/X^{4,0}$
U-Net	32	64	128	256	512
Wide U-Net	35	70	140	280	560

original U-Net architecture. All convolutional layers along a skip pathway ($X^{i,j}$) use k kernels of size 3×3 (or $3 \times 3 \times 3$ for 3D lung nodule segmentation) where $k = 32 \times 2^i$. To enable deep supervision, a 1×1 convolutional layer followed by a sigmoid activation function was appended to each of the target nodes: $\{x^{0,j} \mid j \in \{1, 2, 3, 4\}\}$. As a result, UNet++ generates four segmentation maps given an input image, which will be further averaged to generate the final segmentation map. More details can be founded at github.com/Nested-UNet.

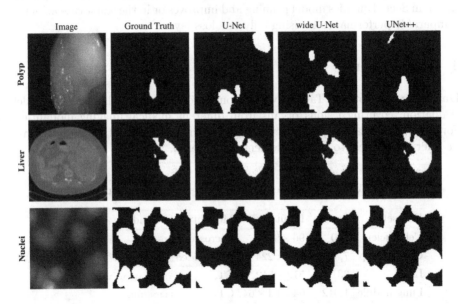

Fig. 2. Qualitative comparison between U-Net, wide U-Net, and UNet++, showing segmentation results for polyp, liver, and cell nuclei datasets (2D-only for a distinct visualization).

Results: Table 3 compares U-Net, wide U-Net, and UNet++ in terms of the number parameters and segmentation accuracy for the tasks of lung nodule segmentation, colon polyp segmentation, liver segmentation, and cell nuclei segmentation. As seen, wide U-Net consistently outperforms U-Net except for liver segmentation where the two architectures perform comparably. This improvement is attributed to the larger number of parameters in wide U-Net. UNet++ without deep supervision achieves a significant performance gain over both U-Net and wide U-Net, yielding average improvement of 2.8 and 3.3 points in

IoU. UNet++ with deep supervision exhibits average improvement of 0.6 points over UNet++ without deep supervision. Specifically, the use of deep supervision leads to marked improvement for liver and lung nodule segmentation, but such improvement vanishes for cell nuclei and colon polyp segmentation. This is because polyps and liver appear at varying scales in video frames and CT slices; and thus, a multi-scale approach using all segmentation branches (deep supervision) is essential for accurate segmen. Figure 2 shows a qualitative comparison between the results of U-Net, wide U-Net, and UNet++.

Model Pruning: Figure 3 shows segmentation performance of UNet++ after applying different levels of pruning. We use UNet++ L^i to denote UNet++ pruned at level i (see Fig. 1c for further details). As seen, UNet++ L^3 achieves on average 32.2% reduction in inference time while degrading IoU by only 0.6 points. More aggressive pruning further reduces the inference time but at the cost of significant accuracy degradation.

Table 3. Segmentation results (IoU: %) for U-Net, wide U-Net and our suggested architecture UNet++ with and without deep supervision (DS).

Architecture	Params	Dataset			
		Cell nuclei	Colon polyp	Liver	Lung nodule
U-Net [9]	7.76M	90.77	30.08	76.62	71.47
Wide U-Net	9.13M	90.92	30.14	76.58	73.38
UNet++ w/o DS	9.04M	**92.63**	**33.45**	79.70	76.44
UNet++ w/ DS	9.04M	92.52	32.12	**82.90**	**77.21**

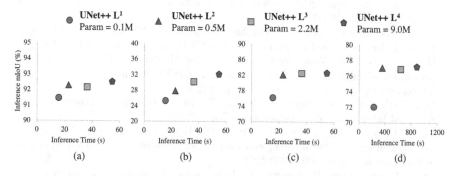

Fig. 3. Complexity, speed, and accuracy of UNet++ after pruning on (a) cell nuclei, (b) colon polyp, (c) liver, and (d) lung nodule segmentation tasks respectively. The inference time is the time taken to process **10k** test images using one NVIDIA TITAN X (Pascal) with 12 GB memory.

5   Conclusion

To address the need for more accurate medical image segmentation, we proposed UNet++. The suggested architecture takes advantage of re-designed skip pathways and deep supervision. The re-designed skip pathways aim at reducing the semantic gap between the feature maps of the encoder and decoder subnetworks, resulting in a possibly simpler optimization problem for the optimizer to solve. Deep supervision also enables more accurate segmentation particularly for lesions that appear at multiple scales such as polyps in colonoscopy videos. We evaluated UNet++ using four medical imaging datasets covering lung nodule segmentation, colon polyp segmentation, cell nuclei segmentation, and liver segmentation. Our experiments demonstrated that UNet++ with deep supervision achieved an average IoU gain of 3.9 and 3.4 points over U-Net and wide U-Net, respectively.

Acknowledgments. This research has been supported partially by NIH under Award Number R01HL128785, by ASU and Mayo Clinic through a Seed Grant and an Innovation Grant. The content is solely the responsibility of the authors and does not necessarily represent the official views of NIH.

References

1. Armato, S.G., et al.: The lung image database consortium (LIDC) and image database resource initiative (IDRI): a completed reference database of lung nodules on CT scans. Med. Phys. **38**(2), 915–931 (2011)
2. Drozdzal, M., Vorontsov, E., Chartrand, G., Kadoury, S., Pal, C.: The importance of skip connections in biomedical image segmentation. In: Carneiro, G., et al. (eds.) LABELS/DLMIA -2016. LNCS, vol. 10008, pp. 179–187. Springer, Cham (2016). https://doi.org/10.1007/978-3-319-46976-8_19
3. Fourure, D., Emonet, R., Fromont, E., Muselet, D., Tremeau, A., Wolf, C.: Residual conv-deconv grid network for semantic segmentation. arXiv preprint arXiv:1707.07958 (2017)
4. He, K., Gkioxari, G., Dollár, P., Girshick, R.: Mask R-CNN. In: 2017 IEEE International Conference on Computer Vision (ICCV), pp. 2980–2988. IEEE (2017)
5. Huang, G., Liu, Z., Weinberger, K.Q., van der Maaten, L.: Densely connected convolutional networks. In: Proceedings of the IEEE Conference on Computer Vision and Pattern Recognition, vol. 1, p. 3 (2017)
6. Lee, C.-Y., Xie, S., Gallagher, P., Zhang, Z., Tu, Z.: Deeply-supervised nets. In: Artificial Intelligence and Statistics, pp. 562–570 (2015)
7. Li, X., Chen, H., Qi, X., Dou, Q., Fu, C.-W., Heng, P.A.: H-DenseUNet: hybrid densely connected UNet for liver and liver tumor segmentation from CT volumes. arXiv preprint arXiv:1709.07330 (2017)
8. Long, J., Shelhamer, E., Darrell, T.: Fully convolutional networks for semantic segmentation. In: Proceedings of the IEEE Conference on Computer Vision and Pattern Recognition, pp. 3431–3440 (2015)
9. Ronneberger, O., Fischer, P., Brox, T.: U-Net: convolutional networks for biomedical image segmentation. In: Navab, N., Hornegger, J., Wells, W.M., Frangi, A.F. (eds.) MICCAI 2015. LNCS, vol. 9351, pp. 234–241. Springer, Cham (2015). https://doi.org/10.1007/978-3-319-24574-4_28

10. Tajbakhsh, N., et al.: Convolutional neural networks for medical image analysis: full training or fine tuning? IEEE Trans. Med. Imaging **35**(5), 1299–1312 (2016)
11. Zhou, Z., Shin, J., Zhang, L., Gurudu, S., Gotway, M., Liang, J.: Fine-tuning convolutional neural networks for biomedical image analysis: actively and incrementally. In: IEEE Conference on Computer Vision and Pattern Recognition (CVPR), pp. 7340–7351 (2017)

Deep Semi-supervised Segmentation with Weight-Averaged Consistency Targets

Christian S. Perone[1] and Julien Cohen-Adad[1,2]([envelope])

[1] NeuroPoly Lab, Institute of Biomedical Engineering, Polytechnique Montreal,
Montreal, QC, Canada
jcohen@polymtl.ca
[2] Functional Neuroimaging Unit, CRIUGM, Universite de Montreal, Montreal,
QC, Canada

Abstract. Recently proposed techniques for semi-supervised learning such as Temporal Ensembling and Mean Teacher have achieved state-of-the-art results in many important classification benchmarks. In this work, we expand the Mean Teacher approach to segmentation tasks and show that it can bring important improvements in a realistic small data regime using a publicly available multi-center dataset from the Magnetic Resonance Imaging (MRI) domain. We also devise a method to solve the problems that arise when using traditional data augmentation strategies for segmentation tasks on our new training scheme.

1 Introduction

In the past few years, we witnessed a large growth in the development of Deep Learning techniques, that surpassed human-level performance on some important tasks [1], including health domain applications [2]. A recent survey [3] that examined more than 300 papers using Deep Learning techniques in medical imaging analysis, made it clear that Deep Learning is now pervasive across the entire field. In [3], they also found that Convolutional Neural Networks (CNNs) were more prevalent in the medical imaging analysis, with end-to-end trained CNNs becoming the preferred approach.

It is also evident that Deep Learning poses unique challenges, such as the large amount of data requirement, which can be partially mitigated by using transfer learning [4] or domain adaptation approaches [5], especially in the natural imaging domain. However, in medical imaging domain, not only the image acquisition is expensive but also data annotations, that usually requires a very time-consuming dedication of experts. Besides that, other challenges are still present in the medical imaging field, such as privacy and regulations/ethical concerns, which are also an important factor impacting the data availability.

According to [3], in certain domains, the main challenge is usually not the availability of the image data itself, but the lack of relevant annotations/labeling

© Springer Nature Switzerland AG 2018
D. Stoyanov et al. (Eds.): DLMIA 2018/ML-CDS 2018, LNCS 11045, pp. 12–19, 2018.
https://doi.org/10.1007/978-3-030-00889-5_2

for these images. Traditionally, systems like Picture Archiving and Communication System (PACS) [3], used in the routine of most western hospitals, store free-text reports, and turning this textual information into accurate or structured labels can be quite challenging. Therefore, the development of techniques that could take advantage of the vast amount of unlabeled data is paramount for advancing the current state of practical applications in medical imaging.

Semi-supervised learning is a class of learning algorithms that can take leverage not only of labeled samples but also from unlabeled samples. Semi-supervised learning is halfway between supervised learning and unsupervised learning [6], where the algorithm uses limited supervision, usually only from a few samples of a dataset together with a larger amount of unlabeled data.

In this work, we propose a simple deep semi-supervised learning approach for segmentation that can be efficiently implemented. Our technique is robust enough to be incorporated in most traditional segmentation architectures since it decouples the semi-supervised training from the architectural choices. We show experimentally on a public Magnetic Resonance Imaging (MRI) dataset that this technique can take advantage of unlabeled data and provide improvements even in a realistic scenario of small data regime, a common reality in medical imaging.

2   Semi-supervised Segmentation Using Mean Teacher

Given that the classification cost for unlabeled samples is undefined in supervised learning, adding unlabeled samples into the training procedure can be quite challenging. Traditionally, there is a dataset $\mathbf{X} = (x_i)_{i \in [n]}$ that can be divided into two disjoint sets: the samples $\mathbf{X}_l = (x_1, \ldots, x_l)$ that contains the labels $\mathbf{Y}_l = (y_1, \ldots, y_l)$, and the samples $\mathbf{X}_u = (x_{l+1}, \ldots, x_{l+u})$ where the labels are unknown. However, if the knowledge available in $p(x)$ that we can get from the unlabeled data also contains information that is useful for the inference problem of $p(y|x)$, then it is evident that semi-supervised learning can improve upon supervised learning [6].

Many techniques were developed in the past for semi-supervised learning, usually creating surrogate classes as in [7], adding entropy regularization as in [8] or using Generative Adversarial Networks (GANs) [9]. More recently, other ideas also led to the development of techniques that added perturbations and extra reconstruction costs in the intermediate representations [10] of the network, yielding excellent results. A very successful method called Temporal Ensembling [11] was also recently introduced, where the authors explored the idea of a temporal ensembling network for semi-supervised learning where the predictions of multiple previous network evaluations were aggregated using an exponential moving average (EMA) with a penalization term for the predictions that were inconsistent with this target, achieving state-of-the-art results in several semi-supervised learning benchmarks.

In [12], the authors expanded the Temporal Ensembling method by averaging the model weights instead of the label predictions by using Polyak averaging

[13]. The method described in [12] is a student/teacher model, where the student model architecture is replicated into the teacher model, which in turn, get its weights updated as the exponential moving average of the student weights according to:

$$\theta'_t = \alpha\theta'_{t-1} + (1 - \alpha)\theta_t \tag{1}$$

where α is a smoothing hyperparameter, t is the training step and θ are the model weights. The goal of the student is to learn through a composite loss function with two terms: one for the traditional classification loss and another to enforce the consistency of its predictions with the teacher model. Both the student and teacher models evaluate the input data by applying noise that can come from Dropout, random affine transformations, added Gaussian noise, among others.

In this work, we extend the mean teacher technique [12] to semi-supervised segmentation. To the best of our knowledge, this is the first time that this semi-supervised method was extended for segmentation tasks. Our changes to extend the mean teacher [12] technique for segmentation are simple: we use different loss functions both for the task and consistency and also propose a new method for solving the augmentation issues that arises from this technique when used for segmentation. For the consistency loss, we use a pixel-wise binary cross-entropy, formulated as

$$C(\theta) = \mathbb{E}_{x \in \mathbf{X}} \left[-y \log(p) + (1 - y) \, log(1 - p) \right], \tag{2}$$

where $p \in [0, 1]$ is the output (after sigmoid activation) of the student model $f(x; \theta)$ and $y \in [0, 1]$ is the output prediction for the same sample from the teacher model $f(x; \theta')$, where θ and θ' are student and teacher model parameters respectively. The consistency loss can be seen as a pixel-wise knowledge distillation [14] from the teacher model. It is important to note that both labeled samples from $\mathbf{X}_l$ and unlabeled samples from $\mathbf{X}_u$ contribute for the consistency loss $C(\theta)$ calculation. We used binary cross-entropy, instead of the mean squared error (MSE) used by [12] because the binary cross-entropy provided an improved model performance for the segmentation task. We also experimented with confidence thresholding as in [15] on the teacher predictions, however, it didn't improve the results.

For the segmentation task, we employed a surrogate loss for the Dice Similarity Coefficient, called the Dice loss, which is insensitive to imbalance and was also employed by [16] on the same segmentation task domain we experiment in this paper. The Dice Loss, computed per mini-batch, is formulated as

$$L(\theta) = -\frac{2\sum_i p_i y_i}{\sum_i p_i + \sum_i y_i}, \tag{3}$$

where $p_i \in [0, 1]$ is the ith output (after sigmoid non-linearity) and $y_i \in \{0, 1\}$ is the corresponding ground truth. For the segmentation loss, only labeled samples from $\mathbf{X}_l$ contribute for the $\mathcal{L}(\theta)$ calculation. As in [12], the total loss used is the weighted sum of both segmentation and consistency losses. An overview detailing the components of the method can be seen in the Fig. 1, while a description of the training algorithm is described in the Algorithm 1.

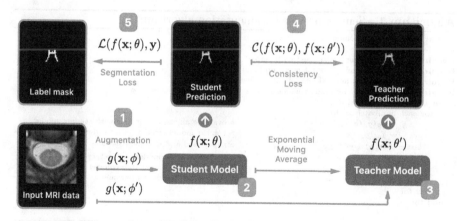

Fig. 1. An overview with the components of the proposed method based on the mean teacher technique. (1) A data augmentation procedure $g(x; \phi)$ is used to perturb the input data (in our case, a MRI axial slice), where ϕ is the data augmentation parameter (i.e. $\mathcal{N}(0, \phi)$ for a Gaussian noise), note that different augmentation parameters are used for student and teacher models. (2) The student model. (3) The teacher model that is updated with an exponential moving average (EMA) from the student weights. (4) The consistency loss used to train the student model. This consistency will enforce the consistency between student predictions on both labeled and unlabelled data according to the teacher predictions. (5) The traditional segmentation loss, where the supervision signal is provided to the student model for the labeled samples.

2.1 Segmentation Data Augmentation

In segmentation tasks, data augmentation is very important, especially in the medical imaging domain where data availability is limited, variability is high and translational equivariance is desirable. Traditional augmentation methods such as affine transformations (rotation, translation, etc.) that change the spatial content of the input data, as opposed to pixel-wise additive noise, for example, are also applied with the exact same parameters on the label to spatially align input and ground truth, both subject to a pixel-wise loss. This methodology, however, is unfeasible in the mean teacher training scheme. If two different augmentations (one for the student and another for the teacher) causes spatial misalignment, the spatial content between student and teacher predictions will not match during the pixel-wise consistency loss.

To avoid the misalignment during the consistency loss, such transformations can be applied with the same parametrization both to the student and teacher model inputs. However, this wouldn't take advantage of the stronger invariance to transformations that can be introduced through the consistency loss. For that reason, we developed a solution that applies the transformations in the teacher in a delayed fashion. Our proposed method is based on the application of the same augmentation procedure $g(x; \phi)$ before the model forward pass only for the student model, and then after model forward pass in the teacher model predictions, making thus both prediction maps aligned for the consistency loss evaluation,

---

Algorithm 1. Semi-supervised segmentation algorithm.

Require: x_i = training samples
Require: y_i = labels for the labeled inputs $i \in \mathbf{Y}_l$
Require: t = global step (initialized with zero)
Require: $w(t)$ = consistency weight ramp-up function
Require: $f_\theta(\cdot)$ = neural network model with parameters θ
Require: $g_\phi(\cdot)$ = stochastic input augmentation procedure with parameters ϕ

    for k in $[1, num\_epochs]$ **do**
        for each minibatch B **do**
            $z_{i \in B} \leftarrow f_\theta(g_\phi(x_{i \in B}))$ ▷ evaluate augmented inputs with student model
            $\tilde{z}_{i \in B} \leftarrow f_{\theta'}(g_{\phi'}(x_{i \in B}))$ ▷ teacher model evaluation w/ different perturbations
            $loss \leftarrow \mathcal{L}(z, y) + w(t)\frac{1}{|B|}\sum_{i \in B} C(z_i, \tilde{z}_i)$ ▷ supervised and unsupervised loss components
            update θ using, e.g., ADAM   ▷ update student model parameters
            $t \leftarrow t + 1$ ▷ increment the global step counter
            $\theta'_t \leftarrow \alpha\theta'_{t-1} + (1 - \alpha)\theta_t$ ▷ update teacher model parameters with using EMA
        end for
    end for

---

while still taking leverage of introducing a much stronger invariance to the augmentation between student and teacher models. This is possible because we do backpropagation of the gradients only for the student model parameters.

3 Experiments

3.1 MRI Spinal Cord Gray Matter Segmentation

In this work, in order to evaluate our technique on a realistic scenario, we use the publicly available multi-center Magnetic Resonance Imaging (MRI) Spinal Cord Gray Matter Segmentation dataset from [17].

Dataset. The dataset is comprised of 80 healthy subjects (20 subjects from each center) and obtained using different scanning parameters and also multiple MRI systems. The voxel resolution of the dataset ranges from $0.25 \times 0.25 \times 2.5$ mm up to $0.5 \times 0.5 \times 5.0$ mm. A sample of one subject axial slice image can be seen in Fig. 1. We split the dataset in a realistic small data regime: only 8 subjects are used as training samples, resulting in 86 axial training slices. We used 8 subjects for validation, resulting in 90 axial slices. For the unlabeled set we used 40 subjects, resulting in 613 axial slices and for the test set we used 12 subjects, resulting in 137 slices. All samples were resampled to a common space of 0.25×0.25 mm.

Network Architecture. To evaluate our technique, we used a very simple U-Net [18] architecture with 15 layers, Batch Normalization, Dropout and ReLU activations. U-Nets are very common in medical imaging domain, hence the architectural choice for the experiment. We also used a 2D slice-wise training procedure with axial slices.

Training Procedure. For the supervised-only baseline, we used Adam optimizer with $\beta_1 = 0.9$ and $\beta_2 = 0.999$, mini-batch size of 8, dropout rate of 0.5, Batch Normalization momentum of 0.9 and L2 penalty of $\lambda = 0.0008$. For the data augmentation, we used rotation angle between -4.5 and 4.5 and pixel-wise additive Gaussian noise sampled from $\mathcal{N}(0, 0.01)$. We used a learning rate $\eta = 0.0006$ given the small mini-batch size, also subject to a initial ramp-up of 50 epochs and subject to a cosine annealing decay as used by [12]. We trained the model for 1600 epochs.

For the semi-supervised experiment, we used the same parameters of the aforementioned supervised-only baseline, except for the L2 penalty of $\lambda = 0.0006$. We used an EMA $\alpha = 0.99$ during the first 50 epochs, later we change it to $\alpha = 0.999$. We also employed a consistency weight factor of 2.9 subject to a ramp-up in the first 100 epochs. We trained the model for 350 epochs.

Results. As we can see in Table 1, our technique not only improved the results on 5/6 evaluated metrics but also reduced the variance, showing a better regularized model in terms of precision/recall balance. The model also showed a very good improvement on overlapping metrics such as Dice and mean intersection over union (mIoU). Given that we exhausted the challenge dataset [17] to obtain the unlabeled samples, a comparison with [16] was unfeasible given different dataset splits. We leave this work for further explorations given that incorporating extra external data would also mix domain adaptation issues into the evaluation.

Table 1. Result comparison for the Spinal Cord Gray Matter segmentation challenge using our semi-supervised method and a pure supervised baseline. Results are 10 runs average with standard deviation in parenthesis where bold font represents the best result. Dice is the Dice Similarity Coefficient and mIoU is the mean intersection over union. Other metrics are self-explanatory.

	Dice	mIoU	Accuracy	Precision	Recall	Specificity
Supervised	67.915	53.679	99.745	57.948	**92.495**	99.775
	(0.313)	(0.327)	(0.005)	(0.788)	**(0.907)**	(0.010)
Semi-supervised	**70.209**	**55.509**	**99.792**	**64.732**	86.112	**99.846**
	(0.229)	**(0.253)**	**(0.003)**	**(0.773)**	(0.936)	**(0.006)**

4   Related Work

Only a few works were developed in the context of semi-supervised segmentation, especially in the field of medical imaging. Only recently, a U-Net was used as auxiliary embedding in [19], however, with focus on domain adaptation and using a private dataset.

In [20], they use a Generative Adversarial Networks (GAN) for the semi-supervised segmentation of natural images, however, they employ unrealistic dataset sizes when compared to the medical imaging domain datasets, along with ImageNet pre-trained networks.

In [21] they propose a technique using adversarial training, but they focus on the knowledge transfer between natural images with pixel-level annotation and weakly-labeled images with image-level information.

5   Conclusion

In this work we extended the semi-supervised mean teacher approach for segmentation tasks, showing that even on a realistic small data regime, this technique can provide major improvements if unlabeled data is available. We also devised a way to maintain the traditional data augmentation procedures while still taking advantage of the teacher/student regularization. The proposed technique can be used with any other Deep Learning architecture since it decouples the semi-supervised training procedure from the architectural choices.

It is evident from these results that future explorations of this technique can improve the results even further, given that even with a small amount of unlabeled samples, we showed that the technique was able to provide significant improvements.

Acknowledgements. Funded by the Canada Research Chair in Quantitative Magnetic Resonance Imaging (JCA), the Canadian Institute of Health Research [CIHR FDN-143263], the Canada Foundation for Innovation [32454, 34824], the Fonds de Recherche du Québec - Santé [28826], the Fonds de Recherche du Québec - Nature et Technologies [2015-PR-182754], the Natural Sciences and Engineering Research Council of Canada [435897-2013], IVADO, TransMedTech, the Quebec BioImaging Network and NVIDIA Corporation for the donation of a GPU.

References

1. He, K., Zhang, X., Ren, S., Sun, J.: Delving deep into rectifiers: Surpassing human-level performance on imagenet classification. In: Proceedings of the IEEE International Conference on Computer Vision, 11–18 December, pp. 1026–1034 (2016)
2. Rajpurkar, P., Hannun, A.Y., Haghpanahi, M., Bourn, C., Ng, A.Y.: Cardiologist-level arrhythmia detection with convolutional neural networks. arXiv preprint (2017)
3. Litjens, G., et al.: A survey on deep learning in medical image analysis. Med. Image Anal. **42**, 60–88 (2017)
4. Yosinski, J., Clune, J., Bengio, Y., Lipson, H.: How transferable are features in deep neural networks? In: Advances in Neural Information Processing Systems (Proceedings of NIPS), vol. 27, pp. 1–9 (2014)
5. Ganin, Y., et al.: Domain-adversarial training of neural networks. J. Mach. Learn. Res. **17**, 1–35 (2016)
6. Olivier, C., Schölkopf, B., Zien, A.: Semi-supervised learning. Interdiscip. Sci. Comput. Life Sci. **1**(2), 524 (2006)

7. Lee, D.H.: Pseudo-label: the simple and efficient semi-supervised learning method for deep neural networks. In: ICML 2013 Workshop: Challenges in Representation Learning, pp. 1–6 (2013)
8. Grandvalet, Y., Bengio, Y.: Semi-supervised learning by entropy minimization. In: Advances in Neural Information Processing Systems - NIPS 2004, vol. 17, pp. 529–536 (2004)
9. Salimans, T., Goodfellow, I., Zaremba, W., Cheung, V., Radford, A., Chen, X.: Improved techniques for training GANs (2016)
10. Rasmus, A., Valpola, H., Berglund, M.: Semi-supervised learning with ladder network, pp. 1–17 (2015). arXiv
11. Laine, S., Aila, T.: Temporal ensembling for semi-supervised learning (2016)
12. Tarvainen, A., Valpola, H.: Mean teachers are better role models: weight-averaged consistency targets improve semi-supervised deep learning results (2017)
13. Polyak, B.T., Juditsky, A.B.: Acceleration of stochastic approximation by averaging. SIAM J. Control. Optim. **30**(4), 838–855 (1992)
14. Hinton, G., Vinyals, O., Dean, J.: Distilling the knowledge in a neural network, March 2015
15. French, G., Mackiewicz, M., Fisher, M.: Self-ensembling for domain adaptation, pp. 1–15 (2017)
16. Perone, C.S., Calabrese, E., Cohen-Adad, J.: Spinal cord gray matter segmentation using deep dilated convolutions, October 2017
17. Prados, F., et al.: Spinal cord grey matter segmentation challenge. NeuroImage **152**, 312–329 (2017)
18. Ronneberger, O., Fischer, P., Brox, T.: U-Net: convolutional networks for biomedical image segmentation. In: Navab, N., Hornegger, J., Wells, W.M., Frangi, A.F. (eds.) MICCAI 2015. LNCS, vol. 9351, pp. 234–241. Springer, Cham (2015). https://doi.org/10.1007/978-3-319-24574-4_28
19. Baur, C., Albarqouni, S., Navab, N.: Semi-supervised deep learning for fully convolutional networks. In: Descoteaux, M., Maier-Hein, L., Franz, A., Jannin, P., Collins, D.L., Duchesne, S. (eds.) MICCAI 2017. LNCS, vol. 10435, pp. 311–319. Springer, Cham (2017). https://doi.org/10.1007/978-3-319-66179-7_36
20. Souly, N., Spampinato, C., Shah, M.: Semi supervised semantic segmentation using generative adversarial network. In: 2017 IEEE International Conference on Computer Vision (ICCV), pp. 5689–5697. IEEE, October 2017
21. Xiao, H., Wei, Y., Liu, Y., Zhang, M., Feng, J.: Transferable semi-supervised semantic segmentation (2017)

Handling Missing Annotations
for Semantic Segmentation
with Deep ConvNets

Olivier Petit[1,2(✉)], Nicolas Thome[1], Arnaud Charnoz[2], Alexandre Hostettler[3], and Luc Soler[2,3]

[1] CEDRIC - Conservatoire National des Arts et Metiers, Paris, France
olivier.petit@visiblepatient.com
[2] Visible Patient SAS, Strasbourg, France
[3] IRCAD, Strasbourg, France

Abstract. Annotation of medical images for semantic segmentation is a very time consuming and difficult task. Moreover, clinical experts often focus on specific anatomical structures and thus, produce partially annotated images. In this paper, we introduce SMILE, a new deep convolutional neural network which addresses the issue of learning with incomplete ground truth. SMILE aims to identify ambiguous labels in order to ignore them during training, and don't propagate incorrect or noisy information. A second contribution is SMILEr which uses SMILE as initialization for automatically relabeling missing annotations, using a curriculum strategy. Experiments on 3 organ classes (liver, stomach, pancreas) show the relevance of the proposed approach for semantic segmentation: with 70% of missing annotations, SMILEr performs similarly as a baseline trained with complete ground truth annotations.

Keywords: Medical images · Deep learning
Convolutional Neural Networks · Incomplete ground truth annotation
Noisy labels · Missing labels

1 Introduction

Fully automatic semantic segmentation of medical images is a major challenge. Over the last few years, Deep Learning and Convolutional Neural Networks (ConvNets) have reached outstanding performances on various visual recognition tasks [9]. Regarding semantic segmentation on natural images, state-of-the-art performances are currently obtained with Fully Convolutional Neural Networks (FCNs) [1,3]. Consequently, several attempts have been made to apply those methods on medical images [11,15,16]. In challenges like Liver Tumor Segmentation Challenge (LiTS), leading methods are based on FCNs [5,10].

Electronic supplementary material The online version of this chapter (https://doi.org/10.1007/978-3-030-00889-5_3) contains supplementary material, which is available to authorized users.

© Springer Nature Switzerland AG 2018
D. Stoyanov et al. (Eds.): DLMIA 2018/ML-CDS 2018, LNCS 11045, pp. 20–28, 2018.
https://doi.org/10.1007/978-3-030-00889-5_3

However, training deep ConvNets requires large amount of data with clean annotations. The annotation process is an extremely time consuming task for semantic segmentation, which requires pixel-level labeling. This challenge is amplified in the medical field, where highly qualified professionals are needed. In this paper, we focus on abdomen 3D CT-scans from an internal dataset with more than 1000 patients, each volume containing about a hundred of 512×512 images. The segmentation masks have been realized by clinical experts but they have focused on specific organs or anatomical structures, *e.g.* liver pathologies. As a consequence, the collected labels intrinsically contain missing annotations, as illustrated in Fig. 1.

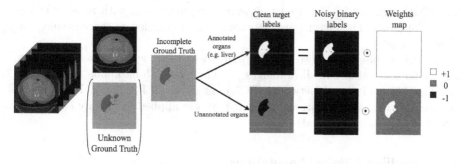

Fig. 1. Our 3D CT-scan dataset is labeled by clinical experts who focused on certain organ pathologies, *e.g.* liver. The ground truth annotations are therefore incomplete. We define ambiguity maps to train binary class predictors, which ignore incorrect background labels.

Several learning methodologies can be used to address the aforementioned missing annotations issue. Weakly Supervised Learning (WSL) can be used to leverage coarse annotations, *e.g.* global image or volume labels. WSL is generally closely connected to Multiple Instance Learning [4], and has been used for WSL segmentation of natural images [13,14] and medical data [7]. However, performing pixel-wise prediction from global labels is known to be a challenging task, making WSL approaches generally substantially inferior to their fully supervised counterparts. Since missing annotations are incorporated to background pixel classes, another option to address this problem is to design models able to incorporate noisy labels, which have been recently applied for semantic segmentation [8,12]. Although interesting, most of these methods rely on the assumption that the ratio of noisy labels remains relatively low, whereas more than 50% of the organs are commonly missing in our context.

In this paper, we introduce SMILE, a new method for Semantic segmentation with MIssing Labels and ConvNEts. Firstly, we design a learning scheme which converts the segmentation of K organ classes into K binary problems, and we define ambiguity maps which allow to train the model with 100% of clean labels (see Fig. 1), while retaining a largely sufficient number of negative samples. The model trained at this first stage is then used for automatically predicting labels for missing organs, using a Curriculum strategy [2] (SMILEr). We perform extensive experiments in an sub-set of our dataset for the segmentation of three organ classes: liver, pancreas and stomach. We show that our approach significantly outperform a strong FCN baseline based on Deeplab [3], especially when the number of missing is large. The final model (SMILEr) trained with only 30% of present organs performs similarly to a baseline trained with complete ground truth annotations.

2   SMILE Model

The SMILE model is dedicated to semantic segmentation with missing labels using ConvNets. The missing organ annotations are labeled as "background", as shown in Fig. 1.

SMILE is based on the strong DeepLab baseline [3], which shows impressive results for natural and medical images [5]. The DeepLab backbone architecture is a Fully Convolutional Networks (FCN), as shown in Fig. 2, *e.g.* Res-Net [6]. In DeepLab, 1×1 convolutions and soft-max are applied to classify each pixel into K (+1, *i.e.* background) classes.

2.1   Handling Missing Annotations

In our context, the main limitation of DeepLab is that background labels sometimes correspond to missing organs. Therefore, back-propagating these background labels may damage training performances by conflicting with pixels where the organ is properly annotated.

SMILE Architecture. To address this problem, we choose to start from the $(K+1)$ multi-class classification formulation, and to classify each organ independently using K binary classifiers. The SMILE architecture is shown in Fig. 2. We use 1×1 convolutions, as in DeepLab, but we apply a sigmoid activation function to predict the presence/absence of an organ at each pixel.

SMILE Training. During training, the K binary models generate K losses at each pixel by computing the binary cross entropy: $L_k(\hat{y}_k, y_k^*) = -(y_k^* \, log(\hat{y}_k) + (1-y_k^*) \, log(1-\hat{y}_k))$. The final loss aggregates these K losses through summation:

$$L(\hat{y}, y^*) = \sum_{k=1}^{K} w_k \, L_k(\hat{y}_k, y_k^*) \tag{1}$$

where $w_k \in \{0; 1\}$ is a binary weight map which select or ignore pixels for class k.

The w_k weights are the core of the SMILE model, which are used to ignore ambiguous annotations during training. We illustrate the rationale of our approach in Fig. 2. We consider a volume where only one organ is annotated. In the baseline DeepLab model, pixels for the other organs in each slice are incorrectly labeled as background, and back-propagated consequently. Contrarily, with SMILE, we only back-propagate labels which are certain. In this example, we can back-propagating positive/negative labels for the annotated organ at every pixels p: we thus have $w_a = 1 \forall p$. On the other hand, for unannotated organs, we only use pixels which are certainly not belonging to the given class for training the binary classifier: $w_u = 1$ for all pixels of the annotated organs. Other pixels are ignored during training, $i.e.$ $w_u = 0$.

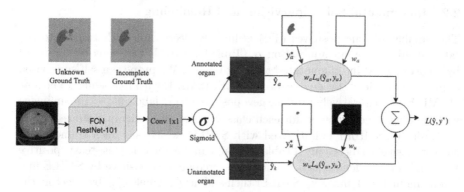

Fig. 2. SMILE architecture and training. The presence of an organ at each pixel is determined by using K independent binary classifiers. During training, a weight w_k for each class enables to ignore ambiguous pixels.

The idea behind SMILE is to only use true positive and true negative labels during training. To formalize this, we consider a given organ class k with its associated binary classification problem. We denote as β_k the ratio of pixels for the organ in all volumes of image slices, and α the ratio of missing labels for this organ in the dataset. Table 1 shows the confusion matrix for the labels used by SMILE and the DeepLab baseline. We can see that they both use the same amount of true positives: $TP = (1 - \alpha) \cdot \beta_k$. For negative examples, however, the baseline uses $FN = \alpha \cdot \beta_k$ false negatives, $i.e.$ the amount of unannotated pixels belonging to the organ. The ratio $\frac{TP}{FN} = \frac{1-\alpha}{\alpha}$ gives a good indication on the influence of the wrong information: with $\alpha > 0.5$, $\frac{TP}{FN} < 1$, which means that the model incorporates more wrong labels than correct ones, dramatically deteriorating its performances.

On the other hand, the baseline learns with more true negatives $(1 - \beta_k)$ than SMILE $(1 - \alpha)(1 - \beta_k) + \epsilon$, where $\epsilon = \sum_{k' \neq k} \beta_{k'}$ corresponds to the other organ labels (see Fig. 2). However, we take advantage on the class unbalance: generally $\beta << 1$, $e.g.$ $\beta = 0.05$, since the organs represent a small proportion of the total volume. As a consequence, even if we remove some background examples, we still have largely enough information to learn it properly.

Table 1. Training label analysis. GT: Ground Truth

(a) Baseline FCN   (b) SMILE

GT \ Used	Pos	Neg
Pos	$(1-\alpha)\cdot\beta_k$	$\alpha\cdot\beta_k$
Neg	0	$1-\beta_k$

GT \ Used	Pos	Neg
Pos	$(1-\alpha)\cdot\beta_k$	0
Neg	0	$(1-\alpha)\cdot(1-\beta_k)+\epsilon$

2.2 Incremental Self-supervision and Relabeling

The number of true positives (TP) is linearly decreasing with respect to the ratio of missing organ annotation α (Table 1). SMILE can thus be improved by recovering TP in unannotated training images. We propose a self-supervised approach to achieve this goal, called SMILEr (SMILE with relabeling). The idea of SMILEr is to iteratively produce new positive target labels $y_{i,t}^* = 1$ in an image with missing annotations $\mathbf{x}_i$ for each class k^1, using a curriculum strategy [2].

Basically, SMILEr is initialized with SMILE, which has been trained with correct positive labels only (Table 1) that can be regarded as "easy positive samples". Let us denote as $\hat{y}_i^+$, the pixels predicted as positive by SMILE in a given unannotated image $\mathbf{x}_i$. SMILEr then add new $\oplus$ labels $y_{i,t}^{*,+}$ by selecting the top scoring pixels among $\hat{y}_i^+$. The model is then retrained with the augmented training set, and the process is iterated T times, by selecting an increasing ratio $\gamma_t = \frac{t}{T}\gamma_{max}$ of top scoring pixels among positives.

The new $\oplus$ labels $y_{i,t}^*$ incorporated at each curriculum iteration are "harder examples", since they are incrementally determined by the model trained with an increased set of auto-supervised positives.

3   Experiments and Results

We perform experiments on a subset of our dataset with complete ground truth annotations for three organs: liver, pancreas and stomach, which gathers 72 3D volume CT-scans. We generate a partially annotated dataset by randomly removing $\alpha\%$ of organs in the volumes independently.

Quantitative Evaluations. We compare our approach to the DeepLab baseline [3] with a varying ratio of missing annotations α. We randomly split training (80%) and testing (20%) data K times, and report averages and standard deviations of Dice scores over the K runs. For SMILEr, we fix $T = 2$ and $\gamma_{max} = 0.66$.

Figure 3 shows the results for the baseline, SMILE and SMILEr, for each organ and on average. As expected, the maximum scores are reached when 100% of the annotations are kept, *i.e.* $\alpha = 0$. When α increases, the performances of the baseline dramatically drop, whereas our approach continues to perform well.

---

[1] We drop the dependence of class in $y_{i,t}^*$ for clarity.

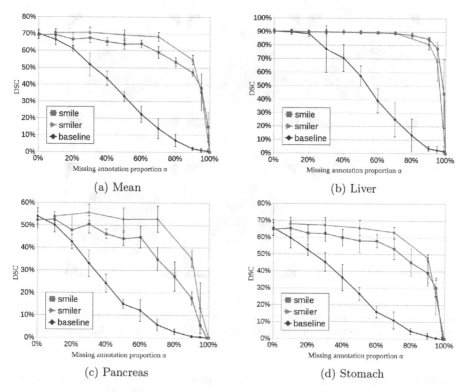

Fig. 3. Dice score versus the proportion of missing annotations α. The baseline is represented in blue, SMILE in red and SMILEr in green. (Color figure online)

For example, SMILE performs similarly as the method trained with complete annotations with $\alpha = 40\%$, whereas the baseline performance is decreased by about 20 points. The gain is even more pronounced for SMILEr which results are comparable to the fully annotated method for $\alpha = 70\%$, whereas the baseline performs very poorly in this regime.

SMILEr Analysis. Figure 3 highlights the fact that the Dice score is better when the organ is bigger. Regarding SMILEr, we can observe that its improvement is especially pronounced for small organs, see for example the large performance boost for pancreas and stomach.

Figure 4 shows how the training evolves during the $T = 3$ curriculum iterations of SMILEr, and with $\gamma_{max} = 1$. At $t = 0$, we show the segmentation of SMILE, blue pixels indicating the new positive labels added for training for the next step. We can see how the segmentation is refined and is nearly perfect at $\gamma_2 = 0.66$ ($t = 2$). It is also interesting to see how the model tends to over predict some labels at $\gamma_3 = 1.0$.

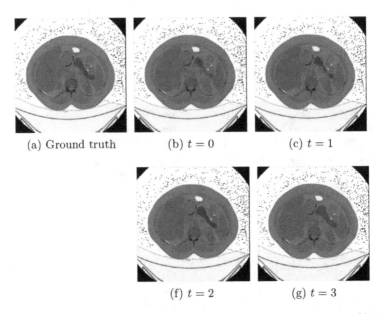

(a) Ground truth   (b) $t = 0$ (c) $t = 1$

(f) $t = 2$ (g) $t = 3$

Fig. 4. SMILEr behaviour with $T = 3$ iterations, $\gamma_{max} = 1.0$ and $\alpha = 50\%$. SMILEr prediction in red, selected $\oplus$ pixels for the next iteration in blue. (Color figure online)

Finally, we give in Fig. 5 the final segmentation for the three organ classes in a test image, for SMILEr and the baseline, at $\alpha = 70\%$. We can notice the incapacity of the baseline, whereas SMILEr successfully segments all organs.

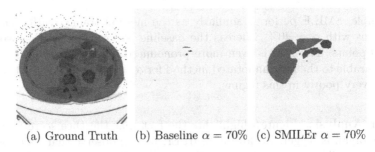

(a) Ground Truth   (b) Baseline $\alpha = 70\%$ (c) SMILEr $\alpha = 70\%$

Fig. 5. Segmentation results for the baseline and SMILEr, with $\alpha = 70\%$. The liver is in blue, the pancreas in red and the stomach in green. (Colou figure online)

4   Conclusions

We introduce a new model, SMILE, dedicated to semantic segmentation with incomplete ground truth. SMILE is based on the use of certain labels for training a first model, which is lately used to incrementally re-label positive pixels.

Experiments show that SMILE can achieve comparable performances to a model trained with complete annotations with only 30% of labels. Future works are the application of SMILE to other organ classes, and the incorporation of uncertainty for selecting the target pixels labels in our curriculum approach.

References

1. Badrinarayanan, V., Kendall, A., Cipolla, R.: SegNet: a deep convolutional encoder-decoder architecture for image segmentation. IEEE Trans. Pattern Anal. Mach. Intell. (2017)
2. Bengio, Y., Louradour, J., Collobert, R., Weston, J.: Curriculum learning. In: Proceedings of the 26th Annual International Conference on Machine Learning, ICML 2009, pp. 41–48 (2009)
3. Chen, L., Papandreou, G., Kokkinos, I., Murphy, K., Yuille, A.L.: Deeplab: semantic image segmentation with deep convolutional nets, atrous convolution, and fully connected CRFs. IEEE Trans. Pattern Anal. Mach. Intell. **40**(4), 834–848 (2018)
4. Dietterich, T.G., Lathrop, R.H., Lozano-Pérez, T.: Solving the multiple instance problem with axis-parallel rectangles. Artif. Intell. **89**(1–2), 31–71 (1997)
5. Han, X.: Automatic liver lesion segmentation using a deep convolutional neural network method. CoRR abs/1704.07239 (2017)
6. He, K., Zhang, X., Ren, S., Sun, J.: Deep residual learning for image recognition. In: 2016 IEEE Conference on Computer Vision and Pattern Recognition, CVPR 2016, Las Vegas, NV, USA, 27–30 June 2016, pp. 770–778 (2016)
7. Hwang, S., Kim, H.-E.: Self-transfer learning for weakly supervised lesion localization. In: Ourselin, S., Joskowicz, L., Sabuncu, M.R., Unal, G., Wells, W. (eds.) MICCAI 2016. LNCS, vol. 9901, pp. 239–246. Springer, Cham (2016). https://doi.org/10.1007/978-3-319-46723-8_28
8. Kraus, O.Z., Ba, L.J., Frey, B.J.: Classifying and segmenting microscopy images with deep multiple instance learning. Bioinformatics **32**(12), 52–59 (2016)
9. Krizhevsky, A., Sutskever, I., Hinton, G.E.: Imagenet classification with deep convolutional neural networks. In: Advances in Neural Information Processing Systems, pp. 1097–1105 (2012)
10. Li, X., Chen, H., Qi, X., Dou, Q., Fu, C., Heng, P.: H-DenseUNet: hybrid densely connected UNet for liver and liver tumor segmentation from CT volumes. CoRR abs/1709.07330 (2017)
11. Liu, H., Feng, J., Feng, Z., Lu, J., Zhou, J.: Left atrium segmentation in CT volumes with fully convolutional networks. In: Cardoso, M.J., et al. (eds.) DLMIA/ML-CDS -2017. LNCS, vol. 10553, pp. 39–46. Springer, Cham (2017). https://doi.org/10.1007/978-3-319-67558-9_5
12. Lu, Z., Fu, Z., Xiang, T., Han, P., Wang, L., Gao, X.: Learning from weak and noisy labels for semantic segmentation. IEEE Trans. Pattern Anal. Mach. Intell. **39**(3), 486–500 (2017)
13. Mordan, T., Durand, T., Thome, N., Cord, M.: WILDCAT: weakly supervised learning of deep ConvNets for image classification, localization and segmentation. In: Computer Vision and Pattern Recognition (CVPR) (2017)
14. Oquab, M., Bottou, L., Laptev, I., Sivic, J.: Is object localization for free? Weakly-supervised learning with convolutional neural networks. In: CVPR (2015)

15. Ronneberger, O., Fischer, P., Brox, T.: U-Net: convolutional networks for biomedical image segmentation. In: Navab, N., Hornegger, J., Wells, W.M., Frangi, A.F. (eds.) MICCAI 2015. LNCS, vol. 9351, pp. 234–241. Springer, Cham (2015). https://doi.org/10.1007/978-3-319-24574-4_28
16. Trullo, R., Petitjean, C., Nie, D., Shen, D., Ruan, S.: Joint segmentation of multiple thoracic organs in CT images with two collaborative deep architectures. In: Cardoso, M.J., et al. (eds.) DLMIA/ML-CDS -2017. LNCS, vol. 10553, pp. 21–29. Springer, Cham (2017). https://doi.org/10.1007/978-3-319-67558-9_3

A Unified Framework Integrating Recurrent Fully-Convolutional Networks and Optical Flow for Segmentation of the Left Ventricle in Echocardiography Data

Mohammad H. Jafari[1(✉)], Hany Girgis[1,2], Zhibin Liao[1], Delaram Behnami[1], Amir Abdi[1], Hooman Vaseli[1], Christina Luong[1,2], Robert Rohling[1], Ken Gin[1,2], Terasa Tsang[1,2], and Purang Abolmaesumi[1]

[1] University of British Columbia, Vancouver, Canada
mohammadj@ece.ubc.ca
[2] Vancouver General Hospital, Vancouver, Canada

Abstract. Accurate segmentation of left ventricle (LV) from echocardiograms is a key step toward diagnosis of cardiovascular diseases. Manual segmentation of the LV done by sonographers or cardiologists can be time-consuming, and its accuracy is subjective to the operator's experience and skill level. Automation of LV segmentation is a challenging task due to a number of factors such as the presence of speckle and a high operator-dependent variability in acquiring echocardiography data. In this paper, we present a method that integrates deep recurrent fully-convolutional networks and optical flow estimation to accurately segment the LV in the apical four-chamber (A4C) view. Our method analyzes the temporal information in echocardiogram cines with the use of convolutional bi-directional long short-term memory units. Furthermore, it uses optical flow motion estimation between consecutive frames to improve the segmentation accuracy. The proposed method is evaluated over an echo cine dataset of 566 patients. Experiments show that the proposed system can reach a noticeably high mean accuracy of 97.9%, and mean Dice score of 92.7% for LV segmentation in A4C view.

Keywords: Fully convolutional network · Recurrent neural network
Convolutional bi-directional LSTM · Deep learning
Video segmentation · Left ventricle segmentation · Echocardiography

1 Introduction

Cardiovascular disease is the foremost cause of mortality worldwide, resulting in an estimated 17.7 million deaths annually [1]. Assessment of left ventricle (LV) function is considered as a key metric to determine the risk of heart disease.

H. Girgis—Joint first authors.

T.Tsang and P. Abolmaesumi—Joint senior authors.

© Springer Nature Switzerland AG 2018
D. Stoyanov et al. (Eds.): DLMIA 2018/ML-CDS 2018, LNCS 11045, pp. 29–37, 2018.
https://doi.org/10.1007/978-3-030-00889-5_4

Echocardiography (echo) is an imaging technique that is often used to inspect cardiovascular function. Segmentation of the LV in echo images is used to derive clinically important measurements such as LV ejection fraction (EF) estimation and wall motion abnormality detection [10]. In particular, the current clinical practice of LV EF estimation requires an expert to manually trace the endocardial border of LV on both end-diastole (ED) and end-systole (ES) frames of an echo cine clip. However, manual LV segmentation is a laborious procedure and its accuracy is often dependent on the operator's experience, resulting in a low test-retest reliability [3].

A number of research groups have attempted to automate the segmentation of LV in echo and also other modalities [3,4,9,11,14,18]. Methods to-date can be categorized into active contour models, deformable templates, level sets, and supervised learning approaches [3,10]. Specifically, in recent years, deep learning [7] has been proposed for segmentation and quantification of LV in computed tomography (CT) and cardiac magnetic resonance imaging (CMR) [9,17,18]. For CT images, Zreik et al. [18] propose a two stage LV segmentation method, where the first stage detects a bounding box containing LV by using Convolutional Neural Networks (CNN), and the second stage performs LV segmentation by using voxel classification within the bounding box. An extensive literature review of methods for LV segmentation in CMR is presented in [9,17]. Specifically, Ngo et al. propose a level-set model, initialized by LV map obtained from a first deep belief network (DBN), and constrained by the location of endocardial and epicardial borders computed by a second DBN. Xue et al. [17] propose a deep network model to quantify LV measurements in CMR as a multi-task relationship learning. In [17], features extracted from cardiac cine using CNNs are fed into two branches of recurrent neural networks, one combined with a Bayesian-based multi-task relationship module for LV quantification, and another branch is ended with a softmax layer to detect the cardiac phase. Most recently, several works investigated deep learning for LV segmentation in echo [4,11,14]. In [11], anatomical priors based on the heart structure are used to regularize training of a deep network for segmentation of LV in 3D ultrasound. Also the works of [4,14] propose to use U-Net and its variations [13] for per frame segmentation of LV in echo cine.

Temporal information encoding is a key research problem in video analysis. Various methods in computer vision have shown that by combining temporal information with shape features, using tools such as recurrent neural networks and optical flow maps, the accuracy of video classification [8], segmentation [16], and interpretation [6] can be improved. Recently, in the area of medical imaging, adaptation of recurrent fully convolutional neural networks have shown promising results for detection of measurement points in echo [15], segmentation of the heart in CMR [12], and 3D biomedical image segmentation [5].

In this paper, we present a deep learning architecture for automatic segmentation of the LV from an entire echo cine. The individual frames of a cardiac echo cine are first processed by a U-Net encoder. The encoded temporal dependency information of the past frames are maintained via stacked bidirectional convolutional LSTM. Furthermore, temporal displacement information of moving objects between the consecutive frames is provided to the network by externally computed optical flow motion vectors. During the training phase, our method only requires LV annotation in ES and ED frames. Therefore, our architecture can be easily trained on most clinically obtained patient data without providing annotation beyond those that are normally recorded as part of standard-of-care in echo. In the test phase, our method can be used to infer accurate LV segmentation for the entire cine loop. Our method is quantitatively evaluated on an echo cine dataset consisting of 648 A4C echo cines that were gathered from 566 patients. We demonstrate that the proposed method can achieve a noticeably high segmentation accuracy of 97.9% with standard deviation of less than 1%.

2   Materials and Method

2.1   Dataset Information and Clinical Background

Our echo imaging data is collected from the Picture Archiving and Communication System at Vancouver General Hospital, with ethics approval of the Clinical Medical Research Ethics Board, in consultation with the Information Privacy Office. Our data consist of a collection of 648 A4C view echo studies from 566 patients, with about 34,000 total number of frames, captured by using Philips iE33 and GE Vivid-i/-7 ultrasound machines. In clinical practice, A4C is one of the primary standard views for LV EF estimation and other cardiac functions analyses. Each study was performed by an expert sonographer, where the LV boundary is traced in two frames (*i.e.*, ED and ES phase frames). The ED phase refers to the cardiac structure at the end of relaxing, *i.e.*, the end of ventricle loading, and the ES phase refers to the cardiac structure at the end of contraction, *i.e.*, the beginning of ventricle filling, respectively. We consider existing annotations at ED and ES phase as ground truth to train our model. In order to evaluate the performance of the model on the entire cine, we sought assistance from an experienced cardiologist, who helped us with annotation of a randomly selected frame between ED and ES frame in our test set. The cardiologist also validated our existing annotation of ED and ES frames by sonographers. An example of sample frames in our dataset and the corresponding cardiologist's annotation of LV segmentation is shown in Fig. 1.

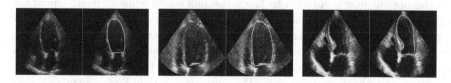

Fig. 1. Examples of sample frames and corresponding annotations.

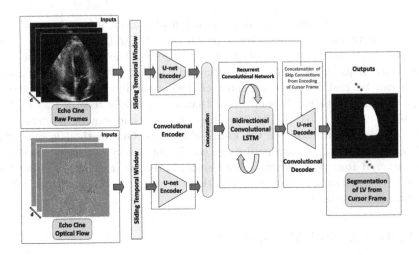

Fig. 2. Block diagram of the proposed architecture to integrate shape, temporal and motion information for LV segmentation in echo cine.

2.2 Network Architecture

The proposed LV segmentation architecture is depicted in Fig. 2, where the individual components of the pipeline are explained below.

Temporal Window: In the first stage, we define a collection of d consecutive frames as a temporal window. This set is fed to the network and the final output would be the segmentation mask of the last frame in the window. The last frame in the temporal window is called the "cursor" frame. The segmentation prediction of the entire cine can be obtained by sliding the model over the temporal dimension, with $stride = 1$.

U-Net Encoder: In the next stage of the network, we use U-Net's [13] encoder schema to process the input echo frames. More specifically, each frame is passed through a number of stacked convolutional layers and pooling layers. A dense representation of the per-frame encoded features is obtained by the end of the encoding stage.

Optical Flow Integration: A second U-Net encoder model is used to process the optical flow motion vector maps between each pair of consecutive frames. We use the optical flow algorithm to track the motion of walls of heart chambers, providing the network with additional information for deriving segmentation. In our method, optical flow is calculated between each two consecutive frames in a temporal window with the use of Horn-Schunck algorithm [2]. Each optical flow input to the network is a two-channel image, showing the direction and distance of movement in both x and y axes. The processed optical flow information goes though a separate U-Net encoder, which is then concatenated with the intensity image encoded representation. Since the speckle motion of background tissue has a much lower velocity than the heart muscle motion, the motion of background tissue can be filtered out by convolutional layers in the U-Net encoder model.

Convolutional LSTM: In the third stage, the concatenated features from echo frames intensity information and optical flow maps are processed by a stack of two convolutional bi-directional recurrent long short term memory (Bi-directional LSTM) layers. Our intention of using convolutional Bi-directional LSTM comes in two-fold: (1) Bi-directional LSTM does not only encode temporal feature from the past context but also from the future context, which has been observed to handle noisy data well in speech recognition, thus making it a good candidate to handle noisy echo data; (2) the convolutional implementation of recurrent neural networks can capture spatio-temporal correlation better than conventional fully-connected recurrent neural networks, which based on our experiments, can be beneficial to localize the segmentation prediction.

U-Net Decoder: During the decoding stage, the representation generated from the Bi-directional LSTM is fed through a pipeline of up-sampling layers in order to obtain the final prediction of segmentation mask, where the architecture of the up-sampling layers is in the reverse order of the U-Net encoder architecture. The skip connections by-pass layers to connect an encoder feature map with corresponding decoder feature map of the same size. In each slide of the temporal window over echo clip, the output segmentation map corresponds to the LV location in the last frame of the temporal window.

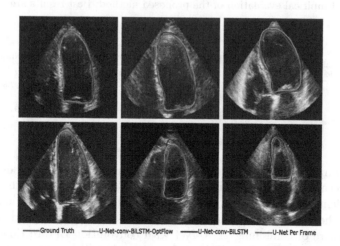

———Ground Truth   ———U-Net-conv-BiLSTM-OptFlow   ———U-Net-conv-BiLSTM   ———U-Net Per Frame

Fig. 3. Example LV segmentation results on six different subjects.

3   Experiments

The echo studies of the 566 patients are randomly assigned into training and test sets, with a split ratio of 80% and 20% of total amount of patients, respectively. This results in 453 patients (with 520 echo studies) in the training set and remaining 113 patients (with 128 echo studies) in the test group. Also, 20% of the training data is held as a validation set for cross-validation of the training hyper-parameters. The echo cine frames are resized to 128 × 128. The network is implemented in Keras with the use of Tensorflow (Google Corp., Mountain View, CA) backend. The network weights are initialized by using a normal distribution. ReLU activation is used in all constitutional layers of the network, and the activation in the prediction layer is a sigmoid function. Dice loss is used as the network's objective function. We use Adam optimizer with the learning rate of $1e - 4$, and batch size of 10. Finally, d in the temporal window is set to 4 frames.

Testing Criteria: Note that in the standard clinical procedure, the LV tracing is routinely done in only the ED and ES frames of the A4C view, therefore we report the Dice score and accuracy on the ED and ES frames. In order to report segmentation accuracy for in-between frames, since developing per-frame ground truth for all echo cine frames is very time consuming, we approximated the full cine segmentation performance by evaluating the performance on a randomly selected frame between the ED and ES frames against an expert manual annotation. This frame is named RF (Random Frame) in Table 1.

Example visual results of the LV tracking by the proposed method compared to the ground truth are shown in Fig. 3. As can be seen, the proposed model accurately detects the LV wall and shape.

Table 1. Empirical evaluation of the proposed method. Best results are in bold.

Method	Dice Score(%)						Accuracy(%)					
	ED		RF		ES		ED		RF		ES	
	Mean	STD	Mean	STD	Mean	STD	Mean	STD	Mean	STD	Mean	STD
U-Net Per Frame	91.2	3.9	90.2	5.3	88.9	4.9	97.2	1.1	97.3	1.0	97.3	0.9
U-Net-conv-BiLSTM	93.3	3.4	92.1	3.8	90.1	8.8	97.8	0.9	97.7	1.0	97.8	1.0
U-Net-conv-BiLSTM-OptFlow	**93.6**	3.0	**92.5**	3.5	**92.1**	4.1	**97.9**	0.9	**97.8**	1.0	**97.9**	1.0

Model Comparison: We compare the performance of the proposed deep learning architecture (*i.e.*, U-Net-conv-BiLSTM-OptFlow) with the off-the-shelf 2D U-Net implementation [14] (*i.e.*, U-Net (Per Frame) in Table 1) that was trained with only the ED and ES frame segmentation ground truth, and also with an architecture of combining 2D U-Net with convolution Bi-directional LSTM (*i.e.*, U-Net-conv-BiLSTM), in Table 1. It is clear that the proposed architecture improves all segmentation metrics. In particular, the combination of U-Net and convolutional Bi-directional LSTM architecture consistently increases the Dice score on all ED, RF and ES frames. Furthermore, the integration of Bi-directional LSTM and optical flow information shows further improvement of segmentation performance. Most importantly, using optical flow information increases the robustness of LV tracking in echo data given the standard deviation of the reported results. Paired t-tests indicate there is a statistically significant difference between every pairs of the compared network architectures for both Dice

Score and Accuracy ($p < 0.05$). Also, in terms of area under the Receiver Operating Characteristic Curve (AUC), our analysis show U-Net per frame has substantially lower AUC (AUC = 0.94) than U-Net-conv-BiLSTM and U-Net-conv-BiLSTM-OptFlow (AUC = 0.97 for both methods). In addition, it can be seen in Fig. 3 that per frame U-Net can be misled by image artifacts and reduction in image quality. Both U-Net-conv-BiLSTM and U-Net-conv-BiLSTM-OptFlow, which utilize temporal information, show more consistent segmentation results.

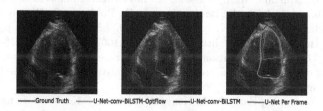

Fig. 4. Sample failed case of our method. Left to right: input echo frame, ground truth by cardiologist, and segmentation by the compared methods.

4   Conclusion and Discussion

Accurate LV segmentation in echocardiograms is an important component to diagnose critical cardiovascular disease. In this work, we present a method based on deep recurrent fully convolutional networks and optical flow for LV tracking in A4C echo cine data. We use convolutional Bi-directional LSTM to encode temporal information from a short number of frames. We also use optical flow information as an additional input to improve the segmentation accuracy and robustness. The proposed model is evaluated on an echo dataset consist of 648 echo studies from 566 patients, and shows advantageous over two compared models. Sample visual comparison of our proposed method can be seen in Fig. 3. The first row in Fig. 3 shows sample cases where all of the three compared methods provide an acceptable tracking of LV. The second row of Fig. 3 shows samples where U-Net per frame has been mislead by artifacts in echo data. Also, poor quality of captured echo in the cursor frame has resulted in high errors by per frame U-Net. This is while incorporating temporal and motion information in U-Net-conv-BiLSTM-Optflow results in a more smooth and accurate tracking of LV. The sample in the right column of the second row in Fig. 3 shows a case where adding information of optical flow has been advantageous comparing the blue contour (U-Net-conv-BiLSTM) with the green segmentation (U-Net-conv-BiLSTM-OptFlow). A sample failed case of our proposed method (U-Net-BiLSTM-OptFlow) is shown in Fig. 4. Captured echo with a low quality throughout the whole cine could be more challenging in terms of accurate segmentation of LV, as is the case with the shown sample. Low quality echo misses the location of the heart wall chambers and makes it hard to annotate LV even for expert human. Future work will include using the proposed architecture to automatically estimate various cardiac measurements, including the Left Ventricle Ejection Fraction.

References

1. World health organization. http://www.who.int/mediacentre/factsheets/fs317/en/
2. Achmad, B., Mustafa, M.M., Hussain, A.: Inter-frame enhancement of ultrasound images using optical flow. In: Badioze Zaman, H., Robinson, P., Petrou, M., Olivier, P., Schröder, H., Shih, T.K. (eds.) IVIC 2009. LNCS, vol. 5857, pp. 191–201. Springer, Heidelberg (2009). https://doi.org/10.1007/978-3-642-05036-7_19
3. Carneiro, G.: The segmentation of the left ventricle of the heart from ultrasound data using deep learning architectures and derivative-based search methods. IEEE Trans. Image Process. **21**(3), 968–982 (2012)
4. Chen, H., Zheng, Y., Park, J.-H., Heng, P.-A., Zhou, S.K.: Iterative multi-domain regularized deep learning for anatomical structure detection and segmentation from ultrasound images. In: Ourselin, S., Joskowicz, L., Sabuncu, M.R., Unal, G., Wells, W. (eds.) MICCAI 2016. LNCS, vol. 9901, pp. 487–495. Springer, Cham (2016). https://doi.org/10.1007/978-3-319-46723-8_56
5. Chen, J., et al.: Combining fully convolutional and recurrent neural networks for 3d biomedical image segmentation. In: NIPS, pp. 3036–3044 (2016)
6. Li, Z.: Videolstm convolves, attends and flows for action recognition. Comput. Vis. Image Underst. **166**, 41–50 (2018)
7. Litjens, G.: A survey on deep learning in medical image analysis. Med. Image Anal. **42**, 60–88 (2017)
8. Ng, J.Y.H., et al.: Beyond short snippets: Deep networks for video classification. In: 2015 IEEE Conference on Computer Vision and Pattern Recognition (CVPR), pp. 4694–4702 (2015)
9. Ngo, T.A.: Combining deep learning and level set for the automated segmentation of the left ventricle of the heart from cardiac cine magnetic resonance. Med. Image Anal. **35**, 159–171 (2017)
10. Noble, J.A., Boukerroui, D.: Ultrasound image segmentation: a survey. IEEE Trans. Med. Imaging **25**(8), 987–1010 (2006)
11. Oktay, O.: Anatomically constrained neural networks (ACNNs): application to cardiac image enhancement and segmentation. IEEE Trans. Med. Imaging **37**(2), 384–395 (2018)
12. Poudel, R.P.K., Lamata, P., Montana, G.: Recurrent fully convolutional neural networks for multi-slice MRI cardiac segmentation. In: Zuluaga, M.A., Bhatia, K., Kainz, B., Moghari, M.H., Pace, D.F. (eds.) RAMBO/HVSMR -2016. LNCS, vol. 10129, pp. 83–94. Springer, Cham (2017). https://doi.org/10.1007/978-3-319-52280-7_8
13. Ronneberger, O., Fischer, P., Brox, T.: U-Net: convolutional networks for biomedical image segmentation. In: Navab, N., Hornegger, J., Wells, W.M., Frangi, A.F. (eds.) MICCAI 2015. LNCS, vol. 9351, pp. 234–241. Springer, Cham (2015). https://doi.org/10.1007/978-3-319-24574-4_28
14. Smistad, E., et al.: 2D left ventricle segmentation using deep learning. In: 2017 IEEE International Ultrasonics Symposium (IUS), pp. 1–4 (2017)

15. Sofka, M., Milletari, F., Jia, J., Rothberg, A.: Fully convolutional regression network for accurate detection of measurement points. In: Cardoso, M.J., et al. (eds.) DLMIA/ML-CDS -2017. LNCS, vol. 10553, pp. 258–266. Springer, Cham (2017). https://doi.org/10.1007/978-3-319-67558-9_30
16. Valipour, S., et al.: Recurrent fully convolutional networks for video segmentation. In: 2017 IEEE Winter Conference on Applications of Computer Vision (WACV), pp. 29–36 (2017)
17. Xue, W.: Full left ventricle quantification via deep multitask relationships learning. Med. Image Anal. **43**, 54–65 (2018)
18. Zreik, M., et al.: Automatic segmentation of the left ventricle in cardiac CT angiography using convolutional neural networks. In: 2016 IEEE 13th International Symposium on Biomedical Imaging (ISBI), pp. 40–43 (2016)

Multi-scale Residual Network with Two Channels of Raw CT Image and Its Differential Excitation Component for Emphysema Classification

Liying Peng[1], Lanfen Lin[1(✉)], Hongjie Hu[2], Huali Li[2],
Qingqing Chen[2], Dan Wang[2], Xian-Hua Han[3], Yutaro Iwamoto[3],
and Yen-Wei Chen[3]

[1] College of Computer Science and Technology, Zhejiang University,
Hangzhou, China
llf@zju.edu.cn
[2] Department of Radiology, Sir Run Run Shaw Hospital, Hangzhou, China
[3] College of Information Science and Engineering, Ritsumeikan University,
Kusatsu, Japan

Abstract. Automated tissue classification is an essential step for quantitative analysis and treatment of emphysema. Although many studies have been conducted in this area, there still remain two major challenges. First, different emphysematous tissue appears in different scales, which we call "inter-class variations". Second, the intensities of CT images acquired from different patients, scanners or scanning protocols may vary, which we call "intra-class variations". In this paper, we present a novel multi-scale residual network with two channels of raw CT image and its differential excitation component. We incorporate multi-scale information into our networks to address the challenge of inter-class variations. In addition to the conventional raw CT image, we use its differential excitation component as a pair of inputs to handle intra-class variations. Experimental results show that our approach has superior performance over the state-of-the-art methods, achieving a classification accuracy of 93.74% on our original emphysema database.

Keywords: Emphysema classification · Multi-scale
Differential excitation component

1 Introduction

Emphysema is a major component of chronic obstructive pulmonary disease (COPD), which is emerging as a worldwide health problem. Generally, as shown in Fig. 1, emphysema can be classified into three subtypes: centrilobular emphysema (CLE) that generally appears as scattered small low attenuation areas; paraseptal emphysema (PSE) which is shown as low attenuation areas aligned in a row along a visceral pleura [1]; and panlobular emphysema (PLE) that usually manifests as a wide range low attenuation region with fewer and smaller lung vessels [1]. They have different pathophysiological significance [2]. Hence, classification and quantification of emphysema are important.

© Springer Nature Switzerland AG 2018
D. Stoyanov et al. (Eds.): DLMIA 2018/ML-CDS 2018, LNCS 11045, pp. 38–46, 2018.
https://doi.org/10.1007/978-3-030-00889-5_5

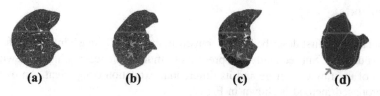

Fig. 1. (a) Normal tissue (NT). (b) CLE. (c) PSE. (d) PLE.

Much research has been conducted to classify the lung tissue of different emphysema subtypes. One common way is based on the local intensity distribution, such as kernel density estimation (KDE) [3]. Another class of approaches describes the morphology of emphysema using texture analysis techniques [1, 4–6]. In the last years, some attempts have revealed the potential of deep learning techniques on lung disease classification, but it has been applied in only two studies [7, 8] for emphysema classification. The networks in these two studies are very preliminary, using two or three convolutional layers, so they are not able to capture the high-level features. Since the classification of emphysema mainly depends on features of texture and intensity, there still remain two major challenges. (1) "inter-class variations": as can be seen in Fig. 1, different emphysematous tissue appears in different scales. Since existing methods ignore the scales of different emphysema which are useful clues for diagnosing emphysema, it is highly desirable to develop new models that can take full advantage of the information from multiple scales. (2) "intra-class variations": in clinical practice, the intensities of CT images acquired from different patients, scanners or scanning protocols may vary [9]. The variation in CT images will affect the classification accuracy of emphysema, so it is necessary to design models which are robust to such variability. In addition, existing methods for emphysema classification are limited to extracting low-level features or mid-level features, which have limited abilities to distinguish different patterns.

In this paper, we focus on the supervised classification of emphysema. We propose a novel deep learning method using the multi-scale residual network (MS-ResNet) [16] with two channels of the raw CT image and its differential excitation component. In contrast to previous works, our proposed method discovers high-level features that can better characterize the emphysema lesions. We incorporate multi-scale information into our networks to address the challenge of inter-class variations. Moreover, to handle intra-class variations, we first transform the raw image data into the differential excitation domain of human perception based on weber's law, which is robust to intensity variability. Then we use the raw CT images and the transformed images as different channels of the inputs of networks. The experiments show that our method can achieve higher classification accuracy than the state-of-the-art methods. Based on the classification results, we calculate the area percentage of each class (CLE%, PLE%, PSE%, respectively). Then, we show the relationship between the quantitative results (area percentages) and the forced expiratory volume in one second dividing with a predicted value ($FEV_{1\%}$), which is the primary indicator of pulmonary function tests (PFTs).

2 Methods

In this section, we first describe how to transform the raw CT image into the differential excitation domain. Subsequently, we present our multi-scale residual network with two channels of the raw CT image and its differential excitation component. An overview of the proposed method is shown in Fig. 2.

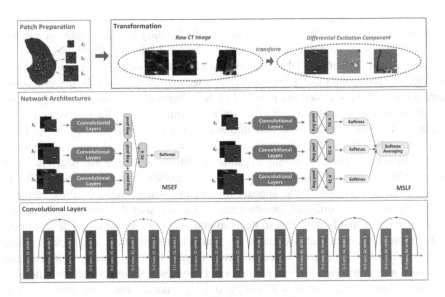

Fig. 2. Overview of the proposed approach

2.1 Differential Excitation Component

Ernst Heinrich Weber, an experimental psychologist in the 19th century, observed that the ratio of the perceived change in stimulus to the initial stimulus is a constant [10], which is well-known as Weber's law and can be defined as $\Delta I/I = \alpha$, where ΔI denotes the perceived change in stimulus, I denotes the initial stimulus, and α is referred to as the Weber fraction for detecting changes in stimulus.

Inspired by Weber's law, which shows that human perception of a pattern depends not only on the absolute intensity of the stimulus but also on the relative variance of the stimulus, we transform the raw image into the differential excitation domain of human perception which is robust to intensity variability [10]. In order to do so, we first compute the difference between a focused pixel and its neighbors, which can be formulated as

$$\Delta I_c = \sum_{i=0}^{p-1} (\Delta I_c^i) = \sum_{i=0}^{p-1} (I_c^i - I_c) \qquad (1)$$

where I_c is the intensity at position x_c, $I_c^i (i = 0, 1, \ldots, p - 1)$ is intensity of the ith neighbor of c, and p is the number of neighbors. The differential excitation component of the focused pixel c is defined as

$$E_c = \arctan[\frac{\Delta I_c}{I_c + \lambda}] = \arctan[\sum_{i=0}^{p-1} \frac{(I_c^i - I_c)}{I_c + \lambda}] \tag{2}$$

where λ is a constant which avoids the situation in which there is zero intensity. λ is set to one in our experiments.

2.2   MS-ResNet with Raw and Excitation Channels

MS-ResNet. Due to the inter-class variations of emphysema, one target category tends to be identified on a certain scale and the most suitable scales for different target classes may vary. That is, we cannot find the best scale for all cases. Thus, it is essential to incorporate information from different scales into our deep neural networks [16].

For a baseline, we build a 20-layer ResNet [11], which has been shown to achieve the excellent performance on image classification. For the sake of adapting it to our problem (small inputs and only 4 classes), we remove the pooling layer and modify the configuration for some layers. Figure 2 (bottom) presents the details of our ResNet. As shown in Fig. 2 (top), for each annotated pixel, we can extract patches with different scales from its neighborhood. The label assigned to each patch is the same as label of the central pixel. Note that, in this paper, different scales mean various sizes of inputs. Figure 2 (middle) presents two ways for fusing information from different scales: multi-scale early fusion (MSEF) and multi-scale late fusion (MSLF). For the MSEF, we employ the independent convolutional layers for each scale. The outputs of average pooling layers are combined and fed into a 4-way shared fully connected layer with softmax to compute a cross entropy classification loss. For the MSLF, we train three separate networks, each focusing on a certain scale. During the fusion step, we first sum up the values of probability vectors yielded by different networks, and then compute the average of them.

Fused Representation of Raw Image and its Differential Excitation Component. As mentioned in Introduction part, there exists the challenge of intra-class variations for emphysema classification. As shown in Fig. 2 in order to reduce the impact of intensity variability, we first transform the raw image data into the differential excitation domain of human perception, which is robust to intensity variability. Then we use the raw CT images and their differential excitation components as different channels of the inputs of networks.

3 Experimental Results

3.1 Materials

Our dataset contains 101 HRCT volumes. The first part of our dataset includes 91 HRCT volumes annotated manually by two experienced radiologists and checked by one experienced chest radiologist. Four types of patterns were annotated: CLE, PLE, PSE, and non-emphysema (NE) which corresponds to tissue without emphysema. This part of dataset is used for evaluation of classification accuracy shown in Sect. 3.2. Since the first part of dataset does not include complete pulmonary function evaluations, we collected additional 10 HRCT volumes from patients who have a complete pulmonary function evaluation for a quantitative analysis of emphysema shown in Sect. 3.3. All data came from two hospitals and were acquired using seven types of CT machines with a slice collimation of 1 mm–2 mm, a matrix of 512 × 512 pixels, and an in-plane resolution of 0.62 mm–0.71 mm.

3.2 Evaluation of Classification Accuracy

Experimental Setup. Our classification experiments are conducted on 91 annotated subjects (the first part of dataset): 59 subjects (about 720,000 patches) for training, 14 subjects (about 140,000 patches) for validation, and 18 subjects (about 160,000 patches) for testing. A 20-layer ResNet is chosen as the baseline in this work (we found 8-layer, 32-layer, 44-layer, and 56-layer ResNet decrease the performance, compared to 20-layer ResNet, on our data). We have done extensive experiments for selecting patch sizes and the experimental results show that the most suitable scales (patch sizes) for different target categories are different: for non-emphysema tissue, the inputs of 27 × 27 generate the best result; for CLE, the best scale is 41 × 41; for PLE and PSE, the highest classification accuracy is obtained with inputs of size 61 × 61. Therefore, patches of sizes 27 × 27, 41 × 41, and 61 × 61 are selected as inputs of the multi-scale neural networks.

Single Scale versus Multiple Scales. In this section, to investigate the effect of fusing multi-scale information on the classification accuracy, we use only raw images as inputs of networks. As shown in Table 1, both MSEF model and MSLF model outperform the single-scale models (27 × 27, 41 × 41, and 61 × 61). To test the statistical significance of the classification accuracy differences between single-scale models and multi-scale models, we calculated the classification accuracy of each patient, and then employed t-test. The results of analysis confirmed the statistically significant (p-value < 0.05) superior performance of the multi-scale models against all single-scale models. Fusion of multi-scale information leads to higher accuracy, so we can conclude that the multi-scale methods are beneficial compared to the single scale setting.

Single Channel versus Multiple Channels. This part compares the classification accuracy between the single-channel models (use only raw images as inputs) and the multi-channel models (use raw CT images and their differential excitation components

Table 1. The comparison between the single-scale models and the multi-scale models.

	27×27	41×41	61×61	MSEF	MSLF
NE	93.19%	91.77%	86.04%	**94.05%**	91.98%
CLE	86.85%	88.87%	86.50%	**91.17%**	89.02%
PLE	83.61%	92.18%	**95.06%**	89.48%	93.78%
PSE	87.35%	89.52%	95.52%	**95.89%**	92.36%
Avg.	87.77%	90.58%	90.81%	**92.68%**	91.80%

as different channels of inputs). As shown in Table 2, for both single-scale setting and multi-scale setting, the multi-channel models offer superior performance to the single-channel models (p-value < 0.05).

Table 2. The comparison between the single-channel models and the multi-channel models.

	27×27	41×41	61×61	MSEF	MSLF
Single-channel	87.77%	90.58%	90.81%	92.68%	91.80%
Multi-channel	**89.39%**	**91.47%**	**91.84%**	**93.74%**	**92.90%**

Comparison to the State-of-the-Art Methods. In this section, our approaches are compared to other state-of-the-art methods. The comparison between our methods and the machine learning (ML) methods for emphysema classification is provided in the first five rows. The results prove the superior performance of our methods that significantly outperform the rest by 14% to 20%. The rest of Table 3 shows a comparison to other deep learning methods. Since existing deep learning methods for emphysema classification [7, 8] are very primary using only two or three convolutional layers, we also compare our approaches with other CNNs for interstitial lung disease (ILD) classification [12, 14]. The results show that our approaches have superior performance over other deep learning methods.

3.3 Emphysema Quantification

In this section, based on the classification results, we quantify the whole lung area of 10 subjects (the second part of dataset with complete pulmonary function evaluations) by calculating the area percentage of each class (CLE%, PLE%, PSE%, respectively), and show the relationship between the quantitative results (area percentages) and the forced expiratory volume in one second dividing with a predicted value ($FEV_{1\%}$), which is the primary indicator of pulmonary function tests (PFTs). Some visual results of full lung classification are shown in Fig. 3. It can be seen that, auto-annotations (or classification results) of proposed method are similar to annotations of radiologists (manual annotations). The relationship between the quantitative results (area percentages) and $FEV_{1\%}$ of 10 subjects are shown in Table 4. According to [15], $FEV_{1\%}$ is an effective indicator that indicates both functional and symptomatic impairment of COPD. Symptoms arise in individuals in relation to a relative loss of FEV_1. More specifically,

Table 3. The comparison of classification accuracy (Acc.) to the state-of-the-art approaches.

ML methods	Acc.
LBPINT [1]	78.67%
Texton-based [4]	79.06%
KDE [3]	76.67%
Sparse representation [5]	72.96%
JWRIULTP [6]	79.31%
DL methods	Acc.
Karabulut [7]	65.51%
Pei [8]	72.34%
AlexNet-TL [12]	81.79%
GoogLeNet-TL [12]	85.75%
Wang [13]	73.62%
Anthimopoulos [14]	85.00%
Proposed method	**93.74%**

$FEV_{1\%}$ can reflect the severity of airflow obstruction in the lungs. The lower value of FEV1% means the more severe the airflow obstruction in the lungs. Our results show that a larger CLE% (or PLE%) corresponds to a lower $FEV_{1\%}$ (the more severe the airflow obstruction in the lungs). From our experiments, we found there is no relationship between PSE% and $FEV_{1\%}$. According to the literature [1], PSE is often not associated with significant symptoms or physiological impairments, which is in close agreement with our experimental results.

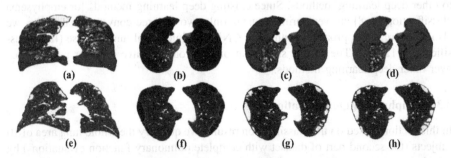

Fig. 3. Examples of the classification results. Each row represents a subject. (a), (e) Classification results in coronal view. (b), (f) Typical original HRCT slices from subjects of (a), (e), respectively. (c), (g) Auto-annotated mask of our proposed method. (d), (h) Manual annotated mask of radiologists. Green mask: CLE lesions. Blue mask: PLE lesions. Yellow mask: PSE lesions.

Table 4. Relationship between quantitative results and $FEV_{1\%}$.

	CLE%	PLE%	PSE%	$FEV_{1\%}$
Case #1	13.120%	11.311%	0.002%	57.000%
Case #2	1.464%	0.002%	0.004%	77.200%
Case #3	16.878%	4.962%	0.000%	36.000%
Case #4	1.138%	1.437%	15.546%	76.100%
Case #5	10.207%	38.158%	0.161%	20.500%
Case #6	0.124%	0.000%	0.001%	81.000%
Case #7	0.057%	0.003%	0.000%	86.000%
Case #8	0.000%	42.368%	0.000%	25.000%
Case #9	13.244%	5.860%	1.769%	53.000%
Case #10	4.467%	0.622%	0.812%	69.000%

4 Conclusions

In this paper, we proposed a novel deep learning approach for emphysema classification, using the multi-scale ResNet with two channels of raw CT image and its differential excitation component. Our proposed approach achieved a classification accuracy of 93.74%, which is superior to the state-of-the-art methods.

Acknowledgements. This work was supported in part by the National Key R&D Program of China under the Grant No. 2017YFB0309800, in part by the Science and Technology Support Program of Hangzhou under the Grant No. 20172011A038, and in part by the Grant-in Aid for Scientific Research from the Japanese Ministry for Education, Science, Culture and Sports (MEXT) under the Grant Nos. 18H03267 and No. 17H00754.

References

1. Sørensen, L., et al.: Quantitative analysis of pulmonary emphysema using local binary patterns. IEEE Trans. Med. Imaging **29**(2), 559–569 (2010)
2. Lynch, D.A., et al.: CT-definable subtypes of chronic obstructive pulmonary disease: a statement of the fleischner society. Radiology **277**(1), 192–205 (2015)
3. Mendoza, C.S., et al.: Emphysema quantification in a multi-scanner HRCT cohort using local intensity distributions. In: ISBI 2012, pp. 474–477 (2012)
4. Gangeh, M.J., Sørensen, L., Shaker, S.B., Kamel, M.S., de Bruijne, M., Loog, M.: A texton-based approach for the classification of lung parenchyma in CT images. In: Jiang, T., Navab, N., Pluim, J.P.W., Viergever, M.A. (eds.) MICCAI 2010. LNCS, vol. 6363, pp. 595–602. Springer, Heidelberg (2010). https://doi.org/10.1007/978-3-642-15711-0_74
5. Jie, Y., et al.: Texton and sparse representation based texture classification of lung parenchyma in CT images. In: EMBC 2016, pp. 1276–1279 (2016)
6. Liying, P., et al.: Joint weber-based rotation invariant uniform local ternary pattern for classification of pulmonary emphysema in CT images. In: ICIP 2017, pp. 2050–2054 (2017)
7. Karabulut, E.M., et al.: Emphysema discrimination from raw HRCT images by convolutional neural networks. In: ELECO 2015, pp. 705–708 (2015)

8. Pei, X.: Emphysema classification using convolutional neural networks. In: Liu, H., Kubota, N., Zhu, X., Dillmann, R., Zhou, D. (eds.) ICIRA 2015. LNCS (LNAI), vol. 9244, pp. 455–461. Springer, Cham (2015). https://doi.org/10.1007/978-3-319-22879-2_42
9. Cheplygina, V., et al.: Transfer learning for multi-center classification of chronic obstructive pulmonary disease. JBHI (2018)
10. Xianhua, H., et al.: Integration of spatial and orientation contexts in local ternary patterns for HEp-2 cell classification. Pattern Recognit. Lett. **82**, 23–27 (2016)
11. Kaiming, H., et al.: Deep residual learning for image recognition. In: CVPR 2016, pp. 770–778 (2016)
12. Shin, H.C., et al.: Deep convolutional neural networks for computer-aided detection: CNN architectures, dataset characteristics and transfer learning. IEEE Trans. Med. Imaging **35**(5), 1285–1298 (2016)
13. Qian, W., et al.: Multiscale rotation-invariant convolutional neural networks for lung texture classification. JBHI **22**, 184–195 (2017)
14. Anthimopoulos, M., et al.: Lung pattern classification for interstitial lung diseases using a deep convolutional neural network. IEEE Trans. Med. Imaging **35**(5), 1207–1216 (2016)
15. Jakeways, N., et al.: Relationship between FEV1 reduction and respiratory symptoms in the general population. Eur. Respir. J. **21**(4), 658–663 (2003)
16. Liying, P., et al.: Classification of pulmonary emphysema in CT images based on multi-scale deep convolutional neural networks. In: ICIP (2018, in Press)

TreeNet: Multi-loss Deep Learning Network to Predict Branch Direction for Extracting 3D Anatomical Trees

Mengliu Zhao[✉] and Ghassan Hamarneh

School of Computing Science, Simon Fraser University, Burnaby, Canada
{mengliuz,hamarneh}@sfu.ca

Abstract. Calculation of blood vessel or airway direction is important for the task of tree tracking in 3D medical images. However, most existing works treat branch direction estimation as only a by-product of vesselness or tubularness computation. In this work, we propose a deep learning framework for predicting tracking directions of anatomical tree structures. We modify the deep V-Net architecture with extra layers and leverage a novel multi-loss function that encodes direction as well as cross sectional plane information. We evaluate our method on both 3D synthetic and 3D clinical pulmonary CT datasets. On the synthetic dataset, we outperform state of the art methods by at least 10% in direction estimation accuracy. For the clinical dataset, we outperform competing methods by 1–4% in mean direction accuracy and 4–10% in corresponding standard deviation.

1 Introduction

Tree extraction is a crucial task in 3D medical image analysis, and accurately extracted circulatory and respiratory trees can be further utilized in surgery planning, registration and tree space analysis [1–3]. However, the automation and accuracy of tree extraction still remains an open problem due to the natural complexity and variability of the topologies of anatomical tree structures [4], the various imaging reconstruction artifacts [5], varying image intensities along branches, the similarity between tubular structure lumen and background tissue lumen, and the changing geometry due to different pathologies [6–8].

One major category of tree extraction algorithms is based on iterative tracking, which usually starts from a given seed point near the root of the tree, predicts the direction of the branch to track along it, detects bifurcations to spawn children trackers, and progresses down the tree hierarchy to smaller branches until some stopping criteria are met [9]. Although there have been several works that tackle the important bifurcation detection step of the tracker [10,11], very few are specifically designed to determine the direction of the branch at a given point. Most works simply treat the problem of direction estimation as a by-product of vesselness or tubularness calculation [12–14].

© Springer Nature Switzerland AG 2018
D. Stoyanov et al. (Eds.): DLMIA 2018/ML-CDS 2018, LNCS 11045, pp. 47–55, 2018.
https://doi.org/10.1007/978-3-030-00889-5_6

Most existing methods on vesselness (with explicit/implicit direction prediction) rely on certain assumptions made on the geometry of tubular structures. Most Hessian based vessel enhancement filters, e.g., Frangi et al. [15] and Jerman et al. [13,14], assumed the vessels were elongated structures. Cetin et al. [10] measured intensity distribution within an oriented cylinder-sphere combined model and constructed a corresponding tensor representation to optimize for vessel directions, however, their success relied on a good match between the cylinder and the actual vessel shape. Law et al. [12] used a gradient based tensor to model oriented flux flow and the vessel direction was also approximated by the eigenvector – intrinsically their assumption of vessel shapes were still straight tubes. However, in clinical datasets, especially those exhibiting various pathologies or abnormalities such as narrowing (e.g., in COPD [6]), aneurysms [7], and high tortuosity (which might indicate diseases like arterial hypertension and strokes [8]), the aforementioned shape assumptions might no longer hold true, which results in incorrect direction estimates.

In contrast to the above deterministic methods, stochastic and learning based tracking methods provide more flexibility by adjusting the prediction retrospectively during the tracking process, or by using prior information learnt from the training data [16]. Lee et al. [17] proposed to use particle filtering to track vessel contours slice by slice, with the per-slice contour obtained by the Chan-Vese model. Lesage et al. [18] also proposed to use particle filtering method, but in contrast, utilized geometric flow, image features, as well as radius and direction prior distributions to perform Bayesian inference. In these tracking processes, vessel directions were found implicitly by subtracting neighboring points along the detected centerlines. On the other hand, a significant number of machine learning based methods ignore directional information completely by focusing on pixel-wise classification [9,19,20].

The fast development of deep learning methods provides vast opportunities in exploring the structures in 3D images from coarse to fine scales [21], however, limited work has been done on analyzing 3D vasculature images, and none of them estimated tree branch directions. Mirikharaji et al. [22] proposed to use an artificial neural network trained on 2D patches to learn the probability map of airway bifurcation locations; instead of tracking new branches, they connected the bifurcations by minimal paths to form the whole tree. Fu et al. [23] proposed to combine a convolutional neural network architecture with a conditional random field model to achieve a smooth binary segmentation for retinal vessels, but their method was only performed on 2D retinal images and no vessel direction was estimated. Chen et al. [24] proposed to use a convolutional autoencoder for voxel-wise cerebral arteries segmentation while completely ignoring directional information.

We claim the following contributions are made in this paper: (i) The proposed method, which extends V-Net [21], is the first tree branch direction prediction deep learning method; (ii) The proposed multi-loss function is novel and specially designed for tracking 3D tubular structures; (iii) The proposed model is trained and tested in a branch-specific way, which takes advantage of the "anatomical tree statistics" [16, 25] and fully utilizes statistical and geometrical information.

2 Methodology

Architecture: Our proposed deep learning architecture is an improvement of V-Net [21]. The choice of V-Net is two-fold: (i) its encoding-decoding process propagates contextual information into higher resolution layers – in our case, the context information is the tubularity of the neighboring points; and, (ii) our multi-loss function (introduced below) relies on cross sectional plane information, so the prediction process implicitly involves plane segmentation and reconstruction. We rescale all input volumes to $64 * 64 * 64$ voxels with histogram equalization. We use batch normalization and add three extra fully connected layers (FCs, with output channels 1024, 64 and 4) at the end of the V-Net and output a 4-element vector $<v, R>$ where v predicts the direction of the vessel in the center of the input cube, and a radius R that serves as intermediate input in training the loss layer. The overall methodology is illustrated in Fig. 1a.

At Testing Time: A region of interest (ROI, or 3D patch, which we use in the context interchangeably) is generated and input into the network (as shown in red dotted box in Fig. 1a), and the output is the predicted vector of the corresponding branch (shown as $\overrightarrow{v_{gt}}$ in Fig. 1b).

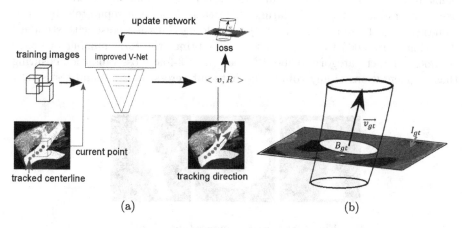

Fig. 1. (a): The proposed architecture and tracking process. (b): Illustration of B_{gt}, $\overrightarrow{v}_{gt}$ and I_{gt} in Eq. 1.

Loss Function: We define the following multi-loss function:

$$L(\boldsymbol{v}_{dt}^i, R_{dt}^i) = \omega_1 L_{dir} + \omega_2 L_{mask} + \omega_3 L_{image} + \omega_4 L_{radius} \tag{1}$$
$$L_{dir}(\boldsymbol{v}_{dt}^i, R_{dt}^i) = -|\boldsymbol{v}_{gt}^i \cdot \boldsymbol{v}_{dt}^i|^2, \quad L_{mask}(\boldsymbol{v}_{dt}^i, R_{dt}^i) = ||B_{gt}^i - B_{dt}^i||_{L_2}^2$$
$$L_{image}(\boldsymbol{v}_{dt}^i, R_{dt}^i) = ||I_{gt}^i - I_{dt}^i||_{L_2}^2, \quad L_{radius}(\boldsymbol{v}_{dt}^i, R_{dt}^i) = |R_{gt}^i - R_{dt}^i|^2$$

where i is the training index, gt refers to ground truth value, dt refers to model prediction. I^i_{gt} and I^i_{dt} are corresponding gt and predicted cross sectional planes (going through the center voxel). B^i_{gt} and B^i_{dt} are the ground truth and predicted (using radius R^i_{dt} and circular expression) branch masks on the cross sectional planes, R^i_{gt} and R^i_{dt} are the ground truth and predicted radii, as illustrated in Fig. 1b. The four terms L_{dir}, L_{image}, L_{mask}, L_{radius} capture the errors in, respectively, direction estimation, cross sectional image plane reconstruction, branch internal area estimation and radius estimation. We normalize L_{image} and L_{mask} by the patch cube size and set the weights empirically to $\omega_1 = \omega_2 = \omega_3 = \omega_4 = 1$. The total loss is optimized over v^i_{dt} and R^i_{dt}. Since accurate direction prediction leads to accurate cross section plane prediction, using multiple loss terms should theoretically increase the direction prediction accuracy.

Tree Tracking: We follow the tracking procedure in [9], which starts from a given seed point in a branch and tracks along vessel/airway detected by the proposed architecture. Additional tracking details are given in Sect. 3.

3   Evaluation

Synthetic Dataset: We use three different types of synthetic dataset to mimic pathologies such as narrowing and aneurysms, and high tortuosity [6–8]: (i) Occlusion, (ii) Torus and (iii) Leakage. Examples are shown in Fig. 2. We augment the data by rotating the volumes along each axis randomly between $[0, 60°]$, using two radius values, translating along each dimension separately by three values ($[-1, 0, 1]$, so 9 cases in total) and adding Gaussian noise with standard deviation from 0.005 to 0.1 (20 cases). This brings the total number of image volumes per each category to 360. We then run a 3-fold cross validation ensuring that augmentations of any volume are not split across the train and test sets.

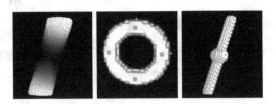

Fig. 2. Synthetic examples (noise free).

Clinical Dataset: The clinical dataset is from the Extraction of Airways from CT (EXACT) 2009 challenge[1]. Sixteen training volumes with binary segmentations were provided by the organizers. We extracted two categories of data: (1) ROIs, each is a cuboid containing one of the following 7 anatomical structures: trachea, right main bronchi (RMB), left main bronchi (LMB), right

---

[1] http://image.diku.dk/exact/index.php.

superior lobar bronchus (RSLB), right intermediate bronchus (RIB), left superior lobar bronchus (LSLB) and left inferior lobar bronchus (LILB); (2) patches, each is a cube randomly sampled from the branch centerlines, with radii twice the mean radii of the branch, intensities normalized to $[0, 1]$, and augmented by adding Gaussian noise with standard deviation $[0.01, 0.04]$ with step size $= 0.01$. We perform a 4-fold cross validation on the patients for training and testing.

Competing Methods: We compare with 4 state-of-the-art algorithms: (i) OOF [12]; (ii) Tensor [10]; (iii) Jerman [13,14]; (iv) Particle filtering [17]. Since particle filtering doesn't directly predict the vessel direction, we use a primitive tracking method to first trace the branch centerline, then estimate the directions. For multiscale methods, the scale ranges are set according to mean branch scales learnt from the dataset, and all other parameters are set according to the original paper (for airways, i.e., dark-on-bright, some parameters are inverted accordingly). Note that although (i) and (ii) are not direction prediction methods per se, they leverage direction estimates to filter branches, which makes the comparison fair.

Tracking Details: Both the proposed method and the competing ones use the same initial seeds, which are selected from the ground truth branch centerlines. By calculating the mean radii $\bar{R}$ of the corresponding branch, the ROI radii are set automatically as $2\bar{R}$.

Evaluation Metrics: Two metrics are used to evaluate the results. For the tracking method, we use the asymmetric distance function proposed in [9] to compare the ground truth centerline to the extracted centerline:

$$D(C_1, C_2) = \{ \min_{s_2 \in C_2} dist(s_1, s_2) | \forall s_1 \in C_1 \} \tag{2}$$

where $dist(s_1, s_2)$ is 3D Euclidean distance between voxels s_1 and s_2, C_1 the ground truth centerline and C_2 the detected centerline (by either the proposed method or particle filtering). $D(C_1, C_2)$ returns a set of distance values for all the points on C_1, so a smaller mean value and standard deviation would indicate a better result. For other competing methods, since they return a per-voxel direction estimate, we use the following symmetric accuracy metric:

$$accu(\boldsymbol{v}_1, \boldsymbol{v}_2) = \boldsymbol{v}_1 \cdot \boldsymbol{v}_2 \tag{3}$$

where $\boldsymbol{v}_1$ and $\boldsymbol{v}_2$ are the branch direction vectors to be compared.

Experiments: The evaluation result on the synthetic dataset is shown in Table 1. We can see a marked improvement in the proposed method over the competing ones by at least 10% in mean direction accuracy. For the Occlusion category, all competing methods performed poorly, since all these methods assume that the foreground is always luminous. For the Torus category, we can see the Tensor method [10] performing the worst, as it modeled the blood vessel as cylindrical tubes, which were very different from the torus shapes in the given

Table 1. Three fold cross validation result on synthetic dataset.

	Year	Occlusion	Torus	Leakage
OOF [12]	2008	0.11 (0.07)	0.69 (0.28)	0.21 (0.12)
Tensor [10]	2015	0.47 (0.1)	0.48 (0.037)	0.89 (0.03)
Jerman [13, 14]	2016	0.44 (0.46)	0.62 (0.48)	0.45 (0.07)
Proposed with L_{dir} only		0.95 (0.06)	0.96 (0.09)	0.97 (0.04)
Proposed w/o L_{image}		0.90 (0.07)	0.95 (0.12)	0.94 (0.04)
Proposed w/o L_{mask}		0.93 (0.07)	0.93 (0.13)	0.97 (0.04)
Proposed w/o L_{radius}		0.94 (0.07)	0.93 (0.10)	0.97 (0.05)
Proposed		**0.97 (0.02)**	**0.97 (0.06)**	**0.99 (0.04)**

images. On the contrary, the Tensor method performed much better than other competing methods on the Leakage category, as a long cylinder might overcome the small leakage (but not good enough to overcome the occlusion) and found the correct direction. It is worth noting that, although the Jerman filter could achieve good enhancement results at tortuous and bulging branches [13,14], the filter was not designed to deal with the direction estimation task.

We observe that by removing only one of the loss terms (other than L_{dir}) actually performs worse than using only L_{dir}. This is not surprising when we remember that the cross sectional plane and the direction together serve as the Frenet frame, so removing one term would invalidate the frame representation. Since L_{image} contains the most information on the cross sectional plane, removing it leads to the worst performance. The improvement in prediction accuracy of the multi-loss function supports our hypothesis that all four terms contribute to the result, given their complementary nature.

Figure 3a shows an example where an airway centerline tree is extracted using our proposed method (red curves) and compared to the ground truth tree centerlines (yellow curves). Figure 3b shows a qualitative comparison between the tracking result, along branch LIB, between the particle filtering and the proposed method. The mean and standard deviation of distance errors of each branch are shown in Fig. 4. The proposed method achieves a lower error mean and standard deviation on every anatomical branch.

The results in Table 2 are consistent with the synthetic data results. The proposed method outperforms all the competing methods on all branches.

We run our experiments on a Nvidia GTX GeForce 12 GB TITAN GPU, and the processing time per patch at testing stage is 0.04 s.

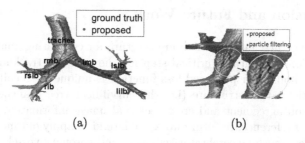

Fig. 3. (a): Whole tree extracted. (b): Centerlines tracked by proposed algorithm and competing particle filtering algorithm on LIB. (Color figure online)

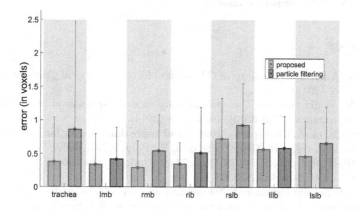

Fig. 4. Distance error bar between GT centerlines and detected centerlines.

Table 2. Direction accuracy (mean and standard deviation) on airway branches of different levels.

	Level 1	Level 2		Level 3			
	Trachea	LMB	RMB	LILB	LSLB	RSLB	RIB
OOF [12]	0.19 (0.18)	0.24 (0.24)	0.29 (0.26)	0.30 (0.24)	0.42(0.31)	0.40 (0.31)	0.43 (0.28)
Tensor [10]	0.86 (0.15)	0.60 (0.20)	0.78 (0.15)	0.68 (0.22)	0.34 (0.29)	0.33 (0.26)	0.82 (0.13)
Jerman [13,14]	0.91 (0.17)	0.93 (0.16)	0.90 (0.18)	0.87 (0.22)	0.87 (0.17)	0.86 (0.21)	0.88 (0.18)
Proposed	**0.92 (0.11)**	**0.95 (0.07)**	**0.93 (0.08)**	**0.89 (0.15)**	**0.91 (0.08)**	**0.90 (0.11)**	**0.90 (0.10)**

4 Conclusion and Future Work

We proposed the first deep learning architecture for estimating anatomical tree branch directions, which is a critical step for the common tracking-based tree extraction methods. Our proposed loss function is unique in that it follows the geometry of the target structure (i.e. the curvilinear tree branches) by using branch direction agreement and cross sectional image information, based on a Frenet frame of reference. In future work, we intend to apply our model on other anatomical trees, such as cerebral vasculature and coronary vessels.

Acknowledgements. We thank NVIDIA Corporation for the donation of Titan X GPUs used in this research and the Natural Sciences and Engineering Research Council of Canada (NSERC) for partial funding.

References

1. Foruzan, A.H., et al.: Analysis of CT images of liver for surgical planning. Analysis **2**(2), 23–28 (2012)
2. Baka, N., et al.: Oriented Gaussian mixture models for nonrigid 2D/3D coronary artery registration. TMI **33**(5), 1023–1034 (2014)
3. Feragen, A., et al.: Tree-space statistics and approximations for large-scale analysis of anatomical trees. In: Gee, J.C., Joshi, S., Pohl, K.M., Wells, W.M., Zöllei, L. (eds.) IPMI 2013. LNCS, vol. 7917, pp. 74–85. Springer, Heidelberg (2013). https://doi.org/10.1007/978-3-642-38868-2_7
4. Kelch, I.D., et al.: Organ-wide 3D-imaging and topological analysis of the continuous microvascular network in a murine lymph node. Sci. Rep. **5**, 16534 (2015)
5. Rodriguez, A., et al.: CT reconstruction techniques for improved accuracy of lung CT airway measurement. Med. Phys. **41**(11), 111911 (2014)
6. Wiggs, B.R., et al.: A model of airway narrowing in asthma and in chronic obstructive pulmonary disease. Am. Rev. Respir. Dis. **145**, 1251–1258 (1992)
7. Baráth, K., et al.: Anatomically shaped internal carotid artery aneurysm in vitro model for flow analysis to evaluate stent effect. Am. J. Neuroradiol. **25**(10), 1750–1759 (2004)
8. Han, H.C.: Twisted blood vessels: symptoms, etiology and biomechanical mechanisms. J. Vasc. Res. **49**(3), 185–197 (2012)
9. Zhao, M., Hamarneh, G.: Bifurcation detection in 3D vascular images using novel features and random forest. In: ISBI, pp. 421–424 (2014)
10. Cetin, S., Unal, G.: A higher-order tensor vessel tractography for segmentation of vascular structures. TMI **34**(10), 2172–2185 (2015)
11. McIntosh, C., Hamarneh, G.: Vessel crawlers: 3D physically-based deformable organisms for vasculature segmentation and analysis. In: CVPR, vol. 1, pp. 1084–1091 (2006)
12. Law, M.W.K., Chung, A.C.S.: Three dimensional curvilinear structure detection using optimally oriented flux. In: Forsyth, D., Torr, P., Zisserman, A. (eds.) ECCV 2008. LNCS, vol. 5305, pp. 368–382. Springer, Heidelberg (2008). https://doi.org/10.1007/978-3-540-88693-8_27
13. Jerman, T., et al.: Enhancement of vascular structures in 3D and 2D angiographic images. TMI **35**(9), 2107–2118 (2016)

14. Jerman, T., et al.: Blob enhancement and visualization for improved intracranial aneurysm detection. IEEE Trans. Vis. Comput. Graph. **22**(6), 1705–1717 (2016)
15. Frangi, A.F., Niessen, W.J., Vincken, K.L., Viergever, M.A.: Multiscale vessel enhancement filtering. In: Wells, W.M., Colchester, A., Delp, S. (eds.) MICCAI 1998. LNCS, vol. 1496, pp. 130–137. Springer, Heidelberg (1998). https://doi.org/10.1007/BFb0056195
16. Zhao, M., et al.: Leveraging tree statistics for extracting anatomical trees from 3D medical images. In: CRV, pp. 131–138 (2017)
17. Lee, S.H., et al.: Enhanced particle-filtering framework for vessel segmentation and tracking. Comput. Methods Programs Biomed. **148**, 99–112 (2017)
18. Lesage, D., et al.: Medial-based Bayesian tracking for vascular segmentation: application to coronary arteries in 3D CT angiography. In: ISBI, pp. 268–271 (2008)
19. Khorshed, R., Celso, C.: Machine learning classification of complex vasculature structures from in-vivo bone marrow 3D data. ISB I, 1217–1220 (2016)
20. Zhou, J., et al.: Vascular structure segmentation and bifurcation detection. In: ISBI, pp. 872–875 (2007)
21. Milletari, F., Navab, N., Ahmadi, S.-A.: V-net: Fully convolutional neural networks for volumetric medical image segmentation. In: 2016 Fourth International Conference on 3D Vision (3DV), pp. 565–571. IEEE (2016)
22. BenTaieb, A., Hamarneh, G.: Uncertainty driven multi-loss fully convolutional networks for histopathology. In: Cardoso, M.J., et al. (eds.) LABELS/CVII/STENT -2017. LNCS, vol. 10552, pp. 155–163. Springer, Cham (2017). https://doi.org/10.1007/978-3-319-67534-3_17
23. Fu, H., Xu, Y., Lin, S., Kee Wong, D.W., Liu, J.: DeepVessel: retinal vessel segmentation via deep learning and conditional random field. In: Ourselin, S., Joskowicz, L., Sabuncu, M.R., Unal, G., Wells, W. (eds.) MICCAI 2016. LNCS, vol. 9901, pp. 132–139. Springer, Cham (2016). https://doi.org/10.1007/978-3-319-46723-8_16
24. Chen, L., et al.: 3D intracranial artery segmentation using a convolutional autoencoder. In: IEEE International Conference on Bioinformatics and Biomedicine (2017)
25. Mirikharaji, Z., Zhao, M., Hamarneh, G.: Globally-optimal anatomical tree extraction from 3d medical images using pictorial structures and minimal paths. In: Descoteaux, M., Maier-Hein, L., Franz, A., Jannin, P., Collins, D.L., Duchesne, S. (eds.) MICCAI 2017. LNCS, vol. 10434, pp. 242–250. Springer, Cham (2017). https://doi.org/10.1007/978-3-319-66185-8_28

3D Deep Affine-Invariant Shape Learning for Brain MR Image Segmentation

Zhou He, Siqi Bao, and Albert Chung[✉]

Department of Computer Science and Engineering,
The Hong Kong University of Science and Technology, Kowloon, Hong Kong
achung@cse.ust.hk

Abstract. Recent advancements in medical image segmentation techniques have achieved compelling results. However, most of the widely used approaches do not take into account any prior knowledge about the shape of the biomedical structures being segmented. More recently, some works have presented approaches to incorporate shape information. However, many of them are indeed introducing more parameters to the segmentation network to learn the general features, which any segmentation network is able learn, instead of specifically *shape* features. In this paper, we present a novel approach that seamlessly integrates the shape information into the segmentation network. Experiments on human brain MRI segmentation demonstrate that our approach can achieve a lower Hausdorff distance and higher Dice coefficient than the state-of-the-art approaches.

1 Introduction

A variety of approaches have been adopted to address the challenging problem of 3D medical image segmentation, such as 3D U-Net [1] and V-Net [4], which have been proven to be highly effective. These approaches, however, simply transplant the 2D image semantic segmentation algorithms to a 3D medical image analysis context. They have little awareness to the fact that 3D medical structures of the same class, unlike objects in 2D natural images, in general have similar shapes. For example, for a 2D natural image segmentation task on the class of 'person', different persons could be very different in shape since a person may have different poses when being photographed, e.g., arms opened/closed, sitting/standing, etc. For the segmentation on biomedical structures such as human caudate nucleus, all caudate nuclei have very similar shape with little structural variation. However, this information is rarely used in deep learning-based 3D medical image segmentation. While some recent literature has introduced some approaches to leverage shape information, many of them are merely introducing more hyperparameters to the network to increase its capacity, while not actually using exactly the *shape* information.

In this paper, we present a novel approach which incorporates the information about the shape of the segmentation target into the loss function of a general

D. Stoyanov et al. (Eds.): DLMIA 2018/ML-CDS 2018, LNCS 11045, pp. 56–64, 2018.
https://doi.org/10.1007/978-3-030-00889-5_7

3D segmentation network. This shape information is deep-learned from a fully convolutional network, whose feature map of the final layer (defined as the **shape signature**) captures the important global shape information. We first pre-train this shape-learning network by ground truth label maps that have undergone different affine transformations, and then have the weights of this network fixed. This shape-learning network will then be able to capture the essential shape information that is invariant to affine transformation. Afterwards, when training the segmentation network, the prediction label map and ground truth label map will both be fed into the pre-trained shape-learning network, and the Euclidean distance between their shape signatures will quantify the dissimilarity in shape between the segmentation prediction and ground truth. This shape loss is then added to the loss function of the segmentation network to facilitate the training.

Our main contributions are summarized as follows:

1. Designed a novel shape-learning network that is able to capture the affine-invariant global shape information in the final feature map;
2. Incorporated the shape dissimilarity information to the segmentation network, making it shape-aware;

2   Related Work

We start by reviewing related prior works on general medical image segmentation, and the utilization of shape information.

2.1   Medical Image Segmentation

Deep learning-based image semantic segmentation became highly successful since the emergence of Fully-convolutional Network (FCN) [3]. This approach has later been adapted to a biomedical image segmentation setting with the novel design of U-Net [7], which contains skip connections between the contracting path and expanding path so that the intricate details in biomedical images can be kept. Recently, U-Net has been modified to accommodate 3D volumes by replacing all the 2D convolutions and convolution transposes by their 3D counterparts, as described in 3D U-Net [1]. Apart from the change in network architecture, some other adaptations have been made to make CNNs more compatible with medical image segmentation. For instance, in V-Net [4], the loss function is derived from Dice coefficient which is a common metric in medical image segmentation.

2.2   The Utilization of Shape Information in Segmentation

Some prior works claimed to have leveraged the shape information of biomedical structures for segmentation purpose. [6] introduced an autoencoder known as Shape Regularization Network (SRN) that regularizes the segmentation result to make it conform to the shape it should have. Its functions include eliminating any noisy part from the general shape, or filling up any holes in the preliminary segmentation result. A more recent work Anatomically Constrained Neural

Networks (ACNN) [5] used an autoencoder to learn the shape by training that autoencoder to reconstruct a label map itself, and used the Euclidean distance between the bottleneck layers of the autoencoder to quantify the dissimilarity in shape.

A commonality among these prior works is that they introduce another network which is trained to capture the shape information, and this network is then used to guide the segmentation network. However, the shape learner in SRN and ACNN are both learning the general features of a 3D structure, including position, volume, shape, etc., instead of specifically learning the *shape*. Inspired by these issues, we propose an approach to learn the essential shape information that is invariant to affine transformations.

3   Methodology

3.1   Overview

While the term *shape* may have many definitions in different settings, in the medical image segmentation setting here, we define it to be the intrinsic properties of the 3D biomedical structures that are invariant to spatial affine transformations, including rotation, translation and scaling, etc. The network architecture used in our approach is composed of two parts, where the first part is to capture the shape information, and the second part to use it.

Concretely, the first part, defined as **shape-learning network**, is a 3D fully convolutional neural network (ConvNet), with the input being the raw binary 3D label map of the biomedical structure being segmented, and the output being a one-channel low-resolution feature map (hereafter referred to as **shape signature**). The second part, defined as **shape-guided segmentation network**, is a segmentation network with the architecture modeled after the 3D U-Net [1] and loss function being the sum of Dice loss and shape loss. The role of the shape-learning network is to learn the **shape signature** of a 3D binary label map, and this information would later become a part of the loss function of the segmentation network. The architecture of the shape-learning network is shown in Fig. 1, while the complete illustration showing the full network architecture is attached at Fig. 2.

3.2   Shape-Learning Network

The first step is to train the shape-learning network. In every iteration of training, we feed the shape-learning network with two binary label maps which are the **same structure** from the **same subject** that have gone through **different affine transformations**. Since these two label maps come from the same subject's same structure under different affine transformations, we call them an *affine pair*, and argue that they contain exactly the **same shape information**. If the network was able to capture shape information well, the difference between the shape signatures of these two label maps from the same *affine pair* should be small. We therefore compute the Euclidean distance between the shape signatures of these two label maps, and use this difference in Euclidean distance as loss and propagate the loss through the entire network and to update the network weights.

Let the ground truth label map be $M \in \mathbb{R}^{w \times h \times d}$ and the shape signature be $\hat{M} \in \mathbb{R}^{w' \times h' \times d'}$ where w', h', d' are much smaller than w, h, d respectively, the shape-learning network is essentially a non-linear mapping from M to $\hat{M}$, namely $\hat{M} = g_\theta(M)$, where θ is the weights in the convolutional layers of this network. Given this shape-learning network g_θ, the shape loss between two binary label maps $M_1, M_2 \in \mathbb{R}^{w \times h \times d}$ is therefore

$$\mathcal{L}_{shape}(M_1, M_2) = \|g_\theta(M_1) - g_\theta(M_2)\|_2$$

Training this shape-learning network therefore essentially means finding the θ that satisfies

$$\theta = \underset{\theta}{\arg\min}\, \mathcal{L}_{shape}(M_1, M_2)$$

where M_1 and M_2 are two instances of the same structure in the same subject, that have gone through different random affine transformation. After the training is finished, given a label map M, $g_\theta(M)$ gives the shape signature of this label map.

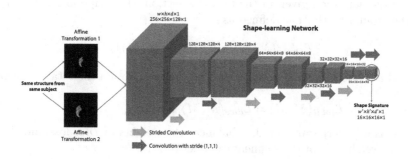

Fig. 1. Architecture of the shape-learning network.

3.3   Shape-Guided Segmentation Network

After the training of the shape-learning network is finished, we then train the segmentation network which is responsible for generating the segmentation label map. The segmentation network is a mapping f from the input (the raw voxels of brain MR image) I to the segmentation result $\tilde{M}$ defined as $\tilde{M} = f_W(I)$ where W is the weights of the segmentation network. The difference between the segmentation result $\tilde{M}$ and ground truth label map M is first measured by the Dice loss defined as

$$\mathcal{L}_{dice}(M, \tilde{M}) = 1 - \frac{2\sum_i M_i \tilde{M}_i}{\sum_i M_i + \sum_i \tilde{M}_i}$$

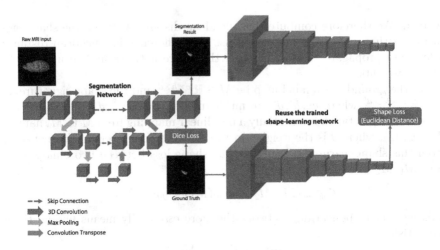

Fig. 2. Diagram of the full network architecture. The segmentation network, following a 3D U-Net architecture, is shown on the left, and the pre-trained shape-learning network that extracts the shape signature is shown on the right. Number of channels is not reflected on this diagram for brevity.

And by the definition given in the previous section, the shape loss between $\tilde{M}$ and the ground truth M is defined as

$$\mathcal{L}_{shape}(M, \tilde{M}) = \|g_\theta(M) - g_\theta(\tilde{M})\|_2$$

After adding the shape loss term to the Dice loss, we obtain the total loss which is

$$\mathcal{L}_{total}(M, \tilde{M}) = \mathcal{L}_{dice}(M, \tilde{M}) + \alpha \mathcal{L}_{shape}(M, \tilde{M})$$

where α is a hyperparameter that balances the weights of Dice loss and shape loss. The weights W of the segmentation network is

$$W = \underset{W}{\mathrm{argmin}}\, \mathcal{L}_{total}(M, \tilde{M})$$

and the segmentation network can be trained by the Stochastic Gradient Descent (SGD) with backpropagation since the entire pipeline is differentiable end-to-end.

4   Experiments

4.1   Experimental Setup

Experiments have been implemented on the human left and right caudate nucleus, as well as left and right hippocampus in the LONI Probabilistic Brain Atlas (LPBA40) dataset [8], which is a publicly available series of maps of human brain anatomic regions. The Magnetic Resonance (MR) images in the native space are used as raw input, while the label maps in the delineation space are the ground truth labels.

All MRI inputs and their corresponding labels are preprocessed and cropped to a region of $256 \times 256 \times 128$ in size, which is identical for every subject. Raw MRI inputs are preprocessed so that the original 12-bit image representation is normalized to a mean of 0.0 and standard deviation of 1.0. The label maps are further preprocessed for left and right caudate nuclei respectively, so that the label maps of both structures are binary three-dimensional arrays. Data augmentation operations on the training data include randomly rotating the object in 3D space up to $8°$, randomly scaling the object from 0.85 times to 1.15 times, as well as randomly translating the object. Left and right caudate nucleus and left and right hippocampus are all processed separately and are ran in separate experiments. Note that these transformations are also used in preparing an affine pair when training the shape-learning network, which requires the same structure to go through two random affine transformations.

4.2   Training the Shape-Learning Network

We first train the shape-learning network, and demonstrate why it is able to capture the essential shape information in the shape signature layer. The shape-learning network was trained with *affine pairs*, where the binary label maps have both gone through a random affine transformation that was employed in the data augmentation step. On each structure, we train for 200 iterations with batch size 1 and learning rate 1×10^{-4} on Adam Optimizer [2]. Experimental results illustrated in Table 1 demonstrate that the average difference in shape signature between affine pairs of the same subject's same structure is much lower than the average shape difference between pairs from different subjects. Therefore, a well-trained shape-learning network is able to capture a structure's essential shape information that is invariant to affine transformations.

Table 1. Average shape loss of 50 random *affine pairs* of the four biomedical structures tested, when the pairs are drawn from the same subject or a different subject.

	Same subject	Different subjects
Left Caudate	**0.120**	0.316
Right Caudate	**0.083**	0.210
Left Hippocampus	**0.251**	0.787
Right Hippocampus	**0.088**	0.277

4.3   Training the Segmentation Network

After finish training the shape-learning network, we freeze its weights and train the segmentation network. The experiments were also run with a batch size of 1, with the optimizer being Adam Optimizer [2] and the learning rate being 1×10^{-4}. The weight of shape loss α was chosen experimentally to be 0.1, and the models of left and right caudate nucleus and left and right hippocampus are first trained without shape loss for 800 iterations, and then trained with shape loss for another 400 iterations. To prevent the shape loss term from being extremely large, we experimentally set it to be capped at 1.0. As ablation experiments, we also run experiments with the same set of hyperparameters and the same dataset with a 3D U-Net model as a comparison. Note that the 3D U-Net here refers to the U-shape network in [1] trained with only Dice loss. Experimental results of Dice coefficient and Hausdorff distance on left and right caudate nucleus of 3D U-Net and our method are listed in Table 2, while the visual results are shown in Fig. 3.

Table 2. Performance of segmentation, evaluated on both Dice coefficient (Dice) and Hausdorff distance (HD).

Structure	Metric	3D U-Net	Our method
Left Caudate	Dice	0.831	**0.835**
	HD	5.472	**5.299**
Right Caudate	Dice	0.782	**0.820**
	HD	6.369	**5.004**
Left Hippocampus	Dice	0.771	**0.793**
	HD	20.170	**5.843**
Right Hippocampus	Dice	0.732	**0.759**
	HD	54.553	**29.878**

The Dice coefficient and Hausdorff distance in the tables are both metrics to evaluate the similarity between a segmentation result and its ground truth label map. A higher Dice coefficient and a lower Hausdorff distance both means greater similarity. It's shown that our approach achieves better results than 3D U-Net in terms of both Dice coefficient and Hausdorff distance. In the visual results, it is shown that our approach, compared with 3D U-Net, captures the intricate shape details better. In both examples in Fig. 3, 3D U-Net cannot segment the sharp part in the lower part of a caudate nucleus while our method is able to.

Since all experiment settings except loss function are the same for 3D U-Net and our method, the better performance of our method is due to the incorporation of shape information. Concretely, the shape loss measures the difference in shape signature, while shape signature extracted by a network trained to minimize the difference in shape signature between two *affine pairs* of the same subject. Therefore, when the difference in shape signature is used as a part of segmentation network's loss function, it naturally guides the segmentation network to produce segmentation results that comply with the shapes they should have, thus having better results both quantitatively and visually.

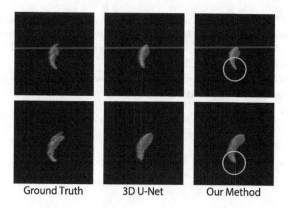

Ground Truth 3D U-Net Our Method

Fig. 3. Visual results of our approach compared with 3D U-Net.

5 Conclusion

We present a novel approach that incorporates shape information into the task of 3D medical image segmentation, by training an shape-learning network that learns the shape signature of the target to be segmented. We run experiments on the public LPBA40 dataset on the brain structure of caudate nucleus and hippocampus. Experimental results show that our approach leads to better results than 3D U-Net in terms of both Dice coefficient and Hausdorff distance.

References

1. Çiçek, Ö., Abdulkadir, A., Lienkamp, S.S., Brox, T., Ronneberger, O.: 3D U-Net: learning dense volumetric segmentation from sparse annotation. In: Ourselin, S., Joskowicz, L., Sabuncu, M.R., Unal, G., Wells, W. (eds.) MICCAI 2016. LNCS, vol. 9901, pp. 424–432. Springer, Cham (2016). https://doi.org/10.1007/978-3-319-46723-8_49
2. Kingma, D.P., Ba, J.: Adam: a method for stochastic optimization. arXiv preprint arXiv:1412.6980 (2014)
3. Long, J., Shelhamer, E., Darrell, T.: Fully convolutional networks for semantic segmentation. In: IEEE CVPR, pp. 3431–3440 (2015)
4. Milletari, F., Navab, N., Ahmadi, S.A.: V-net: fully convolutional neural networks for volumetric medical image segmentation. In: 3DV, pp. 565–571. IEEE (2016)
5. Oktay, O., et al.: Anatomically constrained neural networks (ACNN): application to cardiac image enhancement and segmentation. In: IEEE TMI (2017)
6. Ravishankar, H., Venkataramani, R., Thiruvenkadam, S., Sudhakar, P., Vaidya, V.: Learning and incorporating shape models for semantic segmentation. In: Descoteaux, M., Maier-Hein, L., Franz, A., Jannin, P., Collins, D.L., Duchesne, S. (eds.) MICCAI 2017. LNCS, vol. 10433, pp. 203–211. Springer, Cham (2017). https://doi.org/10.1007/978-3-319-66182-7_24

7. Ronneberger, O., Fischer, P., Brox, T.: U-Net: convolutional networks for biomedical image segmentation. In: Navab, N., Hornegger, J., Wells, W.M., Frangi, A.F. (eds.) MICCAI 2015. LNCS, vol. 9351, pp. 234–241. Springer, Cham (2015). https://doi.org/10.1007/978-3-319-24574-4_28
8. Shattuck, D.W., et al.: Construction of a 3D probabilistic atlas of human cortical structures. NeuroImage **39**(3), 1064–1080 (2008)

Automatic Detection of Patients with a High Risk of Systolic Cardiac Failure in Echocardiography

Delaram Behnami[1(✉)], Christina Luong[1,2], Hooman Vaseli[1], Amir Abdi[1], Hany Girgis[2], Dale Hawley[2], Robert Rohling[1], Ken Gin[1,2], Purang Abolmaesumi[1], and Teresa Tsang[1,2]

[1] University of British Columbia, Kelowna, Canada
delaramb@ece.ubc.ca
[2] Vancouver General Hospital, Vancouver, BC, Canada

Abstract. Heart disease is the global leading cause of death. A key predictor of heart failure and the most commonly measured cardiac parameter is left ventricular ejection fraction (LVEF). Despite available segmentation technologies, experienced cardiologists often rely on visual estimation of LVEF for a swift assessment. In this paper, we present a direct dual-channel LVEF estimation approach that mimics cardiologists' visual assessment for detecting patients with high risk of systolic heart failure. The proposed framework consists of various layers for extracting spatial and temporal features from echocardiography (echo) cines. A data set of 1,186 apical two-chamber (A2C) and four-chamber (A4C) echo cines were used in this study. LVEF labels were assigned based on risk of heart failure: high-risk for LVEF $\leq$ 40% and low-risk for 40% < LVEF $\leq$ 75%. We validated the proposed framework on 237 clinical exams and achieved a success rate of 83.1% for risk-based LVEF classification. Our experiments suggests the fusion of the two apical views improves the performance, compared to single-view networks, especially A2C. The proposed solution is promising for segmentation-free detection of high-risk LVEF. Direct LVEF estimation eliminates ventricle segmentation, and can hence be a useful tool for formal echo and point-of-care cardiac ultrasound.

1 Introduction

Heart disease is the leading cause of death globally, claiming the lives of over 8.5 million people in year 2015 alone [17]. Left ventricular ejection fraction (LVEF) is an important cardiac parameter and the key predictor for prognosis in most cardiac conditions, including valve disease, coronary artery disease, and heart failure [3]. Formally, LVEF is defined as the ratio between the amount of blood pumped out of the left ventricle (LV) every systole and the maximum amount

---

D. Behnami and C. Luong—Joint first authors.

P. Abolmaesumi and T. Tsang—Joint senior authors.

ⓒ Springer Nature Switzerland AG 2018
D. Stoyanov et al. (Eds.): DLMIA 2018/ML-CDS 2018, LNCS 11045, pp. 65–73, 2018.
https://doi.org/10.1007/978-3-030-00889-5_8

of blood in LV at the end of diastole. The most common imaging modality for measuring LVEF is echocardiography (echo) [3]. Echo is non-ionizing, accessible, low-cost, real time, and therefore ideal for studying the cardiac anatomy and function. In 2D echo, LVEF is conventionally quantified using the biplane method of disks, a.k.a. Simpson's rule [3]. This method calculates LVEF through LV volume estimation in end-systolic (ES) and end-diastolic (ED) frames, from apical two-chamber (A2C) and apical four-chamber (A4C) views. This segmentation-based routine is time-consuming and challenging with the presence of noise and unclear endocardial boundaries. Furthermore, studies suggest manual measurement of LVEF suffers from intra- and inter-user variability, especially among novice cardiologists [2,5]. To assist with automation of LV segmentation, several solutions have become commercially available [19]. A number of research groups have also proposed semi-automatic and automatic LV segmentation techniques, including recent machine learning and deep learning approaches [6,8,14,15,21]. Though promising for LV volume estimation in a given frame, these methods can lack robustness for LVEF prediction. This is due to dependence of LVEF on accurate LV tracing in ED and ES.

Clinically, LVEF is often measured through direct visual estimation [13]. Experienced cardiologists can eyeball LVEF from echo cine loops based on the wall motion and atrio-ventricular plane displacements [13]. Studies suggest direct visual estimation of LVEF is closely correlated to quantitative segmentation-based techniques [10]. Though this is the preferred choice of experts for quick LVEF assessment, visual estimation is a highly reader-dependent technique, leading inexperienced novice imagers to hesitate to use it [3,13]. Moreover, eyeballing LVEF is not a reliable option for other clinicians with limited echo training.

Direct estimation of LV volume and LVEF in cardiac magnetic resonance (MR) images has been explored by several groups [9,12,20,22]. Nevertheless, to the best of our knowledge, direct LVEF assessment has not been previously investigated in echo images. It is worth noting that LVEF estimation in echo is inherently a much more difficult problem compared to MR for several reasons. First, variability in acquiring standard echo imaging planes introduces greater variance in the appearance of the LV anatomy in 2D echo images. Moreover, the

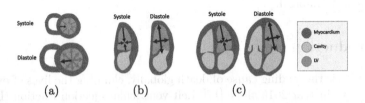

Fig. 1. Comparison of LV motion in ES and ED phases of SAX (a), A2C (b) and A4C (c). Deformations, movements of chambers and valves are more complex in A2C and A4C (used in echo) compared to SAX (used in MR), causing LVEF assessment to be more difficult in echo.

short-axis (SAX) view, used for LVEF estimation in MR (Fig. 1(a)), captures a much simpler cardiac motion and field-of-view compared to the views used in echo (Fig. 1(b) and (c)). Other challenges in echo include variable image quality and image settings, which also add to the complexity of a machine learning-based solution for direct LVEF assessment.

In this paper, we introduce a deep network that mimics the clinicians' eye-balling technique in echo to help classify exams as high-risk (LVEF ≤ 40%) or low-risk (40% < LVEF ≤ 75%). The following contributions are made: (1) Our approach directly estimates LVEF from echo cine loops, eliminating the need for LV segmentation and detection of key cardiac frames. LV segmentation can be challenging due to the high variability in echo image quality and image settings, as well as variability in the operator's experience in obtaining the correct echo standard views; (2) We propose a dual-stream framework for A2C and A4C views, consisted of view-specific spatial feature extraction blocks as well as shared recurrent neural network (RNN) layers. (3) We report the performance of several state-of-the-art networks and empirically show that for all the dual-view framework perform equally or better than a single apical view in classification of low-risk vs. high-risk LVEF.

2 Material

LVEF Labels: Our objective is to distinguish between the low-risk and high-risk LVEF classes. Let $\mathbf{Y}_{Simpson's}$ and $\mathbf{Y}_{Binary}$ denote the Simpson's rule-based gold standard LVEF measurement and derived risk-based binary labels, respectively. We define $\mathbf{Y}_{Binary}$ such that $\mathbf{Y}_{Binary} = 1$ for $\mathbf{Y}_{Simpson's} \leq 40\%$, and $\mathbf{Y}_{Binary} = 0$ for $40\% < \mathbf{Y}_{Simpson's} \leq 75\%$. Figure 2 visualizes the clinical labels in the database ($\mathbf{Y}_{Simpson's}$ and $\mathbf{Y}_{Eyeballed}$) and the derived risk-based binary labels used in the present classification network ($\mathbf{Y}_{Binary}$). Cases with $\mathbf{Y}_{Simpson's} > 75\%$ are excluded from this study due to the very limited number of samples.

Database: Ethics approval was obtained from our local regulatory authority to access a database of clinical echo exams and corresponding diagnostic reports at a tertiary care center. We searched the report database for echo exams that satisfied the following criteria: (1) The segmentation-based ($\mathbf{Y}_{Simpson's}$) and segmentation-free ($\mathbf{Y}_{Eyeballed}$) LVEF labels are recorded in the report database, and in agreement; (2) Correspondences can be found between the echo cines and diagnostic report based on the study identification information; (3) A2C and A4C views are both available. Also, in this paper, we focus the studies acquired

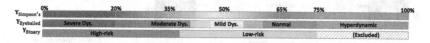

Fig. 2. LVEF labels used in the main database ($\mathbf{Y}_{Simpson's}$, $\mathbf{Y}_{Eyeballed}$) and for classification in this paper.

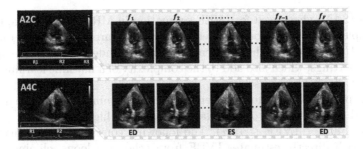

Fig. 3. Examples of synchronized A2C and A4C echo cines. Cines are temporally resampled between R_1^{AXC} to R_2^{AXC}, and effectively synchronized.

using the same family of ultrasound machines (Philips iE33). A total of 1,186 samples with the above criteria were gathered; 541 high-risk and 645 low-risk cases. The dataset was divided in a 4 : 1 ratio for training and test.

Echo Data and Preparation: 2D frames of 800×600 pixels are cleaned using a binary beam-shaped mask, cropped around the beam area, and downsized to 128×128 pixels. Temporally, frames are sampled from one full visible cycle in each cine loop AXC, where AXC $\in \{\text{A2C}, \text{A4C}\}$. To extract one cycle from each AXC cine, we find the of R peaks in its available electrocardiograms (ECG) and trim the cine to frames R_1^{AXC} to R_2^{AXC}. An equal number of $F = 25$ frames are uniformly sampled from each sequence (Fig. 3).

3 Methods

We propose the network in Fig. 4 for binary LVEF classification. This network is consisted of spatial feature extraction (FE) blocks as well as RNN-based layers for temporal learning.

Dual-view Spatial Feature Learning: We rely on CapsuleNet [18] and DenseNets [11] for frame feature extraction (FE), as they have been recently

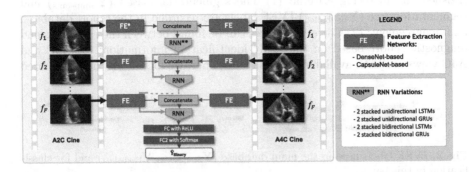

Fig. 4. Architecture of proposed multi-view classification network for LVEF estimation.

proved successful in spatial feature learning. Initially, sampled synchronous A2C and A4C frames are fed into FE blocks. The flattened output of an FE for a frame t is a feature vector $\mathbf{X}_{m,t}^{AXC}$ of length $M \times 1$; $m = 1 : M$. In the dual-view framework, $\mathbf{X}_{m,t}^{A2C}$ and $\mathbf{X}_{m,t}^{4XC}$ are then concatenated to form a dual-view feature vector $\mathbf{X}_{m,t}^{A2C+A4C}$ of length $2M \times 1$. For an exam with two streams and sequence length of F frames, a feature matrix $\mathbf{X}_{m,t}^{A2C+A4C}$ of size $2M \times F$ is constructed, where $t = 1 : F$. $\mathbf{X}_{m,t}^{A2C+A4C}$ is a dense representation of the cardiac cycle based on two views.

RNNs for Temporal Encoding: The other key components in the network are the RNN blocks, which enable sequential and temporal learning. We investigated various RNNs, including cascades of uni- and bi-directional Long Short Term Memory (LSTM) and Gated Recurrent Unit (GRU). The RNN blocks take in $\mathbf{X}_{m,t}^{A2C+A4C}$ at F separate time steps and output an array of the learned sequential features. This output is further pushed to a cascade of two fully connected (FC) layers, with ReLU and Softmax activation functions, respectively.

Training: The proposed architecture is implemented in Python using Keras with TensorFlow backend [4]. Dropout and batch normalization layers are used after FE blocks to prevent overfitting. The start points of the sampled frames are selected at random within the range R_1^{AXC} to R_2^{AXC}. Augmented data is created on the fly via randomly generated transforms, including rotation, scaling, cropping and gamma transformation on the intensities.

4   Results

Quantitative results obtained in this study are demonstrated in Fig. 5. The highest performance is achieved using the dual-view approach with DenseNets and bidirectional GRUs. Figure 6 depicts this network's performance on a few examples of A2C+A4C image pairs.

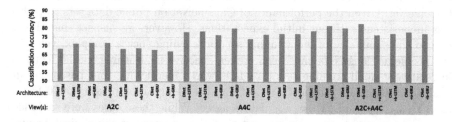

Fig. 5. LVEF classification accuracy using DenseNet (DNet) and CapsuleNet (CNet) as the spatial FE, and various and RNN versions on A2C, A4C and A2C+A4C views.

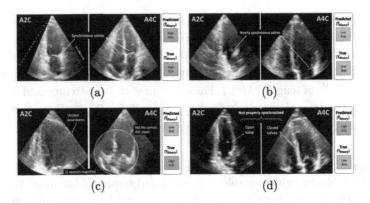

Fig. 6. Performance of DenseNets and bidirectional GRU on a few A2C+A4C pairs. Cardiac echo quality and proper synchronization of views affect the model performance.

5   Discussion and Conclusion

In this paper, we introduced a new framework based on DenseNet, CapsuleNet and RNN layers for estimating LVEF from echo cines in A2C and A4C standard echo views. Our results suggest that A2C alone is a less reliable view for LVEF estimation, while A4C alone appears to be a much more robust option with the current framework. However, the most accurate results is achieved by combining both apical views. This observation is also aligned with anecdotal clinical evidence, where A2C views are more difficult to obtain over A4C, and are more likely to be foreshortened [16], hence LVEF estimation from A2C can be less reliable. LSTM and GRU often performed equivalently, although the highest accuracy was obtained using GRU blocks. The results also consistently suggest that bidirectional recurrent layers are equivalent to or better than unidirectional ones. The optimal deep model, consisted of DenseNet + bidirectional GRU, achieved a success rate of 83.1% on the test set for detecting high-risk LVEF. We observed that DenseNet achieved a higher accuracy, compared to CapsuleNet. Given the performance of CapsuleNet on public data sets [18], this was inconsistent with our initial expectations. However, we suspect that this is due to the small size of our training set for learning such a complex, yet subtle, problem. DenseNets have been proven effective for learning spatial features in relatively small training sets [11]. It is worth mentioning that based on our analysis of the main diagnostic report database, only an approximate 70.1% of the ($\mathbf{Y}_{\text{Simpson's}}$) and ($\mathbf{Y}_{\text{Eyeballed}}$) labels agree. While these cases were excluded from the presented study, we suspect that the accuracy of the clinical ground truth labels may be similarly compromised to some extent.

A key pattern recognized from the results is the link between model performance, the quality of apical images, and view synchronization (Fig. 6). Misclassified images generally have unclear LV boundaries, which causes a great deal of variance in the appearance of the heart and its motion. Also, despite the automatic and manual view classification, confusion between the four apical views

(A2C, three-chamber, A4C and five-chamber) appears to remain a challenge and a potential source of error (*e.g.*, Fig. 6(c)). Thus, a bottom-up approach for improving LVEF accuracy can be through improving the quality of the input data. Abdi *et al.* recently proposed a deep-learning solution for automatic estimation of echo quality [1], which can be used to provide feedback to ultrasound operators for improving the quality of data acquisition.

A resolvable limitation of the proposed solution is the dependence on ECG, for phase detection and synchronization. ECG is not available in point-of-care. Moreover, visual inspection of the results revealed correlation between misclassification and apparent improper synchronization (see *e.g.*, Fig. 6(d), which shows asynchronous A2C and A4C views based on the valve state). We believe improving the phase detection can contribute to achieving more accurate results. Alternatively, a cine-based cardiac phase detection can be implemented into the network. A possible solution has been proposed by Dezaki *et al.* [7] for A4C images, which can be similarly extended to A2C. This method is capable of automatically identifying ES and ED, which could be used to achieve potentially richer temporal sampling of systolic and diastolic phases.

One possible option to eliminate phase-dependence altogether is through having two separate RNN streams; one per A2C and A4C views. This decouples the two views from one another, enabling the use of potentially informative cines in full. However, this architecture causes a large sudden increase in the network size, and is still less successful for LVEF estimation based on our experiments thus far. This is most likely because the inputs of the RNN blocks, *i.e.* the frame feature vectors, are denser and richer when constructed from two complimentary views, allowing for more effective temporal learning. This may change should we increase our training set.

While a binary risk-based LVEF classification tool could assist with immediate decision making in point-of-care, it suffers from a flaw: it imposes a sharp boundary on the true regression labels ($Y_{Simpson's}$). This can be amended by adding a medium-risk class, or more classes of $Y_{Eyeballed}$. We plan to include exams from other ultrasound machines to obtain enough data for this multi-class classification.

Given that LV localization appears to be the key step in some LVEF estimation approaches proposed for cardiac MR [12], another question worth exploring is whether LV localization helps with LVEF accuracy in echo. While the motion of the atria and right ventricle can contain subtle information about LVEF, excluding them decreases variance from the neighbouring chambers. Existing encoder-decoder segmentation networks can be modified and used to localize, track and accordingly crop LV throughout the cine.

References

1. Abdi, A.H., et al.: Quality assessment of echocardiographic cine using recurrent neural networks: feasibility on five standard view planes. In: Descoteaux, M., Maier-Hein, L., Franz, A., Jannin, P., Collins, D.L., Duchesne, S. (eds.) MICCAI 2017. LNCS, vol. 10435, pp. 302–310. Springer, Cham (2017). https://doi.org/10.1007/978-3-319-66179-7_35

2. Bresser, P., De Beer, J., De Wet, Y.: A study investigating variability of left ventricular ejection fraction using manual and automatic processing modes in a single setting. Radiography **21**(1), e41–e44 (2015)

3. Cameli, M., Mondillo, S., Solari, M., et al.: Echocardiographic assessment of left ventricular systolic function: from ejection fraction to torsion. Heart Fail. Rev. **21**(1), 77–94 (2016)

4. Chollet, F., et al.: Keras (2015). https://github.com/keras-team/keras

5. Cole, G.D., Dhutia, N.M., Shun-Shin, M.J., et al.: Defining the real-world reproducibility of visual grading of left ventricular function and visual estimation of left ventricular ejection fraction: impact of image quality, experience and accreditation. Int. J. Cardiovasc. Imaging **31**(7), 1303–1314 (2015)

6. Deo, R.C., Zhang, J., Hallock, L.A., et al.: An end-to-end computer vision pipeline for automated cardiac function assessment by echocardiography. CoRR (2017). http://arxiv.org/abs/1706.07342

7. Dezaki, F.T., et al.: Deep residual recurrent neural networks for characterisation of cardiac cycle phase from echocardiograms. In: Cardoso, M., et al. (eds.) DLMIA/ML-CDS -2017. LNCS, vol. 10553, pp. 100–108. Springer, Cham (2017). https://doi.org/10.1007/978-3-319-67558-9_12

8. Dong, S., Luo, G., Sun, G., et al.: A left ventricular segmentation method on 3D echocardiography using deep learning and snake. In: 2016 Computing in Cardiology Conference (CinC), pp. 473–476. IEEE (2016)

9. Gu, B., Shan, Y., Sheng, V.S., et al.: Sparse regression with output correlation for cardiac ejection fraction estimation. Inf. Sci. **423**, 303–312 (2018)

10. Gudmundsson, P., Rydberg, E., Winter, R., et al.: Visually estimated left ventricular ejection fraction by echocardiography is closely correlated with formal quantitative methods. Int. J. Cardiol. **101**(2), 209–212 (2005)

11. Huang, G., Liu, Z., Weinberger, K.Q., et al.: Densely connected convolutional networks. In: IEEE CVPR (2017)

12. Kabani, A.W., El-Sakka, M.R.: Ejection fraction estimation using a wide convolutional neural network. In: Karray, F., Campilho, A., Cheriet, F. (eds.) ICIAR 2017. LNCS, vol. 10317, pp. 87–96. Springer, Cham (2017). https://doi.org/10.1007/978-3-319-59876-5_11

13. Kim, C., Hur, J., Kang, B.S., et al.: Can an offsite expert remotely evaluate the visual estimation of ejection fraction via a social network video call? J. Dig. Imaging **30**(6), 718–725 (2017)

14. Leclerc, S., Grenier, T., Espinosa, F., Bernard, O.: A fully automatic and multi-structural segmentation of the left ventricle and the myocardium on highly heterogeneous 2D echocardiographic data. In: 2017 IEEE International Ultrasonics Symposium (IUS), pp. 1–4. IEEE (2017)

15. Ngo, T.A., Lu, Z., Carneiro, G.: Combining deep learning and level set for the automated segmentation of the left ventricle of the heart from cardiac cine magnetic resonance. Med. Image Anal. **35**, 159–171 (2017)

16. Nosir, Y., Vletter, W.B., Boersma, E., et al.: The apical long-axis rather than the two-chamber view should be used in combination with the four-chamber view for accurate assessment of left ventricular volumes and function. Eur. Heart J. **18**(7), 1175–1185 (1997)

17. Organization, W.H.: Global health observatory (GHO) data (2017). http://www.who.int/gho/mortality_burden_disease/causes_death/top_10/en/

18. Sabour, S., Frosst, N., Hinton, G.E.: Dynamic routing between capsules. In: Advances in Neural Information Processing Systems, pp. 3859–3869 (2017)

19. Wood, P.W., Choy, J.B., Nanda, N.C., et al.: Left ventricular ejection fraction and volumes: it depends on the imaging method. Echo **31**(1), 87–100 (2014)

20. Xue, W., Lum, A., Mercado, A., Landis, M., Warrington, J., Li, S.: Full quantification of left ventricle via deep multitask learning network respecting intra- and inter-task relatedness. In: Descoteaux, M., Maier-Hein, L., Franz, A., Jannin, P., Collins, D.L., Duchesne, S. (eds.) MICCAI 2017. LNCS, vol. 10435, pp. 276–284. Springer, Cham (2017). https://doi.org/10.1007/978-3-319-66179-7_32

21. Zhang, J., Gajjala, S., Agrawal, P., et al.: A web-deployed computer vision pipeline for automated determination of cardiac structure and function and detection of disease by two-dimensional echocardiography. arXiv:1706.07342 (2017)

22. Zhen, X., Wang, Z., Islam, A., et al.: Multi-scale deep networks and regression forests for direct bi-ventricular volume estimation. Med. Image Anal. **30**, 120–129 (2016)

MTMR-Net: Multi-task Deep Learning with Margin Ranking Loss for Lung Nodule Analysis

Lihao Liu[1(✉)], Qi Dou[1], Hao Chen[1,3], Iyiola E. Olatunji[2], Jing Qin[4], and Pheng-Ann Heng[1]

[1] Department of Computer Science and Engineering,
The Chinese University of Hong Kong, Sha Tin, Hong Kong
lhliu@cse.cuhk.edu.hk
[2] Department of Systems Engineering and Engineering Management,
The Chinese University of Hong Kong, Sha Tin, Hong Kong
[3] Imsight Medical Technology Co., Ltd., Shenzhen, China
[4] Center for Smart Health, School of Nursing,
The Hong Kong Polytechnic University, Kowloon, Hong Kong

Abstract. Lung cancer is the leading cause of cancer deaths worldwide. Early diagnosis of lung nodules is of great importance for therapeutic treatment and saving lives. Automated lung nodule analysis requires both accurate lung nodule benign-malignant classification and attribute score grading. However, this is quite challenging due to the considerable difficulty of nodule heterogeneity modelling and limited discrimination capability on ambiguous cases. To meet these challenges, we propose a **Multi-T**ask deep learning framework with a novel **M**argin **R**anking loss (referred as MTMR-Net) for automated lung nodule analysis. The relatedness between lung nodule classification and attribute score regression is explicitly explored in our multi-task model, which can contribute to the performance gains of both tasks. The results of different tasks can be yielded simultaneously for assisting the radiologists in diagnosis interpretation. Furthermore, a siamese network with a novel margin ranking loss was elaborately designed to enhance the discrimination capability on ambiguous nodule cases. We validated the efficacy of our MTMR-Net on the public benchmark LIDC-IDRI dataset. Extensive experiments demonstrated that our approach achieved competitive classification performance and more accurate attribute scoring over the state-of-the-arts.

1 Introduction

Lung cancer has been the leading cause of cancer deaths worldwide. In the year 2018, the estimated death cases of lung cancer will account for approximately 26% of all cancer deaths in the United States [1]. Early diagnosis of lung cancer is crucial in the future treatment of lung cancer patient, because its five-year survival rate is lower than 20% when it promotes to a late stage. Lung cancer usually refers to small malignant lung nodules (with the diameter in the

© Springer Nature Switzerland AG 2018
D. Stoyanov et al. (Eds.): DLMIA 2018/ML-CDS 2018, LNCS 11045, pp. 74–82, 2018.
https://doi.org/10.1007/978-3-030-00889-5_9

range of 3–30 mm), which can be detected on the chest computed tomography (CT) scans. However, distinguishing the nodules between benign and malignant is quite difficult even for experienced radiologists [2]. Because there are various potential malignancy-related characteristics (e.g., spiculation), these characteristics should be taken into consideration during the diagnosis process.

Computer-aided diagnosis techniques have been proven to be helpful for radiologists in decision making and hold the potential to improve diagnostic accuracy in distinguishing small benign nodules from malignant ones [3]. With the powerful representation capability, deep neural networks are capable of learning more complicated diagnosis patterns from labeled data. Hence, it could assist the automated lung nodule analysis. Recently, several deep learning based methods have been proposed for computer-aided diagnosis of lung nodules. Xie et al. [6] proposed a multi-model ensemble method that considered overall appearance, nodule shape and voxel value of each nodule slice simultaneously to achieve high classification accuracy. Chen et al. [5] introduced a multi-task regression model to explore the internal relationship among the semantic features. Instead of considering these two tasks independently, Hussein et al. [13] proposed a 3D CNN-based multi-task model to implicitly explore the relationship between malignancy classification and attribute score regression tasks. Although achieving state-of-the-art performance, these previous methods either independently or "jointly but implicitly" tackled the benign-malignant classification and attribute score regression tasks, instead of jointly analyzing and explicitly exploring their correlations for more convincing and interpretable diagnosis.

In this paper, we propose a novel **Multi-T**ask deep learning framework with a new **M**argin **R**anking loss (called MTMR-Net) for automated lung nodule analysis. We build a bi-branch model which not only predicts nodule malignancy but also outputs regressed scores of eight attribute characteristics. The relatedness between two highly-correlated tasks is explicitly learned in our model, and both tasks can benefit from each other through the proposed architecture. Furthermore, we propose a novel margin ranking loss based on siamese network architecture to perform comparison while scoring nodules to model their heterogeneity. This enables the network to be more accurate on recognizing marginal lung nodules by referring to lung nodules with different labels but close malignancy scores. We validated our proposed framework on the public LIDC-IDRI dataset and achieved competitive classification accuracy over the state-of-the-arts. In addition, compared with previous approaches which can only output a binary classification result, our proposed model can provide more cues and evidence for radiologists by simultaneously yielding the scores of the attributes when making diagnosis.

2   Method

Our proposed MTMR-Net consists of two components. First, we propose a multi-task deep learning model for nodule analysis, which is composed of lung nodule classification task and attribute score regression task. Second, to further discriminate the marginal nodules, we present a new margin ranking loss to train the model in order to enhance the distinguishing capability among marginal cases.

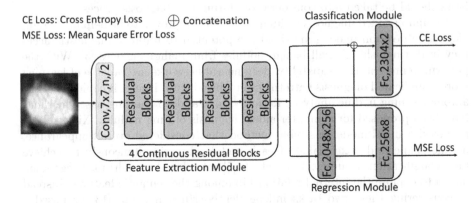

Fig. 1. Multi-task learning framework. Residual blocks used are exactly the same as the residual blocks in original 50-layer residual network [7]. Besides classification branch, an additional regression branch is added to predict 8 attributes scores. The "CE Loss" and "MSE Loss" denote cross entropy loss and mean square error loss, respectively.

2.1   Multi-task Learning for Lung Nodule Analysis

Benign-Malignant Classification. The multi-task model is fine-tuned from a 50-layer residual network [7]. We keep the feature extraction module of the original residual network. However, in the classification module, we concatenated the extracted feature maps with an additional feature map (feature map from regression module) before the last fully-connected layer, as shown in Fig. 1. We formulate the task as a classification problem rather than a regression problem, considering that a definite diagnosis can provide more intuitive information to experts. Therefore, we use cross entropy loss (CE Loss) for backward propagation in the classification module, which is defined as:

$$\mathcal{L}_{cls} = -\frac{1}{N} \sum_i log \; p_i^c \left(y_i^c | x_i; W_{cls}, W_s \right), \tag{1}$$

where x_i and p_i^c are the input image and output probability from the classification module, while $y_i^c \in \{0, 1\}$ is the ground truth of lung nodule classification label, W_s and W_{cls} are the weights of shared feature extraction path and nodule classification task, respectively. N is the total number of training samples.

Nodule Attribute Score Regression. Motivated by the clinical observation that radiologists analyze the characteristics of attributes for malignancy assessment, we hypothesize that exploring the correlation between malignancy classification and attributes scoring would help to further improve the discrimination capability for lung nodule analysis. Therefore, besides the classification task, we also add a regression module for attributes score prediction in the network. Before the last fully-connected layer for final regression, we explicitly extract attributes features using another fully-connected layer following the shared feature extraction module, as shown in Fig. 1. In addition, rather than using these attributes features solely for regression task, we concatenate the malignant feature in the classification module with the attributes features. The concatenation between malignancy feature map and attributes feature map enables more attributes information guidance in the nodule classification task. For the attributes score regression task, we used mean square error loss (MSE Loss) during the training process, which is defined as:

$$\mathcal{L}_{reg} = \frac{1}{N} \sum_i ||\hat{y_i^r}(x_i; W_s, W_{reg}) - y_i^r||_2^2, \tag{2}$$

where $y_i^r \in \mathbb{R}^{1 \times n}$ is the output of regression task of network, while $\hat{y_i^r} \in \mathbb{R}^{1 \times n}$ is the ground truth of attribute scores. $n = 8$, for using eight semantic attributes.

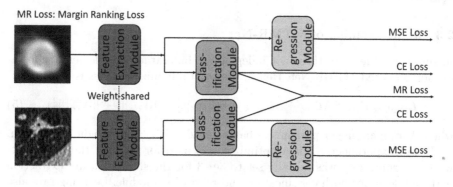

Fig. 2. Siamese model based on two shared-weight proposed multi-task model. "MR Loss" means margin ranking loss. All 3 modules (feature extraction, classification, regression) are weight-shared in two branches of siamese network.

2.2 Margin Ranking Loss for Discriminating Marginal Nodules

Despite multiple correlated supervision information is employed in our deep neural network, we still observe there exists misclassification on marginal lung nodules. To tackle the similar misclassification problem, Kong et al. [8] used siamese network to enhance model's discrimination capability on ambiguous cases. Inspired by Kong et al. [8], we perform the same architecture with a novel margin ranking loss while scoring nodules to model nodules' heterogeneity. Siamese network is well-known for using two shared-weight feature extraction branches in its network architecture. It enables the network to train in a pairwise mode, see Fig. 2, which can enhance classification accuracy by applying comparison and referring. Besides, a novel margin ranking loss is designed for capturing the ranking relationship between different training samples:

$$\mathcal{L}_{rank} = \frac{1}{2N} \sum_{i,j} max\left(0, \gamma - \delta\left(p_i^c, p_j^c\right) * \left(t_i^c - t_j^c\right)\right), \tag{3}$$

$$\delta\left(p_i^c, p_j^c\right) = \begin{cases} 1, & p_i^c \geq p_j^c \\ -1, & p_i^c < p_j^c \end{cases}, \tag{4}$$

where $t_i^c \in [0,1], t_j^c \in [0,1]$ denotes the ground truth malignancy score for the ith, jth training sample, respectively. While $p_i^c \in [0,1], p_j^c \in [0,1]$ are the ith, jth training sample's predicted malignancy probability, respectively. $\delta\left(p_i^c, p_j^c\right)$ is the indicator function. γ is the margin parameter.

If the predicted scores' ranking is the same as ground truth scores' ranking (e.g., $t_i^c \geq t_j^c, p_i^c \geq p_j^c$), then the loss is 0. Otherwise, the loss is penalized during the training process (e.g., $t_i^c \geq t_j^c, p_i^c < p_j^c$). Applying this mechanism into a siamese network can easily explore and model the difference between marginal lung nodules by adjusting the margin parameter γ.

2.3   Joint Training of MTMR-Net

In summary, there are three not independent but rather complementary losses for our proposed MTMR-Net. Hence, the total minimization loss is defined as:

$$\mathcal{L}_{total} = \mathcal{L}_{cls} + \lambda\mathcal{L}_{reg} + \beta\mathcal{L}_{rank} + \eta(||W_s||_2^2 + ||W_{cls}||_2^2 + ||W_{reg}||_2^2), \tag{5}$$

where λ, β, η are hyper-parameters balancing $\mathcal{L}_{cls}$, $\mathcal{L}_{reg}$ and weight decay term.

In our experiments, Adam optimizer was used for training the entire network. Learning rate was initially set to 3e−3 for the shared feature extraction part and 3e−5 for both classification and regression module. Learning rate also periodically annealed by 0.1. We trained our model for 150 epochs using the pytorch. After using grid-search for finding hyper-parameters, we set 3 parameters for controlling the weights for λ, β, η as 1, 5e−1, 1e−3, respectively, and the marginal parameter γ was chosen as 1e−1.

3   Experiments

3.1   Dataset and Preprocessing

We validated the proposed MTMR-Net on the LIDC-IDRI dataset, which consisted of 1018 CT scans [9] and 1422 lung nodules (972 benign lung nodules and 450 malignant lung nodules). The nodules were rated from 1 to 5 by four experienced radiologists signifying the degree of malignancy in an increasing order. For benign-malignant classification task, nodules with average score less than

3 and greater than 3 were labeled as benign and malignant, respectively. Nodules with average score of 3 were left out in our experiments as all other works did [4–6]. Besides malignancy, eight semantic attributes (i.e., subtlety, calcification, sphericity, margin, spiculation, texture, lobulation and internal structure) were also scored in the LIDC-IDRI dataset. The higher the score is, the more obvious the characteristic is. Most features were rated in the range of 1–5, while the internal structure and calcification were given scores in the range of 1–4 and 1–6, respectively. We rescaled the average score labels from 1–5, 1–6, 1–4 to 0–1 for normalization before training.

We divided the dataset into training (90%) and testing (10%) sets following the setting in [4], which is well calculated so the sampled training and testing dataset has similar distribution. We cropped an adaptive patch region according to the diameter and position of the nodule and resized the patch to 224×224 using bilinear interpolation. In addition, we employed random cropping, horizontal flipping, and vertical flipping as data augmentations. In [12], Dou et al. employed 3D CNN to preserve more spatial information. Instead, we use 2D CNN to explore each slice's malignancy and semantic attribute score, and then averaged the probability scores of slices enclosing nodule to get the final results as mentioned in [6]. This method may lose some spatial information, but the average operation can effectively prevent overfitting.

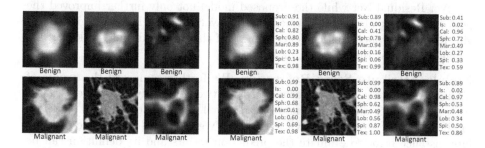

Fig. 3. Left part: classification outputs from previous work's model [4,6]. Right part: classification outputs with attribute score from MTMR-Net. Sub, Is, Cal, Sph, Mar, Lob, Spi, Tex denotes subtlety, internal structure, calcification, sphericity, margin, spiculation, lobulation and texture, respectively. Score for each attribute is rescaled to the range of 0–1. The higher the score is, the more obvious the characteristic is.

3.2 Results and Evaluation Comparison

Benign-Malignant Classification. We compared the proposed model with several state-of-the-art methods and performed an ablation analysis of the proposed model. The results are reported in Table 1. We employed four commonly used metrics for the comparison: accuracy, specificity, sensitivity and area under curve (AUC); the definitions of these metrics can be found in [6]. As shown

Table 1. Performance of lung nodule classification methods on LIDC-IDRI dataset

Methods	Accuracy (%)	Sensitivity (%)	Specificity (%)	AUC
Anand et al. 2015 [10]	86.3	89.6	86.7	–
Xie et al. 2016 [6]	93.4	**91.4**	94.1	**0.978**
Shen et al. 2017 [11]	87.1	77.0	93.0	0.930
Causey et al. 2017 [4]	93.2	87.9	**98.5**	0.971
50-layer Residual Net	90.1	83.1	97.0	0.950
MTMR-Net (w/o $\mathcal{L}_{reg}$)	91.6	84.6	**98.5**	0.957
MTMR-Net (w/o $\mathcal{L}_{rank}$)	92.3	86.2	97.0	0.946
MTMR-Net	**93.9**	89.2	**98.5**	0.957

in Table 1, our method achieved the best accuracy, sensitivity and comparable specificity, AUC when compared with state-of-the-art methods, demonstrating the effectiveness of exploiting the relatedness of classification task and attribute prediction task as well as the margin ranking loss in improving the classification accuracy. In order to carefully scrutinize the contributions of different components of the proposed model, we further compared the proposed original the 50-layer Residual Net, the MTMR-Net without MSE Loss, and the MTMR-Net without MR Loss. It is observed that both the MTMR-Net without MSE Loss and the MTMR-Net without MR Loss achieve better performance than the 50-layer Residual Net while the proposed model not only further improved the performance but also outperformed the 50-layer Residual Net by a great margin, further corroborating the effectiveness of the proposed multi-task learning scheme as well as the margin ranking loss.

Nodule Attribute Score Regression. We further compared the results of attribute score prediction of our model with two commonly used models, lasso regression model and elastic network, as well as a state-of-the-art method, MTR [5]. The results are shown in Table 2. We employed the metric of absolute distance error to evaluate the prediction results and its definition can be found in [5]. Compared with previous methods, our model achieved significantly lower absolute distance error on most of the features, demonstrating in our multi-task model trained based on the relatedness between these two tasks, while the attribute prediction task can improve the performance of the classification task, in turn, the classification task can also enhance the attribute prediction accuracy.

Figure 3 showed typical results of classification and the corresponding attribute prediction results. Inspiringly, we found our results are quite consistent with those of previous clinical studies. For example, the malignant cases usually have higher calcification, higher lobulation and lower spiculation while internal structure has no influence on malignancy diagnosis. The results also demonstrate that we cannot classify the nodules based solely on one or two attributes. However, we should comprehensively consider more attributes, which has also been stated in many clinical studies. Compared with previous methods without explicitly exploring the relatedness of two tasks, the proposed model can also provide more cues and evidence for diagnosis by simultaneously outputting the

Table 2. Performance of attribute scores prediction. MTR, LASSO, EN are multi-task regression model [5], lasso regression model and elastic network, respectively. Sub, Is, Cal, Sph, Mar, Lob, Spi, Tex shares the same definition as in Fig. 3. The score is calculated on the original unscaled data.

Methods	Features							
	Sub	Is	Cal	Sph	Mar	Lob	Spi	Tex
MTR [5]	0.75	0.04	**0.48**	0.81	0.86	0.87	0.80	0.58
LASSO	1.25	**0.02**	2.18	1.25	1.13	0.95	0.89	1.04
EN	1.20	0.14	1.44	1.09	0.98	0.96	0.86	1.24
MTMR-Net	**0.52**	0.03	0.62	**0.58**	**0.53**	**0.51**	**0.49**	**0.38**

attribute scores, besides better classification accuracy. The proposed method not only can be used in automated lung nodule diagnosis systems, but also it can be employed as a tool for the investigations which aim at revealing the underlying yet complicated relationship between the malignancy of a nodule and its attributes as shown in Fig. 3.

4 Conclusion

In this paper, we presented the MTMR-Net under a multi-task deep learning framework with margin ranking loss for automated lung nodule analysis. The relatedness between lung nodule classification and attribute score regression was explicitly explored with multi-task deep learning, which contributed to the performance gains of both tasks. Furthermore, a novel margin ranking loss was explored to model nodule heterogeneity and encourage the discrimination capability of ambiguous nodule cases. Extensive experiments on the benchmark dataset verified the efficacy of our method and achieved competitive performance over the state-of-the-arts.

Acknowledgement. This project is funded by Hong Kong Innovation and Technology Commission, under ITSP Tier 2 Scheme (Project No. ITS/426/17FP).

References

1. Siegel, R.L., Siegel, R.L., Miller, K.D., Jemal, A.: Cancer statistics, 2018. CA Cancer J. Clin. **67**(1), 7–30 (2018)
2. del Ciello, A., Franchi, P., Contegiacomo, A., Cicchetti, G., Bonomo, L., Larici, A.R.: Missed lung cancer: when, where, and why? Diagn. Interv. Radiol. **23**(2), 118–126 (2017)
3. Kumar, D., Wong, A., Clausi, D.A.: Lung nodule classification using deep features in CT images. In: Computer and Robot Vision (CRV), pp. 133–138 (2015)
4. Causey, J., et al.: Highly accurate model for prediction of lung nodule malignancy with ct scans. Scientific Reports 8(1), 9286 (2018)

5. Chen, S., Qin, J., Ji, X., Lei, B., Wang, T., Ni, D., Cheng, J.Z.: Automatic scoring of multiple semantic attributes with multi-task feature leverage: a study on pulmonary nodules in ct images. IEEE Trans. Med. Imaging **36**(3), 802–814 (2017)
6. Xie, Y., Xia, Y., Zhang, J., Feng, D.D., Fulham, M., Cai, W.: Transferable multi-model ensemble for benign-malignant lung nodule classification on chest CT. In: Descoteaux, M., Maier-Hein, L., Franz, A., Jannin, P., Collins, D.L., Duchesne, S. (eds.) MICCAI 2017. LNCS, vol. 10435, pp. 656–664. Springer, Cham (2017). https://doi.org/10.1007/978-3-319-66179-7_75
7. He, K., Zhang, X., Ren, S., Sun, J.: Deep residual learning for image recognition. In: Proceedings of the IEEE conference on Computer Vision and Pattern Recognition, pp. 770–778 (2016)
8. Kong, S., Shen, X., Lin, Z., Mech, R., Fowlkes, C.: Photo aesthetics ranking network with attributes and content adaptation. In: Leibe, B., Matas, J., Sebe, N., Welling, M. (eds.) ECCV 2016. LNCS, vol. 9905, pp. 662–679. Springer, Cham (2016). https://doi.org/10.1007/978-3-319-46448-0_40
9. Armato III, S.G., et al.: The lung image database consortium (LIDC) and image database resource initiative (IDRI): a completed reference database of lung nodules on CT scans. Med. Phys. **38**(2), 915–931 (2011)
10. Anand, S.V.: Segmentation coupled textural feature classification for lung tumor prediction. In: IEEE International Conference on Communication Control and Computing Technologies (ICCCCT). pp. 518–524 (2010)
11. Shen, W., et al.: Multi-crop convolutional neural networks for lung nodule malignancy suspiciousness classification. Pattern Recogn. **61**, 663–673 (2017)
12. Dou, Q.: 3d deeply supervised network for automated segmentation of volumetric medical images. Med. Image Anal. **41**, 40–54 (2017)
13. Hussein, S., Cao, K., Song, Q., Bagci, U.: Risk stratification of lung nodules using 3D CNN-based multi-task learning. In: Niethammer, M., Styner, M., Aylward, S., Zhu, H., Oguz, I., Yap, P.-T., Shen, D. (eds.) IPMI 2017. LNCS, vol. 10265, pp. 249–260. Springer, Cham (2017). https://doi.org/10.1007/978-3-319-59050-9_20

Active Deep Learning with Fisher Information for Patch-Wise Semantic Segmentation

Jamshid Sourati[1]($\boxtimes$), Ali Gholipour[1], Jennifer G. Dy[2], Sila Kurugol[1],
and Simon K. Warfield[1]

[1] Radiology Department, Boston Children's Hospital, 300 Longwood Avenue,
Boston, MA 02115, USA
jamshid.sourati@childrens.harvard.edu
[2] Department of Electrical and Computer Engineering, Northeastern University,
360 Huntington Avenue, Boston, MA 02115, USA

Abstract. Deep learning with convolutional neural networks (CNN) has achieved unprecedented success in segmentation, however it requires large training data, which is expensive to obtain. Active Learning (AL) frameworks can facilitate major improvements in CNN performance with intelligent selection of minimal data to be labeled. This paper proposes a novel diversified AL based on Fisher information (FI) for the first time for CNNs, where gradient computations from backpropagation are used for efficient computation of FI on the large CNN parameter space. We evaluated the proposed method in the context of newborn and adolescent brain extraction problem under two scenarios: (1) semi-automatic segmentation of a particular subject from a different age group or with a pathology not available in the original training data, where starting from an inaccurate pre-trained model, we iteratively label small number of voxels queried by AL until the model generates accurate segmentation for that subject, and (2) using AL to build a universal model generalizable to all images in a given data set. In both scenarios, FI-based AL improved performance after labeling a small percentage (less than 0.05%) of voxels. The results showed that FI-based AL significantly outperformed random sampling, and achieved accuracy higher than entropy-based querying in transfer learning, where the model learns to extract brains of newborn subjects given an initial model trained on adolescents.

1 Introduction

Image segmentation plays an important role for extracting quantitative imaging markers of disease for improved medical diagnosis and treatment. CNNs have

S. K. Warfield—This work was supported by NIH grants R01 NS079788, R01 EB019483, R01 DK100404, R44 MH086984, BCH IDDRC U54 HD090255, and by a research grant from the Boston Children's Hospital Translational Research Program. A.G. is supported by NIH grant R01 EB018988. S.K. is also supported by CCFA's Career Development Award and AGA-Boston Scientific Technology and Innovation Award.

D. Stoyanov et al. (Eds.): DLMIA 2018/ML-CDS 2018, LNCS 11045, pp. 83–91, 2018.
https://doi.org/10.1007/978-3-030-00889-5_10

been shown to be promising for medical image segmentation [1]. However, they require large training sets to be able to generalize well. In medical applications, labels are often only available for limited subjects who come from a healthy group with a specific age range. Models trained on this population will not perform well in subjects from a different age group (such as newborns or children), subjects imaged on a different scanner or subjects with a specific disease. In order to generalize models, annotating more images is crucial. Due to costly efforts needed for medical annotation, *active learning* (AL) seems imperative enabling us to build generalizable models with the smallest number of additional annotations. Generally speaking, AL aims to select the most informative queries to be labeled among a *pool* of unlabeled samples.

Among AL algorithms used for medical image segmentation, uncertainty sampling has been one of the popular methods [2,3], which queries the most uncertain samples to be labeled. It has recently been used with neural networks, where uncertainty was measured based on sample margins [4] or bootstrapping [5]. For the same purpose, Wang et al. [6] used entropy function but mixed it with weak labels. In addition, more sophisticated objectives such as Fisher information (FI) has theoretically been shown to be beneficial for active learning [7–9]. FI measures the amount of information carried by the observations about the underlying unknown parameter. An earlier work [10] successfully applied FI in medical image segmentation using logistic regression. However, FI based objective functions for AL have not previously been applied to CNN models mainly because of the significantly larger parameter space of deep learning models which leads to intractable computations for evaluating FI.

In this paper, we propose a modified version of FI-based AL for image segmentation with CNN. Modification of FI-based approach is towards making the queries even more informative by making them as diverse as possible. We observe that using the selected queries to fine-tune only the last few layers of a CNN can effectively improve the initial model performance, and thus there is no need for blending with weak labels. Furthermore, we leverage the very efficient backpropagation methods that exist for gradient computation in CNN models to make evaluation of FI tractable. We formulate the proposed diversified FI-based AL for the application of CNN based patch-wise brain extraction and compared it with two baselines, random sampling and entropy-based querying (uncertainty sampling), within two scenarios: semi-automatic segmentation and universal active learning. Our results show that the proposed methods significantly outperform random querying and can effectively improve the performance of a pre-trained model by querying a very small percentage (less than 0.05%) of image voxels. Finally, we show that the FI-based method outperforms entropy-based approach when active querying is used for transfer learning.

2   Methods

We explain our AL method in the context of a single querying iteration, when a parameter estimate $\hat{\theta}$ is already available from an initial labeled data set. We assume that the CNN model is capable of providing us with the class posterior probability $\mathbb{P}(y|\hat{\boldsymbol{\theta}}, \mathbf{x})$. In each iteration, selected queries will be labeled by the expert and the model will be updated. This process repeats using the updated model. Throughout this section, $\mathcal{U} = \{\mathbf{x}_1, ..., \mathbf{x}_n\}$ denotes the unlabeled pool of samples and $Q \subseteq \mathcal{U}$ is the (candidate) query set. The goal in a querying iteration is to generate (no more than) $k > 0$ most informative queries.

2.1 FI-Based AL

Fisher information (FI), defined as $\mathbb{E}_{\mathbf{x},y}\left[\nabla_{\boldsymbol{\theta}} \log \mathbb{P}(y|\mathbf{x}, \boldsymbol{\theta}_0)\nabla_{\boldsymbol{\theta}}^{\top} \log \mathbb{P}(y|\mathbf{x}, \boldsymbol{\theta}_0)\right]$, measures the amount of information that an observation carries about the true model parameter $\boldsymbol{\theta}_0 \in \mathbb{R}^{\tau}$. Trace of (inverse) FI serves as a useful active learning objective [8,9], where it is optimized with respect to a query distribution $\mathbf{q}$ defined over the pool $\mathcal{U}$ (hence q_i is the probability of querying $\mathbf{x}_i \in \mathcal{U}$). Different approximations can be introduced for tractability [7,10]. Here, we follow the algorithm in [11] (originally used for logistic regression), which aims to solve

$$\underset{\mathbf{q}\in[0,1]^n}{\arg\min} \ \operatorname{tr}\left[\mathbf{I}_{\mathbf{q}}(\boldsymbol{\theta}_0)^{-1}\right]. \tag{1}$$

This optimization has a non-linear objective, but it can be reformulated in the form of a semi-definite programming (SDP) problem [12].

2.2 Diversified FI-Based AL

Although (1) takes into account the interaction between different samples, it is not obvious how much diversity it includes within Q. In order to further encourage a well-spread probability mass function (PMF) and more diverse queries, we included an additional covariance-dependent term $-\lambda \operatorname{tr}\left[\operatorname{Cov}_{\mathbf{q}}[\mathbf{x}]\right]$ into the objective, where λ is a positive mixing coefficient. Unfortunately, adding this term to the objective prevents us from forming a linear SDP. In order to keep the tractability, we constrain ourselves to zero-mean PMFs, i.e., $\mathbb{E}_{\mathbf{q}}[\mathbf{x}] = \mathbf{0}$. This constraint makes the covariance term linear with respect to q_i's:

$$\underset{\mathbf{q}\in[0,1]^n}{\arg\min} \ \operatorname{tr}\left[\mathbf{I}_{\mathbf{q}}(\boldsymbol{\theta}_0)^{-1}\right] - \lambda \sum_{i=1}^{n} q_i \, \mathbf{x}_i^{\top} \mathbf{x}_i \quad \text{s.t.} \quad \sum_{i=1}^{n} q_i \, \mathbf{x}_i = \mathbf{0}. \tag{2}$$

Following an approach similar to [11], we can get the following linear SDP:

$$\underset{\mathbf{q}\in[0,1]^n, \mathbf{t}\in\mathbb{R}^{\tau}}{\arg\min} \ t_1 + ... + t_{\tau} - \lambda \sum_{i=1}^{n} q_i \, \mathbf{x}_i^{\top} \mathbf{x}_i$$

$$\text{s.t.} \quad \sum_{\mathbf{x}_i \in \mathcal{U}} q_i \, \mathbf{x}_i = \mathbf{0} \quad \& \quad \begin{bmatrix} \sum_i q_i \, \mathbf{A}_i & \mathbf{e}_j \\ \mathbf{e}_j^{\top} & t_j \end{bmatrix} \succeq 0, \ j = 1, ..., \tau. \tag{3}$$

where $t_1, .., t_\tau$ are auxiliary variables, $\mathbf{e}_j$ is the j-th canonical vector, and $\mathbf{A}_i \in \mathbb{R}^{\tau \times \tau}$ is the conditional FI of $\mathbf{x}_i$, defined as

$$\mathbf{A}_i := \sum_{y=1}^{c} \mathbb{P}(y \,|\, \mathbf{x}_i, \boldsymbol{\theta}_0) \nabla_\theta \log \mathbb{P}(y \,|\, \mathbf{x}_i, \boldsymbol{\theta}_0) \nabla_\theta^\top \log \mathbb{P}(y \,|\, \mathbf{x}_i, \boldsymbol{\theta}_0) \tag{4}$$

Since $\boldsymbol{\theta}_0$ is not known, it is replaced by the available estimate $\hat{\boldsymbol{\theta}}$. Finally, (2) can be slow when n (pool size) and τ (parameter length) are very large, which is usually the case for CNN-based image segmentation. In order to speed up, we moderate both values by (a) downsampling $\mathcal{U}$ by only keeping β most uncertain samples [11,13], and (b) shrinking the parameter space by representing each CNN layer with the average of its parameters. When the querying PMF $\mathbf{q}$ is obtained, k samples will be drawn from it and the distinct samples will be used as the queries.

3 Experimental Results

We applied the proposed method and the baselines for CNN based patch-wise brain extraction. We use tag random for random querying, entropy for entropy-based querying, and Fisher for FI-based querying with $\lambda = 0.25, \beta = 200$. In entropy, we used Shannon entropy as the uncertainty measure. Our data sets contain T1-weighted MRI images of two groups of subjects: (a) 66 adolescents from age 10 to 15, and (b) 25 newborns from the Developing Human Connectome Project [14]. The CNN model used in our experiments is shown in Fig. 1. Inputs are axial patches of size $25 \times 25 \times 1$. The feature vectors $\mathbf{x}_i$ in (3) are extracted from the output of the second FC layer.

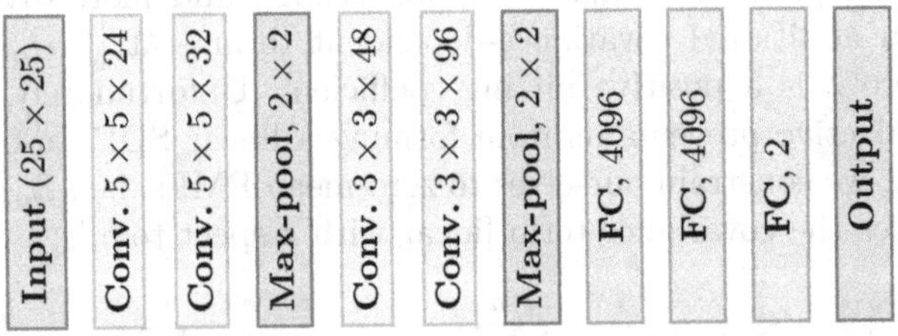

Fig. 1. Architecture of the CNN model used for brain extraction

We first trained an initial model using randomly selected patches from three adolescent subjects and used it to initialize AL experiments, where k is set to 50. Each querying iteration started with an empty labeled data set $\mathcal{L}_0$ and an initial model $\mathcal{M}_0$. At iteration i, $\mathcal{M}_{i-1}$ was used to score samples and select the queries. Labels of the queries were added to $\mathcal{L}_{i-1}$ to form $\mathcal{L}_i$, which was used to update $\mathcal{M}_{i-1}$ by fine-tuning only the FC layers. Accordingly, when computing conditional FI's in (4), we only computed gradients for the FC layers. Next we discuss two general scenarios in evaluating the performance of AL methods.

Table 1. F1 scores of the models obtained from querying iterations of different AL algorithms. The scores of intermediate querying iterations are based on grid samples, whereas the initial and final scores are reported based on full segmentation.

Initial	Adolescents			Newborns		
	85.73 ± 3.91			79.93 ± 2.92		
# Queries	Fisher (%)	entropy (%)	random (%)	Fisher (%)	entropy (%)	random (%)
100	87.11 ± 3.04	86.85 ± 3.29	82.61 ± 5.05	84.26 ± 2.86	83.33 ± 2.84	76.4 ± 6.22
500	90.9 ± 2.07	90.62 ± 2.16	85.28 ± 3.48	86.92 ± 2.37	86.47 ± 2.29	80.75 ± 2.96
1000	92.42 ± 1.76	92.57 ± 1.64	86.71 ± 2.88	88.11 ± 2.23	87.89 ± 2.12	82.12 ± 2.84
1500	93.57 ± 1.37	93.5 ± 1.39	87.78 ± 2.44	89.07 ± 2.02	88.82 ± 2	83.11 ± 2.85
Final	95.21 ± 0.94	95.15 ± 0.9	91 ± 1.48	90.24 ± 1.84	89.88 ± 1.72	86.92 ± 2.2

3.1 Active Semi-automatic Segmentation

Here, the goal is to refine the initial pre-trained model to segment a particular subject's brain by annotating the smallest number of additional voxels from the same subject. For the sake of computational simplicity, we used grid-subsampling of voxels with a fixed grid spacing of 5, resulting in pool of unlabeled samples with size $\sim 200,000$ for adolescent and $\sim 350,000$ for newborn subjects. We evaluated the resultant segmentation accuracy for the specific subject after each AL iteration over grid voxels. We also reported the initial/last segmentations over full voxels after post-processing the segmentations with CRF (for newborns), Gaussian smoothing (with standard deviation 2), morphological closing (with radius 2) and 3D connected component analysis.

Table 1 shows mean and standard deviation of F1 scores in different querying iterations from 25 newborns and 63 adolescents (after excluding three images used in training $\mathcal{M}_0$). This table shows that Fisher and entropy raised the performance significantly higher than random, and increased the initial F1 score by labeling less than 0.05% of total voxels. Whereas, random decreased the average score in the early iterations, which implies potential negative effect of bad query selection. This table shows a slight difference between Fisher and entropy when considering all the images collectively. However, we observed that Fisher actually outperformed entropy in more than 60% of the newborn subjects (16 out of 25), while performing almost equally on the others. Figure 2(a) shows box plots of the difference between F1 scores of Fisher and entropy for these two groups of subjects, where the white boxes are mostly in the positive side.

The improvements in F1 scores are shown for two selected subjects, one from each group, in Figs. 2(b) and (c). Furthermore, in order to visualize how differences in F1 scores may reflect in segmentations, we also showed in Fig. 3 segmentation of a slice of the subject associated with Fig. 2(b). Observe that the pre-trained model from adolescent subjects falsely classified skull as brain, since brains of adolescent and newborn subjects look very different in their T1-weighted contrast. After AL querying, the methods could better distinguish these regions but random and entropy have much more false negatives than Fisher.

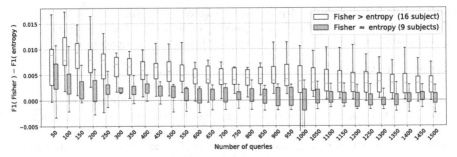

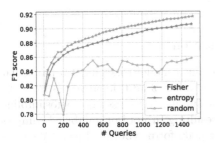 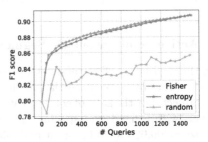

(a) F1 score difference between Fisher and entropy for two groups of newborns

(b) Example subject (Fisher>entropy)   (c) Example subject (Fisher≈entropy)

Fig. 2. F1 scores reported separately for two groups of newborn subjects, when Fisher > entropy and Fisher ≈ entropy. The box-plots consider all subjects in each group, whereas the F1 curves in (b) and (c) are for one sample subject from each group.

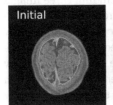 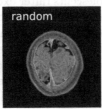 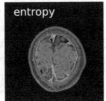 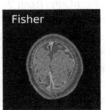

Fig. 3. Segmentation of a slice using $\mathcal{M}_0$ and models obtained in active semi-automatic segmentation of the newborn for which F1 curves are shown in Fig. 2(b). Green boundaries show the ground-truth segmentation and red regions are the resulting brain extraction. (Color figure online)

3.2 Universal Active Learning

In this section, we used FI-based AL sequentially on a subset of new subjects to further improve the initial CNN model in order to achieve a universal model that can be used to segment all other subjects in the same data set. The goal was to show that FI-based querying method is able to result a more generalizable model.

We ran a sequence of FI-based AL over 11 subjects in each data set, such that the initial model of querying iterations over one subject was the final model obtained from the previous subject. The pre-trained model $\mathcal{M}_0$ described above was used to initialize the AL algorithm for the first image. For each subject, we continued running the querying iterations with $k = 50$ until 1,500 queries were labeled. The resulting universal model was then tested on the remaining unused subjects in the data set. Note that for the newborn dataset the problem is a transfer learning scenario, where an initial pre-trained model from the adolescent data set was updated using the proposed AL approach to achieve improved performance in the newborn dataset. Results from test subjects reported in Fig. 4 show that the initial model is significantly improved after labeling a very small portion (less than 0.02%) of the voxels involved in the querying.

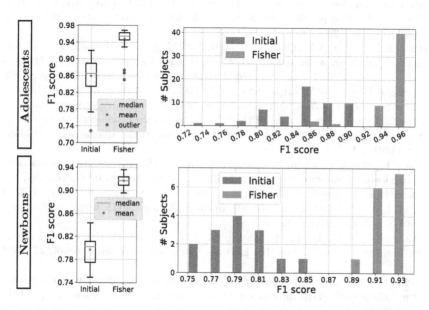

Fig. 4. Statistics of F1 scores of universal models resulting from sequence of FI-based querying over 11 images and the initial model $\mathcal{M}_0$ over the test images of adolescent and newborn subjects. The box-plots and histograms show that except for a few adolescent outliers, the F1 scores are significantly increased by our proposed FI-based AL.

4   Conclusion

In this paper, we presented active learning (AL) algorithms based on Fisher information (FI) for patch-wise image segmentation using CNNs. In these new algorithms a diversifying term was added to the querying objective based on the FI criterion; where efficient FI evaluation was achieved using gradient computations from backpropagation on the CNN model. In the context of brain extraction, the proposed AL algorithm significantly outperformed random querying.

We also observed that FI worked better than entropy in transfer learning, where we actively fine-tuned a pre-trained model to adapt it to segment images from a patient group with different characteristics (age, pathology, scanner) than the source data set. FI-based querying was also successfully applied for creating universal CNN models for both source (adolescent) and target (newborn) data sets, to label minimal new samples while achieving large improvement in performance.

References

1. Litjens, G., et al.: A survey on deep learning in medical image analysis. Med. Image Anal. **42**, 60–88 (2017)
2. Top, A., Hamarneh, G., Abugharbieh, R.: Active learning for interactive 3D image segmentation. In: Fichtinger, G., Martel, A., Peters, T. (eds.) MICCAI 2011. LNCS, vol. 6893, pp. 603–610. Springer, Heidelberg (2011). https://doi.org/10.1007/978-3-642-23626-6_74
3. Pace, D.F., Dalca, A.V., Geva, T., Powell, A.J., Moghari, M.H., Golland, P.: Interactive whole-heart segmentation in congenital heart disease. In: Navab, N., Hornegger, J., Wells, W.M., Frangi, A.F. (eds.) MICCAI 2015. LNCS, vol. 9351, pp. 80–88. Springer, Cham (2015). https://doi.org/10.1007/978-3-319-24574-4_10
4. Zhou, S., Chen, Q., Wang, X.: Active deep networks for semi-supervised sentiment classification. In: Proceedings of the 23rd International Conference on Computational Linguistics: Posters, Association for Computational Linguistics, pp. 1515–1523 (2010)
5. Yang, L., Zhang, Y., Chen, J., Zhang, S., Chen, D.Z.: Suggestive annotation: a deep active learning framework for biomedical image segmentation. In: Descoteaux, M., Maier-Hein, L., Franz, A., Jannin, P., Collins, D.L., Duchesne, S. (eds.) MICCAI 2017. LNCS, vol. 10435, pp. 399–407. Springer, Cham (2017). https://doi.org/10.1007/978-3-319-66179-7_46
6. Wang, K., Zhang, D., Li, Y., Zhang, R., Lin, L.: Cost-effective active learning for deep image classification. IEEE Trans. Circuits Syst. Video Technol. **27**, 2591 (2016)
7. Zhang, T., Oles, F.: The value of unlabeled data for classification problems. In: Proceedings of the 17th International Conference on Machine Learning, pp. 1191–1198 (2000)
8. Chaudhuri, K., Kakade, S.M., Netrapalli, P., Sanghavi, S.: Convergence rates of active learning for maximum likelihood estimation. In: Advances in Neural Information Processing Systems, pp. 1090–1098 (2015)
9. Sourati, J., Akcakaya, M., Leen, T.K., Erdogmus, D., Dy, J.G.: Asymptotic analysis of objectives based on fisher information in active learning. J. Mach. Learn. Res. **18**(34), 1–41 (2017)
10. Hoi, S.C., Jin, R., Zhu, J., Lyu, M.R.: Batch mode active learning and its application to medical image classification. In: Proceedings of the 23rd International Conference on Machine Learning, pp. 417–424. ACM (2006)
11. Sourati, J., Akcakaya, M., Erdogmus, D., Leen, T., Dy, J.G.: A probabilistic active learning algorithm based on fisher information ratio. IEEE Trans. Pattern Anal. Mach. Intell. **40**, 2023–2029 (2017)

12. Vandenberghe, L., Boyd, S.: Semidefinite programming. SIAM Rev. **38**(1), 49–95 (1996)
13. Wei, K., Iyer, R., Bilmes, J.: Submodularity in data subset selection and active learning. In: Proceedings of the 21st International Conference on Machine Learning, vol. 37 (2015)
14. Makropoulos, A., et al.: The developing human connectome project: a minimal processing pipeline for neonatal cortical surface reconstruction. NeuroImage **173**, 88–112 (2018)

Contextual Additive Networks to Efficiently Boost 3D Image Segmentations

Zhenlin Xu[✉], Zhengyang Shen, and Marc Niethammer

Department of Computer Science, UNC Chapel Hill, Chapel Hill, USA
`zhenlinx@cs.unc.edu`

Abstract. Semantic segmentation for 3D medical images is an important task for medical image analysis which would benefit from more efficient approaches. We propose a 3D segmentation framework of cascaded fully convolutional networks (FCNs) with contextual inputs and additive outputs. Compared to previous contextual cascaded networks the additive output forces each subsequent model to refine the output of previous models in the cascade. We use U-Nets of various complexity as elementary FCNs and demonstrate our method for cartilage segmentation on a large set of 3D magnetic resonance images (MRI) of the knee. We show that a cascade of simple U-Nets may for certain tasks be superior to a single deep and complex U-Net with almost two orders of magnitude more parameters. Our framework also allows greater flexibility in trading-off performance and efficiency during testing and training.

1 Introduction

Recently, deep convolution neural networks (CNNs) have shown excellent performance on various computer vision and medical image analysis tasks including semantic segmentation [1]. Early CNN approaches use sliding windows and approach segmentation as many independent classifications, which is inefficient. Fully-convolutional networks (FCN) [2] instead directly operate on full images. Consequentially, FCNs are more efficient and many FCN variants achieve state-of-the-art segmentation performance [3,4]. When dealing with 3D image segmentations, the simplest approach is to treat a 3D volume as a sequence of 2D slices [5] and to segment them independently with a 2D CNN. However, this overlooks correlations across slices. To account for such correlations while avoiding 3D CNNs, triplanar schemes [6] have been proposed which apply 2D CNNs on image slices from three orthogonal planes of an image volume. Naturally, applying a 3D CNN to an image volume can take advantage of the full 3D information, but has high computational cost and memory requirements.

Most existing work on semantic segmentation focuses on improving performance by designing deeper and more complex networks. This, generally results in better performance, but comes at the cost of additional complexity, especially for the segmentation of 3D images. Hence, it would be beneficial to design more

D. Stoyanov et al. (Eds.): DLMIA 2018/ML-CDS 2018, LNCS 11045, pp. 92–100, 2018.
https://doi.org/10.1007/978-3-030-00889-5_11

efficient network architectures for 3D segmentation while *retaining* segmentation performance. Inspired by work that applies an auto-context approach [7] to CNN models [8] and additive learning schemes such as boosting [9], we propose a cascaded 3D semantic segmentation framework composed of a sequence of 3D FCNs with contextual inputs and additive outputs. As an alternative design strategy to a monolithic complex deep FCN, we show that such a sequence of simpler and shallower FCNs achieves performance on par with a more complex network, but using two orders of magnitude less parameters. This approach also allows to trade-off model accuracy with run-time and memory requirements.

Contributions: (1) We show that a cascaded model composed of several simple FCNs can perform as well as a single complex FCN with almost two orders of magnitude more parameters, resulting in better computational efficiency. (2) Our additive model shows better performance than an auto-context approach using contextual input (i.e., segmentations) only without the additive strategy. (3) We provide an analysis to give insight into why the additive output helps refine the segmentation model. (4) Lastly, we evaluate our model on a relatively large knee MRI dataset from the Osteoarthritis Initiative for cartilage segmentation.

2 Methods

In this section we (1) introduce the two components of our cascaded framework: contextual input and additive output; (2) provide an analysis illuminating the effect of additive outputs; and (3) describe the FCNs used to construct the cascaded models in our experiments. Figure 1 illustrates the proposed approach.

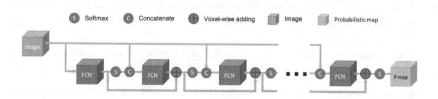

Fig. 1. Schematic diagram of proposed contextual additive model.

2.1 Contextual Additive Networks

Context information is useful for image segmentation [7,10]. Inspired by the auto-context algorithm [7], cascaded models have been proposed that input the *concatenation* of an image and a segmentation (either the resulting labeling itself or the class label probabilities) to subsequent models. The segmentation is generated by a previous model with the image as its only input. Furthermore, residual skip connections [11] are widely used for CNNs. These help the training of deep networks and boost performance. Our contextual additive network is inspired by both approaches. However, instead of using the residual connections across layers inside a neural network, we use them to connect the output of each sub-model to generate the class probability. We use a sequence of such models each also having access to the original input image (see Fig. 1).

Formally, our cascaded model Φ is based on a sequence of FCNs $\{\phi^0, \phi^1, ..., \phi^M\}$, whose parameters are $\Theta = \{\theta^0, \theta^1, ..., \theta^M\}$ respectively. The first FCN, ϕ^0, with parameters θ^0 takes an image x as input and predicts the probability map of all class labels, P^0, by applying softmax to the output of the FCN: $P^0(x; \theta^0) = \sigma(\phi^0(x; \theta^0))$, where σ is the softmax function. For an output $z \in \mathbb{R}^C$ of C classes, the probability of class j is

$$\sigma(z)_j = \frac{e^{z_j}}{\sum_{l=0}^{C-1} e^{z_l}}, \ c \in \{0, \cdots, C-1\}. \tag{1}$$

Subsequent FCNs use the image and the probability map (i.e., the *contextual input*) of the previous FCN as input. However, instead of directly predicting the input to a softmax function to obtain label probabilities these subsequent FCNs (unlike previous work [8]) predict a residual between the previous prediction, added to the output of the previous stage (i.e., the *additive output*) *before* the softmax. The output of the contextual additive model after the M-th FCN is

$$P^M(x; \Theta) = \sigma(\phi^0(x; \theta^0) + \sum_{m=1}^{M} \phi^m(x, P^{m-1}; \theta^m)). \tag{2}$$

Such a cascaded model can be trained by training each additive FCN via:

$$\hat{\theta}^m = \arg \min_{\theta^m} \mathcal{L}(Y, P^m(X; \{\hat{\theta}^0, \cdots, \hat{\theta}^{m-1}, \theta^m\})), \tag{3}$$

where Y denotes the set of label images, X the set of images in the training dataset, and $\mathcal{L}$ is the chosen loss function. Alternatively it can be trained end-to-end by minimizing the sum of the losses for all stages of the model:

$$\hat{\Theta} = \{\hat{\theta}^0, \hat{\theta}^1, ..., \hat{\theta}^M\} = \arg \min_{\Theta} \sum_{m=0}^{M} \mathcal{L}(Y, P^m(X; \{\theta^0, ..., \theta^m\})). \tag{4}$$

Both training strategies work well in our experiments. When applying the trained model one obtains the class label by selecting the most probable label:

$$\hat{y}(x; \hat{\Theta}) = \arg \max_{j} P_j^M(x; \hat{\Theta}), \tag{5}$$

where $\hat{y}$ denotes the label output for input image x and model parameters $\hat{\Theta}$.

2.2   Why an Additive Network is Beneficial

To give insight into the effect of adding model outputs *before* the softmax in the cascade we approximate the loss function to first order. We use the cross-entropy loss for multi-class segmentation which for a single model output, ϕ^0, is

$$\mathcal{L}_{CE}^0 = -\sum_{j=0}^{C-1} y_j \ln(\sigma(\phi_j^0)), \tag{6}$$

where j is the class index and C is the total number of classes. Considering a cascaded model of two FCNs, we assume we trained the first FCN ϕ^0 by optimizing $\mathcal{L}_{CE}^0$. With the additive output of the second model, the loss becomes

$$\mathcal{L}_{CE}^1 = - \sum_{j=0}^{C-1} y_j \ln(\sigma(\phi^0 + \phi^1)_j). \tag{7}$$

We can think of ϕ^1 as a perturbation to ϕ^0. Approximating the loss function (7) around ϕ^0 via a Taylor series expansion results in

$$\mathcal{L}_{CE}^1 \approx - \sum_{j=0}^{C-1} y_j \ln(\sigma(\phi_j^0)) - \sum_{j=0}^{C-1} y_j \sum_{l=0}^{C-1} \frac{\partial \ln \sigma(\phi^0)_j}{\partial \phi_l^0} \phi_l^1$$

$$= \mathcal{L}_{CE}^0 + \sum_{j=0}^{C-1} y_j \sum_{l=0}^{C-1} \Delta \mathcal{L}_{CEj}^1(\phi_l^1 | \phi^0), \tag{8}$$

where $\mathcal{L}_{CE}^0$ only depends on ϕ^0 and can therefore be ignored for sequential training of ϕ^1; $\Delta \mathcal{L}_{CEj}^1(\phi_l^1 | \phi^0)$ captures how the loss depends on the output of the second model for class l, ϕ_l^1, for voxels annotated as class j:

$$\Delta \mathcal{L}_{CEj}^1(\phi_l^1 | \phi^0) = \begin{cases} -(1 - \sigma(\phi_j^0))\phi_j^1 = -(1 - P_j^0)\phi_j^1 \, , \, l = j \\ \sigma(\phi_l^0)\phi_l^1 = P_l^0 \phi_l^1 \qquad\qquad , \, l \neq j \end{cases} \tag{9}$$

Intuitively, when the first model performs well P_j^0 is high and $P_{l,l\neq j}^0$ is low; increasing ϕ_j^1 and decreasing $\phi_{l,l\neq j}^1$ is of low benefit to reduce the loss. When the first model performs badly P_j^0 is low and $P_{l,l\neq j}^0$ is high; increasing ϕ_j^1 and decreasing $\phi_{l,l\neq j}^1$ is of high benefit. I.e., improving the prediction where the first model perform badly is more beneficial than improving already good predictions. In effect, the loss of the additive model naturally weighs each voxel so that it focuses on problematic regions.

2.3   3D Fully Convolution Networks

Many FCN variants exist [3,12]. The U-Net [13] and the 3D U-Net [14] have been popular to segment medical images. U-Nets add skip connections between the encoder/decoder paths to retain high resolution features. We use the 3D U-Net as our elementary FCN because of its good performance. The original 3D U-Net is a dense architecture with four resolution steps in the encoder/decoder paths, and 512 feature channels at the bottleneck, resulting in a total of ~19 million parameters. We also build three simpler U-Nets with fewer feature channels and fewer resolution levels (Fig. 2). The smallest one has only 45,808 parameters.

3   Experiments

For each U-Net, we train a cascaded model of length M, where M is larger for smaller U-Nets as the performance of a model with more complex U-Nets saturates with smaller M. We explore results for end-to-end and sequential training.

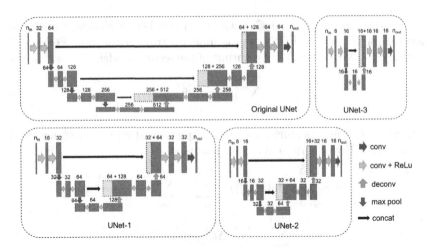

Fig. 2. U-Nets of the cascaded models (# of parameters in parentheses): original U-Net (~19M), U-Net-1 (~1.1M), U-Net-2 (~287K), U-Net-3 (~46K)

We also use only contextual input and only additive output for our cascaded U-Net-3 × 6 model to investigate the impact of our two key techniques. We study memory use and runtime to explore our model's segmentation efficiency.

3.1 Dataset and Preprocessing

We use knee MRIs from the Osteoarthritis Initiative consisting of 176 MR images from 88 patients (2 longitudinal scans per patient). We split the dataset into a training set of 60 patients (120 images), a validation set of 8 patients (16 images) and a test set of 20 patients (40 images). All images are of size $384 \times 384 \times 160$ and resolution $0.36 \times 0.36 \times 0.7\,\mathrm{mm}^3$ per voxel. We normalize the intensities of each image such that the 0.1 percentile and the 99.9 percentile are mapped to $\{0, 1\}$ and clamp values that are smaller to 0 and larger to 1 to avoid outliers. We did not apply bias-field correction, because our exploratory experiments indicated that bias-field correction did not substantially impact segmentation results. For each volume, femoral and tibial cartilage are annotated on sagittal slices. We transform the corresponding 2D polygon annotations to 3D label maps.

Table 1. Models' parameter size and memory consumption in sequential training

Model		Original U-Net	U-Net-1 × 2	U-Net-2 × 3	U-Net-3 × 6
params #		19,065,888	2,294,486	862,185	275,538
Memory (MB)	Train	11116	5836	3190	2434
	Test	10312	7614	4044	2820

3.2   Implementation Details

Due to the high memory demands of 3D convolutions, the full image volume and its network outputs may not fit on a single GPU. Hence, we use overlapping tiles as in the U-Net [13]. We choose image patches of size $128 \times 128 \times 32$ considering the nonuniform voxel resolution and that annotations were drawn sagittally.

During training, we randomly crop 3D patch pairs from image-label pairs. To avoid class imbalances due to the high proportion of background voxels we use three types of patches: any possible patch, patches with more than $r_1\%$ of femoral cartilage voxels, and patches with more that $r_2\%$ tibial cartilage voxels. Patches are randomly sampled at a ratio of $1 : 1 : 2$ ($r_1 = 1$, $r_2 = 2$). We use the Adam [15] optimizer with first moment $\beta_1 = 0.9$, second moment $\beta_2 = 0.999$, and $\epsilon = 1e{-}10$. The learning rate is initialized as $5e{-}4$ and decays at half of the total epochs and at the beginning of the last 50 epochs by 0.2. We train the original U-Net and each sub-network in the sequentially trained cascaded models with 600 epochs. When training a cascaded model of M U-Nets end-to-end, $100 * (M - 1)$ extra epochs were applied to assure convergence. Regarding training time, the cascaded models take less time than the original U-Net (13 h) except U-Net-3 × 6 (17 h for end-to-end training and 20 h for sequential training). During training, we recorded a model's Dice score on the validation dataset and evaluate the model with the best validation score on the separate testing dataset.

Table 2. Segmentation evaluation of contextual additive models using different U-Nets. E.g. U-Net-1 × 2 is a cascaded model of two U-Net-1. Results are for sequential training (end-to-end results in parentheses). Our models can achieve performance on par with the original U-Net with much fewer parameters and lower memory requirements.

Model	Stage	DSC (%)	mIOU (%)
Original U-Net	-	89.08 ± 2.41	86.89 ± 2.56
U-Net-1 × 2	0	$88.88 \pm 2.61\ (88.78 \pm 2.60)$	$86.69 \pm 2.76\ (86.58 \pm 2.74)$
	1	$\mathbf{89.17 \pm 2.55\ (89.31 \pm 2.39)}$	$\mathbf{87.00 \pm 2.71\ (87.15 \pm 2.55)}$
UNet-2 × 3	0	$88.13 \pm 2.55\ (88.31 \pm 2.60)$	$85.88 \pm 2.67\ (86.07 \pm 2.72)$
	1	$88.72 \pm 2.47\ (88.79 \pm 2.34)$	$86.50 \pm 2.61\ (86.58 \pm 2.47)$
	2	$\mathbf{88.74 \pm 2.51\ (89.14 \pm 2.30)}$	$\mathbf{86.53 \pm 2.66\ (86.96 \pm 2.45)}$
UNet-3 × 6	0	$85.00 \pm 3.13\ (83.44 \pm 3.00)$	$82.64 \pm 3.10\ (81.08 \pm 2.90)$
	1	$87.68 \pm 2.66\ (86.83 \pm 2.68)$	$85.40 \pm 2.77\ (84.51 \pm 2.73)$
	2	$88.23 \pm 2.50\ (88.08 \pm 2.57)$	$85.98 \pm 2.62\ (85.83 \pm 2.68)$
	3	$88.57 \pm 2.45\ (88.70 \pm 2.45)$	$86.34 \pm 2.59\ (86.48 \pm 2.59)$
	4	$88.63 \pm 2.42\ (89.01 \pm 2.35)$	$86.40 \pm 2.57\ (86.81 \pm 2.50)$
	5	$\mathbf{88.67 \pm 2.42\ (89.10 \pm 2.35)}$	$\mathbf{86.45 \pm 2.56\ (86.92 \pm 2.50)}$
UNet-3 × 6 (contextual input only)	5	88.23 ± 2.59	85.98 ± 2.71
UNet-3 × 6 (additive output only)	5	87.22 ± 2.78	84.92 ± 2.87

4   Results and Discussion

We quantitatively evaluate the segmentation results of each model and the output at intermediate stages. Table 2 shows average Dice scores (DSC) and the mean Intersection of Union (mIOU) of femoral and tibial cartilage and their standard deviations. We also report the performance of U-Net-3 × 6 models using contextual input or additive output only. The number of model parameters and memory consumption in sequential training (batch size 4) and testing (batch size 8) are given in Table 1. Table 3 shows segmentation results at different stages of the U-Net-3 × 6 cascade.

We observe that our contextual additive networks are more efficient as they use significantly fewer parameters while achieving similar or better performance than using a single more complex U-Net. The original U-Net has for example almost two orders of magnitude more parameters than the U-Net-3 × 6 while resulting in very similar accuracy. We also observe that both the contextual inputs *and* the additive output helps boost the performance in cascaded U-Nets.

Table 3. Segmentation results of end-to-end trained U-Net-3 × 6. Rows are Sagittal, Axial, Coronal views and 3D rendering. Red and green labels represent femoral and tibial cartilage respectively.

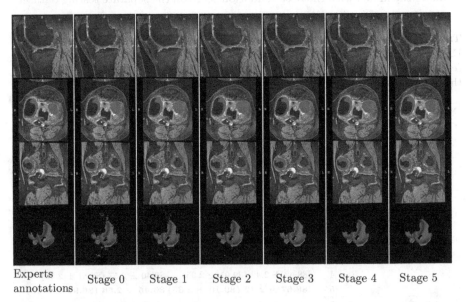

| Experts annotations | Stage 0 | Stage 1 | Stage 2 | Stage 3 | Stage 4 | Stage 5 |

5   Conclusion

We developed a framework of cascaded FCNs with contextual inputs and additive output to boost the performance of 3D semantic segmentation. Our theoretical analysis shows that the additive output focuses the additive model on regions where previous output results were relatively poor. Experiments on a large 3D MRI knee dataset demonstrated that our framework can refine the results of a single U-Net. Importantly, we showed that a cascaded model of simple U-Nets can match the performance of a complex U-Net, while providing better efficiency in terms of using fewer parameters and requiring less memory. Our approach may provide an alternative to improve FCNs for segmentation. Future work will investigate different FCNs as elements of the cascade, e.g. networks with inputs of multiple resolutions, and evaluate performance on different datasets.

References

1. Garcia-Garcia, A., Orts-Escolano, S., Oprea, S., Villena-Martinez, V., Garcia-Rodriguez, J.: A review on deep learning techniques applied to semantic segmentation. arXiv preprint arXiv:1704.06857 (2017)
2. Long, J., Shelhamer, E., Darrell, T.: Fully convolutional networks for semantic segmentation. In: CVPR, pp. 3431–3440 (2015)
3. Chen, L.C., Papandreou, G., Kokkinos, I., Murphy, K., Yuille, A.L.: DeepLab: semantic image segmentation with deep convolutional nets, atrous convolution, and fully connected CRFS. arXiv preprint arXiv:1606.00915 (2016)
4. Milletari, F., Navab, N., Ahmadi, S.A.: V-net: fully convolutional neural networks for volumetric medical image segmentation. In: 3DV, pp. 565–571. IEEE (2016)
5. Chen, H., Qi, X., Yu, L., Dou, Q., Qin, J., Heng, P.A.: DCAN: deep contour-aware networks for object instance segmentation from histology images. Med. Image Anal. **36**, 135–146 (2017)
6. Prasoon, A., Petersen, K., Igel, C., Lauze, F., Dam, E., Nielsen, M.: Deep feature learning for knee cartilage segmentation using a triplanar convolutional neural network. In: Mori, K., Sakuma, I., Sato, Y., Barillot, C., Navab, N. (eds.) MICCAI 2013. LNCS, vol. 8150, pp. 246–253. Springer, Heidelberg (2013). https://doi.org/10.1007/978-3-642-40763-5_31
7. Tu, Z., Bai, X.: Auto-context and its application to high-level vision tasks and 3d brain image segmentation. TPAMI **32**(10), 1744–1757 (2010)
8. Salehi, S.S.M., Erdogmus, D., Gholipour, A.: Auto-context convolutional neural network (auto-net) for brain extraction in magnetic resonance imaging. IEEE Trans. Med. Imaging **36**(11), 2319–2330 (2017)
9. Friedman, J., Hastie, T., Tibshirani, R., et al.: Additive logistic regression: a statistical view of boosting. Ann. Stat. **28**(2), 337–407 (2000)
10. Loog, M., van Ginneken, B.: Supervised segmentation by iterated contextual pixel classification. In: 16th International Conference on Pattern Recognition. Proceedings, vol. 2, pp. 925–928. IEEE (2002)
11. He, K., Zhang, X., Ren, S., Sun, J.: Deep residual learning for image recognition. In: CVPR, pp. 770–778 (2016)
12. Badrinarayanan, V., Kendall, A., Cipolla, R.: SegNet: a deep convolutional encoder-decoder architecture for image segmentation. TPAMI **39**(12), 2481–2495 (2017)
13. Ronneberger, O., Fischer, P., Brox, T.: U-Net: convolutional networks for biomedical image segmentation. In: Navab, N., Hornegger, J., Wells, W.M., Frangi, A.F. (eds.) MICCAI 2015. LNCS, vol. 9351, pp. 234–241. Springer, Cham (2015). https://doi.org/10.1007/978-3-319-24574-4_28

14. Çiçek, Ö., Abdulkadir, A., Lienkamp, S.S., Brox, T., Ronneberger, O.: 3D U-Net: learning dense volumetric segmentation from sparse annotation. In: Ourselin, S., Joskowicz, L., Sabuncu, M.R., Unal, G., Wells, W. (eds.) MICCAI 2016. LNCS, vol. 9901, pp. 424–432. Springer, Cham (2016). https://doi.org/10.1007/978-3-319-46723-8_49
15. Kingma, D.P., Ba, J.: Adam: a method for stochastic optimization. arXiv preprint arXiv:1412.6980 (2014)

Unsupervised Probabilistic Deformation Modeling for Robust Diffeomorphic Registration

Julian Krebs[1,2]([✉]), Tommaso Mansi[2], Boris Mailhé[2], Nicholas Ayache[1], and Hervé Delingette[1]

[1] Inria, Epione Team, Université Côte d'Azur, Sophia Antipolis, France
julian.krebs@inria.fr
[2] Siemens Healthineers, Medical Imaging Technologies, Princeton, NJ, USA

Abstract. We propose a deformable registration algorithm based on unsupervised learning of a low-dimensional probabilistic parameterization of deformations. We model registration in a probabilistic and generative fashion, by applying a conditional variational autoencoder (CVAE) network. This model enables to also generate normal or pathological deformations of any new image based on the probabilistic latent space. Most recent learning-based registration algorithms use supervised labels or deformation models, that miss important properties such as diffeomorphism and sufficiently regular deformation fields. In this work, we constrain transformations to be diffeomorphic by using a differentiable exponentiation layer with a symmetric loss function. We evaluated our method on 330 cardiac MR sequences and demonstrate robust intra-subject registration results comparable to two state-of-the-art methods but with more regular deformation fields compared to a recent learning-based algorithm. Our method reached a mean DICE score of 78.3% and a mean Hausdorff distance of 7.9 mm. In two preliminary experiments, we illustrate the model's abilities to transport pathological deformations to healthy subjects and to cluster five diseases in the unsupervised deformation encoding space with a classification performance of 70%.

1 Introduction

Deformable registration is an essential task in medical image analysis. It describes the process of finding voxel correspondences in a pair of images [9]. Traditional registration approaches aim to optimize a local similarity metric between deformed and target image, while being regularized by various energies [9]. In order to retrieve important properties such as invertible deformation fields, diffeomorphic registration was introduced. Among other parametrizations, one way to parametrize diffeomorphisms are stationary velocity fields (SVF) [1].

In recent years, major drawbacks of these approaches like high computational costs and long execution times have led to an increasing popularity of learning-based algorithms – notably deep learning (DL). One can classify these algorithms

© Springer Nature Switzerland AG 2018
D. Stoyanov et al. (Eds.): DLMIA 2018/ML-CDS 2018, LNCS 11045, pp. 101–109, 2018.
https://doi.org/10.1007/978-3-030-00889-5_12

as supervised or unsupervised. Due to the difficulty of finding ground truth voxel correspondences, supervised methods need to rely on predictions from existing algorithms [11], simulations [8] or both [6]. These methods are either limited by the performance of the used existing algorithms or the realism of simulations. On the other hand, unsupervised approaches make use of spatial transformer layers (STN [3]) to warp the moving image in a differentiable way such that loss functions can operate on the warped image (similarity metric) and on the transformation itself (regularization) [2,4,10]. While unsupervised approaches perform well in minimizing a similarity metric, it remains unclear if the retrieved deformation fields are sufficiently regular which is of high interest for intra-subject registration. Furthermore, important properties like symmetry or diffeormorphisms [9] are still missing in DL-based approaches.

In this paper, we suggest to learn a low-dimensional probabilistic parameterization of deformations which is restricted to follow a prescribed distribution. This stochastic encoding is defined by a latent code vector of an encoder-decoder neural network and it restricts the space of plausible deformations with respect to the training data. By using a conditional variational autoencoder (CVAE [5]), our generative network constrains encoder and decoder on the moving image. After training, the probabilistic encoding can be potentially used for deformation analysis tasks such as clustering of deformations or the generation of new deformations for a given image – similar to the deformations seen during training. Furthermore, we include a generic vector field exponentiation layer to generate diffeomorphic transformations. Our framework contains an STN and can be trained with a choice of similarity metrics. To avoid asymmetry, we use a symmetric local cross correlation criterion. The main contributions are:

- A probabilistic formulation of the registration problem through unsupervised learning of an encoded deformation model.
- A differentiable exponentiation and an user-adjustable smoothness layer that ensure the outputs of neural networks to be regular and diffeomorphic.
- As a proof of concept, first experiments on deformation transport and disease clustering.

2   Methods

The goal of image registration is to find the spatial transformation $\mathcal{T}_z : \mathbb{R}^3 \to \mathbb{R}^3$, parametrized by a d-dimensional vector $z \in \mathbb{R}^d$, which best warps the moving image $\mathbf{M}$ to match the fixed image $\mathbf{F}$. Both images are defined in the spatial domain $\Omega \in \mathbb{R}^3$. Typically, this is done by minimizing an objective function of the form: $\arg\min_z \mathcal{F}(z, \mathbf{M}, \mathbf{F}) = \mathcal{D}(\mathbf{F}, \mathbf{M} \circ \mathcal{T}_z) + \mathcal{R}(\mathcal{T}_z)$ with the image similarity $\mathcal{D}$ of the fixed $\mathbf{F}$ and the warped moving image $\mathbf{M} \circ \mathcal{T}_z$ and a spatial regularizer $\mathcal{R}$. Recent unsupervised DL-based approaches (e.g. [2,4]) mimic the optimization of such an objective function.

Instead, we propose to model the registration probabilistically by parametrizing the deformation as a vector z to follow a prior $p(z)$. To learn this probabilistic space, we define the latent vector of dimensionality d in an encoder-decoder neural network as this z. Given the moving and the fixed image as input, a variational inference method (CVAE [5]) is used to *reconstruct* the fixed by warping the moving image. An exponentiation layer interprets the network's output as velocities v (an SVF) and returns a diffeomorphism ϕ which is used by a dense STN to retrieve the warped image $\mathbf{M}^*$. To enforce an user-adjustable level of deformation smoothness (comparable to [7]), a convolutional Gaussian layer is added before the exponentiation with Gaussian weights according to the variance σ_S^2. During training, the network parameters are updated through backpropagation of the gradients. The network architecture can be seen in Fig. 1a. Finally, registration is done in a single forward path. The trained probabilistic framework can be also used for the sampling of deformations as shown in Fig. 1b.

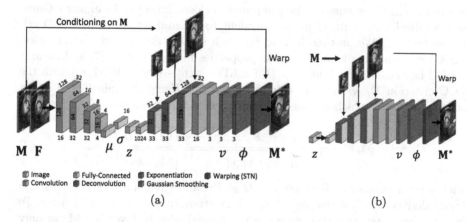

Fig. 1. (a) CVAE registration network during training and registration including diffeomorphic layer (exponentiation). Deformations are encoded in z from which velocities are decoded while being conditioned on the moving image. (b) Decoder network for sampling and deformation transport: Apply z-code conditioned on any new image $\mathbf{M}$.

Learning a Probabilistic Deformation Encoding. Learning a generative model typically involves a latent variable model (as in VAE), where an encoder maps an image to its z-code – a low-dimensional latent vector, from which a decoder aims to reconstruct the original image. Typically, the encoder and decoder are defined as distributions q_ω and p_γ with trainable network parameters ω and γ. The network is trained by maximizing a lower bound on the data likelihood with respect to a prior distribution $p(z)$. We define the prior as multivariate unit Gaussians $p(z) = \mathcal{N}(0, I)$ with the identity matrix I. In CVAE [5], encoder q_ω and decoder p_γ distributions are additionally conditioned on extra information (e.g. classes). We propose to frame image registration as a reconstruction problem in which the moving image $\mathbf{M}$ acts as the conditioning data and is warped to reconstruct or to match the fixed image $\mathbf{F}$. Thus, the decoder reconstructs $\mathbf{F}$ given z and $\mathbf{M}$: $p_\gamma(\mathbf{F} \mid z, \mathbf{M})$. To have z, the encoder serves as an approximation of the intractable true posterior probability of z given $\mathbf{F}$ and $\mathbf{M}$ and is denoted as $q_\omega(z \mid \mathbf{F}, \mathbf{M})$. Since the prior $p(z)$ is defined as multivariate unit Gaussians, the encoder network predicts the mean $\mu \in \mathbb{R}^d$ and diagonal covariance $\sigma \in \mathbb{R}^d$, from which z is drawn: $q_\omega(z \mid \mathbf{F}, \mathbf{M}) = \mathcal{N}(\mu(\mathbf{F}, \mathbf{M}), \sigma(\mathbf{F}, \mathbf{M}))$.

Both distributions can be combined in a two-term loss function [5] where the first term describes the reconstruction loss as the expected negative log-likelihood of $p_\gamma(\mathbf{F} \mid z, \mathbf{M})$. In other words, the reconstruction loss represents a similarity metric between input $\mathbf{F}$ and output $\mathbf{M}^*$. The second term acts as a regularization term on the deformation latent space by forcing the encoded distribution $q_\omega(z \mid \mathbf{F}, \mathbf{M})$ to be close to the prior probability distribution $p(z)$ using a Kullback-Leibler (KL) divergence. The loss function results in:

$$l(\omega, \gamma, \mathbf{F}, \mathbf{M}) = -E_{z \sim q_\omega(\cdot|\mathbf{F}, \mathbf{M})} \left[\log p_\gamma(\mathbf{F} \mid z, \mathbf{M})\right] + KL\left[q_\omega(z \mid \mathbf{F}, \mathbf{M}) \parallel p(z)\right], \quad (1)$$

where the KL-divergence can be computed in closed form [5]. Assuming a Gaussian log-likelihood term of p_γ is equivalent to minimizing a weighted SSD criterion (cf. [5]). We propose instead to use a symmetric local cross-correlation (LCC) criterion due to its favorable properties for registration [7] and assume a LCC Boltzmann distribution $p_\gamma(\mathbf{F} \mid z, \mathbf{M}) \sim \exp(-\lambda \mathcal{D}_{LCC}(\mathbf{F}, \mathbf{M}, v))$ with the LCC criterion $\mathcal{D}_{LCC}$ and the weighting factor λ. Using the velocities v and a small constant ϵ, which is added for numerical stability, we define:

$$\mathcal{D}_{LCC}(\mathbf{F}, \mathbf{M}, v) = \frac{1}{P} \sum_{x \in \Omega} \frac{\overline{\mathbf{F}_x \circ \exp\left(-\frac{v_x}{2}\right) \mathbf{M}_x \circ \exp\left(\frac{v_x}{2}\right)}^2}{\left[\overline{\mathbf{F}_x \circ \exp\left(-\frac{v_x}{2}\right)}\right]^2 \left[\overline{\mathbf{M}_x \circ \exp\left(\frac{v_x}{2}\right)}\right]^2 + \epsilon}, \quad (2)$$

with a total number of P pixels $x \in \Omega$ and where $\bar{}$ symbolizes the local mean image derived by Gaussian smoothing with a strength of σ_G and kernel size k. To help the reconstruction task, we introduce conditioning by involving $\mathbf{M}$ not only as the image to be warped in the STN, but also in the first decoder layers by concatenating down-sampled versions of $\mathbf{M}$ with the filter maps on each scale. The hypothesis is that in order to better optimize the reconstruction loss, the network makes use of the provided extra information of $\mathbf{M}$ such that less anatomical but more deformation information are conveyed by the low-dimensional latent layer, which would make the encoding more geometry-invariant.

Exponentiation Layer: Generating Diffeomorphisms. In the SVF setting, the transformation ϕ is defined as the Lie group exponential map with respect to the velocities v: $\phi(x) = \exp(v)$. For efficient computation, the scaling and squaring algorithm is typically used [1]. In order to generate diffeomorphic transformations ϕ in a neural network, we propose an exponentiation layer that implements this algorithm in a fully differentiable way. To this end, the layer expects a vector field as input (the velocities v) which is scaled with a factor N which we precompute on a subset of the training data according to the formulations in [1]. In the squaring step, the approximated $\phi_0 \approx id + v * 2^{-N}$

(with *id* as a regular grid) is recursively squared, N-times, from $k = 1$ to N: $\phi_k = \phi_{k-1} \circ \phi_{k-1}$. The result is the diffeomorphism $\phi_N \equiv \phi$ [1]. The squaring step requires the composition of two vector fields on regular grids which we realized by linear interpolation. All these computations consist of standard operations that can be added to the computational graph and are auto-differentiable in modern deep learning libraries. This differentiable layer can be added to any neural network which predicts (stationary) velocity fields.

3 Experiments

We evaluate our framework on an intra-subject task of cardiac MRI cine registration where end-diastole frames are registered to end-systole frames (ED-ES) – a very large deformation. Furthermore, we show preliminary experiments evaluating the learned deformation encoding: its potentials for transporting encoded deformations from one subject to another and showing the clustering of diseases in the encoding space. All experiments are in 3-D.

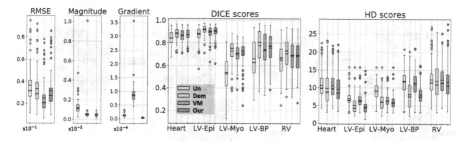

Fig. 2. Comparing registration performance: unregistered (Un), LCC-Demons (Dem), VoxelMorph (VM) and our method in terms of RMSE and mean deformation magnitude and gradient, DICE and 95%-tile Hausdorff distances (HD).

We used 184 short-axis datasets acquired from different hospitals and 150 cases from the Automatic Cardiac Diagnosis Challenge (ACDC) at STACOM 2017[1], mixing congenital heart diseases with images from adults. We used 234 cases for training and for testing the remaining 100 cases from ACDC, that contain segmentation and disease label information from five cardiac diseases. Both information were only used for evaluation purposes. All images were sampled with a spacing of $1.5 \times 1.5 \times 3.15$ mm and cropped to a size of $128 \times 128 \times 32$ voxels. These dimensions were chosen to save computation time and are not a limitation of the framework (validated on different image sizes).

---

[1] https://www.creatis.insa-lyon.fr/Challenge/acdc/index.html.

Implementation Details. The encoder of our neural network consisted of four convolutional layers with strides (2, 2, 2, 1) (Fig. 1a). The bottleneck layers (μ, σ, z) were fully-connected. The decoder had one fully-connected and three deconvolutional layers, where the outputs at each layer were concatenated with sub-sampled versions of **M**. Two convolutional layers and a convolutional Gaussian layer with $\sigma_S = 3$ (kernel size 15) were placed in front of the exponentiation and transformer layer. The latent code size d was set to 16 as a trade off between registration quality and generalizability. This leads to a total of ∼267k trainable parameters. L2 weight decay with a factor of 0.0001 was applied. The numbers of iterations in the exponentiation layer was set to $N = 4$ in all experiments. In training, the strength of the Gaussians for computing the LCC was set to $\sigma_G = 2$ with a kernel size $k = 9$. The loss balancing factor $\lambda = 5000$ was empirically chosen such that encoded training samples roughly had zero means and variances of 1 and the reconstruction loss was optimized. We used the Adam optimizer with a learning rate of 0.0005 and a batch size of one. We performed online data augmentation by randomly shifting, rotating, scaling and mirroring training images. The framework has been implemented using *Keras* with *Tensorflow*. Training took 24 h on a *NVIDIA GTX TITAN X* GPU.

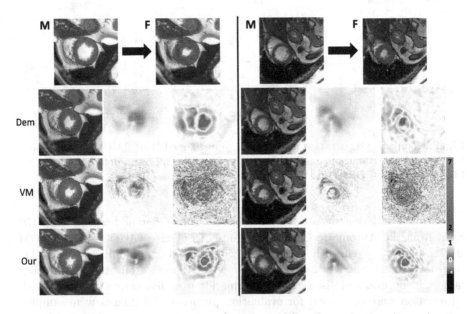

Fig. 3. Two random examples of end-diastole to end-systole registration: (Row 1) original images. The LCC-demons (Dem, Row 2) and VoxelMorph (VM, Row 3) versus our method (Row 4), showing the warped moving image, the deformation field and the Jacobian determinants. All results are in 3-D, showing the central short-axis slices.

Registration Results. We compare our registration algorithm with the LCC-demons [7] with manually tuned parameters (on training images) and the non-diffeomorphic DL-based method VoxelMorph-2 [2] (VM) with a regularization weighting parameter of 1.5, as recommended. As a surrogate measure of registration performance, we used the intensity root mean square error (RMSE), mean DICE score and 95%-tile Hausdorff distance (HD) in mm on the following anatomical structures: myocardium and epicardium of the left ventricle (LV-Epi, LV-Myo), left bloodpool (BP) and heart (Heart). The LCC-demons showed better mean DICE scores (averaged over the five structures, in %) with 79.9 compared to our algorithm with 78.3 and VM with 77.5 (cf. Fig. 2). The Voxel-Morph algorithm reached a very low RMSE of 0.025 compared to ours (0.031) and the demons (0.034), but could not reach the other algorithms in terms of HD with a mean score of 9.4 mm compared to ours with 7.9 mm and the demons with 8.2 mm. Besides these metrics, VM produced very irregular and highly non-diffeomorphic deformation fields since 2.2% of the displacements had a negative Jacobian determinant (cf. in Fig. 3). In general, our approach led to deformation fields with both smaller amplitudes and smaller gradients than the demons and the VM algorithm. Furthermore, our results were more robust as variances were lower for all metrics compared to the demons and lower or comparable to VM. This is also visible in Fig. 3 and further shown by the fact that HD scores are the smallest experienced in the experiments. Average execution time per test case was 0.32 s using the mentioned GPU and an *Intel Xeon CPU E5*, compared to 108 s for the demons on CPU.

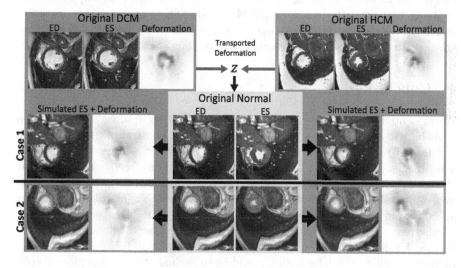

Fig. 4. Transport the z-code of pathological deformations (top row: cardiomyopathy DCM and hypertrophy HCM) to two healthy subjects (bottom rows: Normal). The simulated deformation fields are *similar* compared to the pathological deformations but are adapted to the geometry of the healthy image (e.g. translated).

Deformation Encoding. For evaluating the learned deformation encoding, we show geometry-invariance by transporting a deformation from one subject to another. Therefore, we take a z-code from a pathological subject and condition the decoder on the ED image of healthy subjects (Fig. 1b). More precisely, in Fig. 4 we transported a cardiomyopathy (DCM) and hypertrophy (HCM) deformation to two healthy cases (Normal). One can see the disease-specific deformation (DCM: reduced cardiac contraction) which are different from the healthy transformations. The resulting deformation fields are

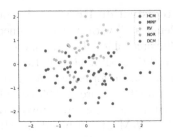

Fig. 5. Distribution of cardiac diseases after projecting 100 z-codes of test images on 2 CCA components.

adapted to the anatomy of the conditioning image and they are translation-invariant.

In a second experiment, we used the encoded z-codes and disease information of our cardiac test set to visualize the structure of the learned space. Therefore, we linearly projected the 16-D z-codes to a 2-D space by using the two most discriminative CCA components (canonical correlation analysis). We used the ACDC classes: dilated cardiomyopathy DCM, hypertrophic cardiomyopathy HCM, myocardial infarction MNF, abnormal right ventricle RV and normal NOR. In Fig. 5, one can see that the classes of the 100 test sets are clustered in the projected space. The five class classification accuracy reaches 70% with 10-fold cross-validation, by using the six most discriminative CCA components and applying support vector machine (SVM) on-top. These results which are solely based on unsupervised deformation z-codes suggest that similar deformations are close to each other in the deformation encoding space.

4   Conclusion

We presented an unsupervised deformable registration approach that learns a probabilistic deformation encoding. This encoding constrains the registration and leads to robust and accurate registration results on a large dataset of cardiac images. Furthermore, an exponentiation layer has been introduced that creates diffeomorphic transformations. The performance of the proposed method was comparable and partially superior to two state-of-the-art algorithms. Our approach produced more regular deformation fields than a DL-based algorithm. Furthermore, first results show, that the probabilistic encoding could potentially be used for deformation transport and clustering tasks. In future work, we plan to further explore the deformation encoding to evaluate these tasks more deeply.

Acknowledgements. Data used in this article were obtained from the EU FP7-funded project MD-Paedigree and the ACDC STACOM challenge 2017.

References

1. Arsigny, V., Commowick, O., Pennec, X., Ayache, N.: A log-euclidean framework for statistics on diffeomorphisms. In: Larsen, R., Nielsen, M., Sporring, J. (eds.) MICCAI 2006. LNCS, vol. 4190, pp. 924–931. Springer, Heidelberg (2006). https://doi.org/10.1007/11866565_113

2. Balakrishnan, G., et al.: An unsupervised learning model for deformable medical image registration. In: Proceedings of the IEEE CVPR, pp. 9252–9260 (2018)

3. Jaderberg, M., Simonyan, K., Zisserman, A., et al.: Spatial transformer networks. In: Advances in Neural Information Processing Systems, pp. 2017–2025 (2015)

4. Yu, J.J., Harley, A.W., Derpanis, K.G.: Back to basics: unsupervised learning of optical flow via brightness constancy and motion smoothness. In: Hua, G., Jégou, H. (eds.) ECCV 2016. LNCS, vol. 9915, pp. 3–10. Springer, Cham (2016). https://doi.org/10.1007/978-3-319-49409-8_1

5. Kingma, D.P., et al.: Semi-supervised learning with deep generative models. In: Advances in Neural Information Processing Systems, pp. 3581–3589 (2014)

6. Krebs, J., et al.: Robust non-rigid registration through agent-based action learning. In: Descoteaux, M., Maier-Hein, L., Franz, A., Jannin, P., Collins, D.L., Duchesne, S. (eds.) MICCAI 2017. LNCS, vol. 10433, pp. 344–352. Springer, Cham (2017). https://doi.org/10.1007/978-3-319-66182-7_40

7. Lorenzi, M., Ayache, N., Frisoni, G.B., et al.: LCC-Demons: a robust and accurate symmetric diffeomorphic registration algorithm. NeuroImage 81, 470–483 (2013)

8. Sokooti, H., de Vos, B., Berendsen, F., Lelieveldt, B.P.F., Išgum, I., Staring, M.: Nonrigid image registration using multi-scale 3D convolutional neural networks. In: Descoteaux, M., Maier-Hein, L., Franz, A., Jannin, P., Collins, D.L., Duchesne, S. (eds.) MICCAI 2017. LNCS, vol. 10433, pp. 232–239. Springer, Cham (2017). https://doi.org/10.1007/978-3-319-66182-7_27

9. Sotiras, A., Davatzikos, C., Paragios, N.: Deformable medical image registration: a survey. IEEE Trans. Med. Imaging 32(7), 1153–1190 (2013)

10. de Vos, B.D., Berendsen, F.F., Viergever, M.A., Staring, M., Išgum, I.: End-to-End unsupervised deformable image registration with a convolutional neural network. In: Cardoso, M.J., et al. (eds.) DLMIA/ML-CDS -2017. LNCS, vol. 10553, pp. 204–212. Springer, Cham (2017). https://doi.org/10.1007/978-3-319-67558-9_24

11. Yang, X., Kwitt, R., Niethammer, M.: Fast predictive image registration. In: Carneiro, G., et al. (eds.) LABELS/DLMIA -2016. LNCS, vol. 10008, pp. 48–57. Springer, Cham (2016). https://doi.org/10.1007/978-3-319-46976-8_6

Rapid Training Data Generation for Tissue Segmentation Using Global Approximate Block-Matching with Self-organizing Maps

Lee B. Reid[(✉)] and Alex M. Pagnozzi

The Australian e-Health Research Centre,
Commonwealth Scientific and Industrial Research Organisation,
Brisbane, QLD, Australia
lee.reid@csiro.au

Abstract. Deep learning techniques for tissue segmentation require large amounts of data for training, testing, and cross-validation. Manually generating such segmentations, however, is extremely time-consuming. This can lead to such techniques being limited to imaging modalities and populations for which ground truths already exist, over-fitting, or the use of data that is not expert-checked and so likely to contain errors. A need exists for a means of accelerating expert tissue-segmentation, such as automated techniques that require little correction and have little reliance on existing atlases. Here, we describe a method which can reliably perform registration-free tissue-segmentation using a single atlas that is only partially complete. This Global Approximate Block-matching method utilizes a self-organizing map, an unorthodox artificial neural network. This network trains quickly only on the provided partial atlas and allows these labels to be propagated throughout the target image via block-matching. Using this technique we segmented brains of 22 subjects and compared its performance to expert ground truths. When provided with an atlas for which only 2% of voxels were labelled, this achieved mean dice similarity coefficients of 0.88 (grey-matter) and 0.92 (white matter). Performance improved as higher amounts of atlas were provided, up to a maximum of 0.93 (grey-matter) and 0.96 (white matter) when a single whole-brain atlas was provided. Although segmentations produced by this technique are sufficiently accurate to be used directly for many purposes, its primary use case may lie in accelerating the creation of expert atlases for deep-learning techniques.

Keywords: Block-matching · Self-organizing map · Segmentation Ground-truth

1 Introduction

Deep learning techniques are gaining popularity for tissue segmentation but require large amounts of data for training, testing, and cross-validation.

© Crown 2018
D. Stoyanov et al. (Eds.): DLMIA 2018/ML-CDS 2018, LNCS 11045, pp. 110–118, 2018.
https://doi.org/10.1007/978-3-030-00889-5_13

Generating data ultimately requires manually delineated segmentations, but this process can take several days to complete per volume if attention to detail is desired. Although data augmentation can artificially boost the quantity of training data, this is unlikely to produce a satisfying dataset for cross-validation and does not necessarily provide the true anatomical variance seen in the population. As a result, segmentation techniques such as deep-learning are at risk of becoming limited to certain magnetic resonance (MR) sequences and populations for which ground truth data already exist. A need exists for a means of accelerating expert tissue-segmentation. One option is to automatically generate segmentations with a method that has little-or-no requirement on existing atlases, and to correct this segmentation as needed. A widely available tool to achieve this is expectation-maximization (EM) segmentation, but its accuracy and ability to self-improve when provided with human-corrected data can be limited.

Block-matching (BM) techniques are typically designed to remove image noise but can also perform tissue segmentation [2]. Such methods typically match similar cubes of voxels (patches) from an atlas to a target image, and compute a 'non-local mean' of these patches. Alternatively, labels from these patches can be averaged (rather than voxel intensities) to generate a probabilistic tissue segmentation. Block matching leverages the small patterns that exist throughout an image, such as the repeated sulcal folding of brain tissue. However, such techniques are unable to take full advantage of this redundancy because exhaustively comparing patches to one another is computationally expensive. To circumvent this, techniques such as volBrain [2] rely on atlas-to-target registration and search only a local area for patches similar to a target. This requires at least one whole-brain atlas with reasonable spatial correspondence to the target image.

Dimensionality reduction is an alternative, or complementary, way to reduce the computational cost of comparing patches exhaustively. The self-organizing map (SOM) is a neural-network based non-linear dimensionality reduction technique [1]. Briefly, SOMs are implemented as a collection of nodes which each have local connectivity, a fixed position in low dimensional space (e.g. forming a 2D grid), and a trainable position in the high-dimensional space. Through competitive learning, rather than backpropagation, SOMs train quickly and provide a smooth projection between high- and low-dimensional spaces. Intuitively, a trained 1D SOM can be thought to optimally 'snake', much as principal components analysis (PCA) draws a straight line, through high dimensional space.

We have developed a 'Global Approximate Block-Matching' (GAB) denoising and segmentation algorithm. GAB requires no spatial correspondence between the atlas and target, nor for the atlas to be completely labelled. This allows a partially segmented image to act as an atlas for another image, or to act as its own atlas, propagating manually segmented labels to non-segmented regions. To achieve this, GAB performs a whole-image search for atlas patches matching each target. To reduce this operation's computational burden, each patch is collapsed into a singular value (SV) through a method such as the SOM. Here, we describe GAB and demonstrate its tissue segmentation performance using incomplete atlases. The accuracy and speed afforded by this method may enable rapid atlas building, in turn enabling deep learning methods to target diverse populations and utilize MR sequences for which training data are not yet available.

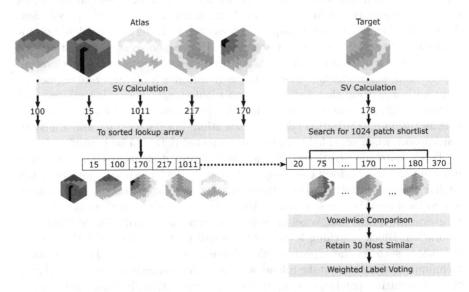

Fig. 1. In Step 1 (top left), the atlas image was split into overlapping $5 \times 5 \times 5$ voxel patches. For each patch, a singular value (SV) was calculated using one of four methods. Patches and their corresponding labels (not shown) were then sorted by these SVs. In Step 2 (right), for each target patch from a target image, an SV was calculated. Using a binary search, 1024 atlas patches with similar SVs were selected as a 'shortlist'. The voxel-wise sum of square differences (SSDs) were calculated for these patches versus the target, and the 30 patches with the most similar SSDs selected, their labels contributing toward final image reconstruction. See the text for details on final image reconstruction.

2   Methods

We tested the ability of GAB and EM to perform a series of three-tissue (cortical grey-matter, cortical white-matter, cerebrospinal fluid) segmentations in MR images. Our dataset consisted of N4 bias-corrected MPRAGE images (0.9 mm isotropic) from 23 participants ($28.8 \pm 1.5y$) acquired in a previous study [4,5]. MR acquisition was approved by the local ethics committee. Participants gave written informed consent. We also utilized the expert (manually corrected) brain masks and expert tissue segmentations for each image generated during this study. GAB does not require that all areas of an atlas have accompanying labels; its segmentation accuracy was tested when provided with an atlas in varying degrees of completion (Fig. 3). Performance was judged by the quantitative similarity between automatically generated and expert generated segmentations.

2.1   The "Global Approximate Block Matching" Method

Images were processed in two steps: independently-applied denoising of both target and atlas images, followed by segmentation of the target image. Both steps used the GAB method. Below we detail how segmentation was performed, followed by a brief explanation as to how this was modified to perform denoising.

The GAB method, summarized in Fig. 1, accepts five images: (1) a target image, such as a T1; (2) a target mask; (3) an atlas image; (4) an atlas mask; and (5) atlas labels. The masked target is linearly intensity scaled to match the histogram of the masked atlas and both are stored as 8-bit unsigned integer images. These images are split into overlapping $5 \times 5 \times 5$ voxel patches within their respective brain masks. For each patch, an SV is calculated from voxel intensities. Atlas patches are then sorted by their SV. To find matching patches to a target, GAB conducts a binary search for the most similar atlas patch, based on target and atlas patch SVs. This approximate best-match, and those patches between 512 positions before and 511 positions after it in the sorted array, constitute a 1024-patch 'shortlist' of items likely to be similar to the target. The voxelwise sum of square differences (SSD) was calculated between the target patch and shortlist to identify the 30 most similar patches to the target. The labels for these patches are multiplied by their patch's weight $(1/(SSD + 10^{-6}))$, filtered by a Gaussian of $\sigma = 1$ voxel, and added to the appropriate label's 'sum' image. These weights are multiplied by this Gaussian and added to a 'weights' image. Upon completion of all block matching, each sum image is divided by the weights image to generate a final tissue probability map. This 'unweighting' is required as each sum image voxel is contributed to by up to 125 block-matching operations, each operation in turn summing 30 weighted patches. A voxelwise maximum likelihood approach converts the probabilistic tissue maps into a hard segmentation.

2.2   Singular Value Calculation

Four GAB variants were tested, differing from one another by their SV calculation method: PCA (ϵ_0), mean voxel intensity, random (SV randomly generated), and SOM. Each SOM was arranged as 4096 nodes equally-spaced in 1D, and trained on up to 10^7 randomly selected patches from the input image. SV calculation using the SOM was performed by locating a patch's continuous position in this array (i.e. between the best matched node and its most similar neighbor) based on voxel-wise SSD. PCA transformations were calculated from the same randomly selected patches. We also re-ran GAB-SOM with an artificially boosted number of atlas patches, providing the algorithm with 48 unique augmentations (all rotations, plus their mirror images) of each labelled atlas patch.

Denoising utilized GAB with two modifications to the method detailed above: (1) patches were $3 \times 3 \times 3$ in size; (2) the target, atlas, and label images were the same, I.E. the method matched patches within the target image to others within that same image. As such, it reconstructed a single low-noise version of the input image, rather than several probabilistic tissue maps. Denoising was always performed with the SOM SV method, the performance of which was not quantified, as it is beyond the intended scope of this paper.

2.3   Expectation Maximization

For a comparator method, we used an Expectation Maximization segmentation algorithm with a modified Markov Random Field implementation. This method was selected as it has previously been reported to perform robustly in the absence of atlas based priors [3]. EM was executed with a single Gaussian per tissue class, initialized with means of 0, 2, and 3 for cerebrospinal fluid (CSF), grey-matter (GM), and white-matter (WM) respectively, each with $\sigma = 1$. These values were selected after empirical testing demonstrated that they produced reliable segmentation performance in a similar dataset acquired on the same scanner. Moderate deviations from this initialization did not meaningfully alter the performance of EM for the current dataset.

2.4   Atlas and Performance Metric

We use the term 'atlas availability' herein to refer to the fraction of an atlas' labels which were made available to the segmentation algorithm. One randomly selected image was assigned as an atlas; the remaining 22 images constituted targets for segmentation. This atlas was converted into a series of 'partially complete' atlases, which were then used by GAB to segment targets. This was performed as follows: (1) $11 \times 11 \times 11$ voxel masks were placed on the atlas in the left temporal lobe, right temporal lobe, and frontal lobe, constituting the atlas labels mask (Fig. 3); (2) for each target image, the whole brain was segmented using only the atlas labels within this masked area and the result saved; (3) the labels mask was dilated with 6 connectivity and cropped to the brain mask. Steps 2 and 3 were repeated until the labels mask was identical to the brain mask, providing segmentations for each image across a range (0.2%–100%) of atlas availabilities. Dice similarity coefficients (DSC) for cortical GM and WM were calculated, within the entire brain mask, for each target segmentation by comparison to that target's corresponding expert segmentation.

3   Results

Methods were implemented in .Net 4.0 and OpenCL 1.2 and ran on a Dual Xeon 8-core E5-2650 node with 128 GB of RAM and 3 Kepler Tesla K20 GPUs. Denoising + segmentation with GAB took 7–11.5 min in total, with processing using more-complete atlases taking longer than with incomplete atlases. EM segmentation ran in <1 min in each case. EM segmentation achieved DSCs of 0.67 ± 0.21 (mean $\pm$ SD; GM) and 0.84 ± 0.19 (WM). All GAB methods except GAB-Random outperformed EM segmentation at atlas availability $\geq 0.8\%$. This accuracy increased markedly until 6% atlas availability, after which

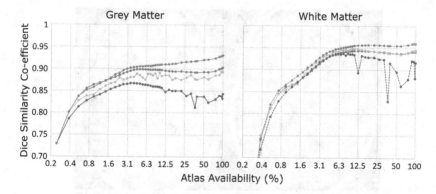

Fig. 2. Dice similarity coefficients for grey (left) and white (right) matter for segmentations generated by GAB, when provided with differing proportions of atlas. GAB methods are color-coded by their SV method as follows: Red, Random; Gold, PCA; Blue, Mean; Green, SOM. All methods achieved a dice similarity coefficient of 0.51 for white matter segmentation at an atlas availability of 0.24%, not shown here. (Color figure online)

Table 1. Dice similarity coefficients for GAB-derived grey matter (GM) and white matter (WM) segmentations at four different atlas availabilities. Each row indicates a different singular-value (SV) calculation method. SOM-48 indicate SOM-based SV calculation, with 48 patch augmentations (see text). All standard deviations were <0.02, except GAB-Random which demonstrated SDs of 0.03 (GM) and 0.02 (WM) at 100% atlas availability.

SV	GM				WM			
	0.9%	2%	6%	100%	0.9%	2%	6%	100%
SOM-48	0.88	0.90	N/A	N/A	0.92	0.88	N/A	N/A
SOM	0.84	0.89	0.91	0.93	0.91	0.85	0.95	0.96
Mean	0.86	0.88	0.90	0.90	0.89	0.86	0.94	0.94
PCA	0.84	0.87	0.87	0.89	0.90	0.85	0.94	0.95
Random	0.84	0.86	0.86	0.84	0.89	0.85	0.94	0.91

a gradual increase was seen (Fig. 2; Table 1). GAB-SOM provided superior segmentation accuracy to other methods, particularly for GM labelling, with more stable results than GAB-PCA or GAB-Random (Fig. 2). When the SOM-based analyses were run with 48 augmentations of each atlas patch, the atlas availability required to achieve a DSC of 0.90 in both tissue classes fell from 3.1% to 1.7%. Such augmentation, however, was infeasible in the current implementation above 3.5% atlas availability because of GPU memory constraints.

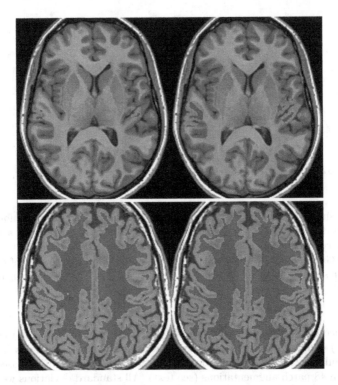

Fig. 3. Top: The atlas cropped to the labels-mask at 0.2% (left) and 2% (right) availability. The third labelled region is not visible in this slice. Bottom: Segmentation results for a representative dataset. The left segmentation was generated using GAB-SOM with 48 augmentations at 2% atlas availability. The right segmentation was generated with GAB-SOM at 100% atlas availability.

4   Discussion

Artificial neural networks such as deep learning can require large amounts of data for training, validation, and cross-validation in order to demonstrate task proficiency. In the case of brain-tissue segmentation, this often means that a large number of whole-brain tissue segmentations are required, but the time cost of generating these accurately can be very high. Here, we have demonstrated a Global Approximate Block-matching method which, unlike most methods, can segment a full brain MR image with reasonable accuracy when provided with an atlas that is predominantly incomplete. We found that this method reliably outperformed EM, an alternative technique with similar advantages, when provided with an atlas for which $\geq 0.8\%$ of voxels had been manually labelled. GAB was most effective when using an SOM for SV calculation, achieving dice coefficients of ≥ 0.9 for both cortical GM and cortical WM when provided with an atlas that was as low as 1.7% complete (Fig. 2). GAB-SOM also demonstrated performance comparable with some deep learning networks when provided with a whole brain atlas [6]. The relative performance of GAB-SOM is likely due to the SOM's highly non-linear nature enabling an effective whole-brain search for similar patches to a target. This is indicated by the relatively poorer performance of GAB when relying on PCA or mean voxel intensity for SV calculation, particularly at moderate atlas availabilities.

One advantage of GAB, for generation of 'ground truth' segmentations, is that it can be used in an iterative strategy in which an image is automatically segmented, then partially manually corrected, in a repeated manner. In such a strategy, a target image would act as its own atlas, and the GAB-based segmentation can be expected to improve with each iteration. This has the potential to drastically lower the time-cost of generating the first 'ground truth' segmentation of a series. For segmentations of subsequent images, GAB is likely to perform a high-quality segmentation, as this first image can be provided as an atlas.

A block-matching segmentation algorithm, volBrain, has previously been described [2]. Presently, volBrain and GAB have different strengths. Whilst volBrain relies on multiple whole-brain atlases in order to perform multi-atlas label fusion, GAB requires only a fraction of an atlas to be provided. This makes GAB a stronger candidate for creating expert segmentations for new populations and imaging modalities. GAB also does not limit patch searches to a local area. This means it is not reliant on image registration, and may perform sensibly when target and atlas anatomy differ meaningfully, such as with pathology. However, unlike volBrain, modifications are likely to be needed for accurate delineation of localized tissues such as the deep grey matter. Potential modifications exist, such as including a patch's location as parameters in the SV calculation, or splitting volumes into regions which are segmented using different partial atlases, but these modifications are yet untested.

In conclusion, we proposed a Global Approximate Block-matching method that relies on the SOM as a powerful dimensionality reduction technique. When provided with minimal training data, this method generates accurate brain tissue segmentations that have little need for manual correction. This technique may prove a useful tool for quickly generating training data sets for deep learning methods targeting imaging modalities and populations for which ground truth data are not widely available.

References

1. Kohonen, T.: Self-organized formation of topologically correct feature maps. Biol. Cybern. **43**(1), 59–69 (1982)
2. Manjon, J.V., Coupe, P.: volBrain: an online MRI brain volumetry system. Front. Neuroinformatics **10**, 30 (2016)
3. Pagnozzi, A.M., et al.: Alterations in regional shape on ipsilateral and contralateral cortex contrast in children with unilateral cerebral palsy and are predictive of multiple outcomes. Hum. Brain Mapp. **3603**, 3588–3603 (2016)

4. Sale, M., Reid, L., Cocchi, L., Pagnozzi, A., Rose, S., Mattingley, J.: Brain changes following four weeks of unimanual motor training: evidence from behavior, neural stimulation, cortical thickness, and functional MRI. Hum. Brain Mapp. **38**(9), 4773–4787 (2017)
5. Tustison, N.J., et al.: N4ITK: improved N3 bias correction. IEEE Trans. Med. Imaging **29**(6), 1310–20 (2010)
6. Wachinger, C., Reuter, M., Klein, T.: DeepNAT: deep convolutional neural network for segmenting neuroanatomy. NeuroImage **170**, 434–445 (2018)

Focal Dice Loss and Image Dilation for Brain Tumor Segmentation

Pei Wang$^{(\boxtimes)}$ and Albert C. S. Chung

Lo Kwee-Seong Medical Image Analysis Laboratory,
Department of Computer Science and Engineering,
The Hong Kong University of Science and Technology, Kowloon, Hong Kong
pei.wang@connect.ust.hk

Abstract. For accurate tumor segmentation in brain magnetic resonance (MR) images, the extreme class imbalance not only exists between the foreground and background, but among different sub-regions of tumor. Inspired by the focal loss [3] that down-weights the well-segmented classes, our proposed Focal Dice Loss (FDL) considers the imbalance among structures of interest instead of the entire image including background. Image dilation is applied to the training samples, which enlarges the tiny sub-regions, bridges the disconnected pieces of tumor structures and promotes understanding on overall tumor rather than complex details. The structuring element for dilation is gradually downsized, resulting in a coarse-to-fine and incremental learning process with the structure of network unchanged. Our experiments on the BRATS2015 dataset achieves the state-of-the-art in Dice Coefficient on average with relatively low computational cost.

1 Introduction

Gliomas are the most frequent primary brain tumors in adults [5], and the accurate segmentation of glioma and its sub-regions is crucial in clinical diagnosis, treatment planning, and post-operation evaluation. However, as shown in Fig. 1, the multiclass segmentation of multimodal brain MR images is very challenging. The major obstacle includes the great variance in terms of tumor size, shape, and location, also the extreme class imbalance.

Recently, deep convolutional neural networks (CNNs) have achieved remarkable performance in automatic brain tumor segmentation. Specifically, Pereira et al. [6] trained a 2D CNN on patches with data augmentation. A 3D CNN with multi-scale and multi-stream architecture is performed on patches extracted by nonuniform sampling [1], and followed by a fully connected conditional random field (CRF) to refine segmentation output [2]. Based on the fully convolutional network (FCN) [4], Shen et al. [7] introduced a boundary-aware network to achieve multi-task learning on 2D image slices. Zhao et al. [12] integrated FNNs and CRFs, and trained on both patches and slices in multiple stages. Additionally, three modes are trained on images of axial, coronal and sagittal views respectively, and combined by voting-based fusion strategy.

© Springer Nature Switzerland AG 2018
D. Stoyanov et al. (Eds.): DLMIA 2018/ML-CDS 2018, LNCS 11045, pp. 119–127, 2018.
https://doi.org/10.1007/978-3-030-00889-5_14

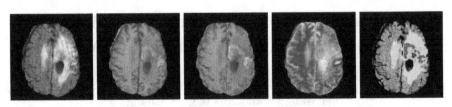

Fig. 1. Different modalities and the ground truth of an HG Tumor. Left to right: Flair, T1, T1c, T2, and expert manually segmented labels: necrosis (red), edema (yellow), non-enhancing tumor (blue), and enhancing tumor (green). (Color figure online)

To sum up, all these methods except [7] operate at the *patch* level, and balance the data by controlling the *sampling rate* [1,2,6,12]. Without prior knowledge, it is hard to extract test patches by the same sampling ratio. Moreover, the end-to-end (image to segmentation map) FCN frameworks like [7] are more computationally efficient comparing to the patch-based methods, but fail to handle the imbalance by nonuniform sampling or data augmentation.

To address the challenges above, we propose the Focal Dice Loss inspired by [3] and apply image dilation. To tackle the extreme class imbalance on image slices, our FDL down-weights the well-segmented classes during training. Instead of taking all classes into consideration like focal loss [3], the FDL emphasizes the imbalance among foreground classes. Meanwhile, dilation is applied to the ground truth of training samples that allows the network to learn the complex details of tumor structure in a coarse-to-fine approach. This differs from dilated convolution [11] that enlarges the receptive fields for convolutional kernels.

Our major contributions are as follows: (1) we propose Focal Dice Loss to address the class imbalance for multimodal brain tumor segmentation, and validated on publicly available dataset; (2) to the best of our knowledge, we are the first to apply image dilation to ground truth labels during training with gradually downsized structuring element, which obtains better high-level understanding; (3) we show that the proposed method achieves the state-of-the-art performance in Dice Coefficient on average, and with high computational efficiency.

2   Methodology

We employ the elegant U-Net that takes the full image context into account. As shown in Fig. 2, each block includes 3 convolutional layers of size 3×3, and each layer followed by ReLU activation and batch normalization. Max-pooling and up-sampling of size 2×2 are adopted in the two paths. Feature maps from the contracting path are concatenated to the ones in the expanding path.

2.1 Focal Dice Loss for Highly Unbalanced Data

Focal loss [3] based on standard cross entropy, is introduced to address the data imbalance of dense object detection. It is worth noticing that for the brain tumor, the class imbalance exists not only between tumor and background, but among different sub-regions of the tumor (e.g., necrosis and edema in Fig. 1 and Table 1). It is stated by Sudre et al. [10] that with the increasing level of data imbalance, loss functions based on overlap measurements are more robust than weighted cross entropy. Our experiments in the next session also support this argument. Therefore, Dice Coefficient is adopted to focus on the tumor sub-regions.

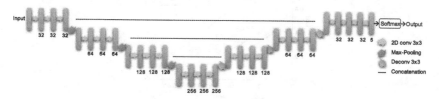

Fig. 2. Network Architecture: U-Net.

Balanced Dice Loss. The Dice Coefficient (DICE), also called the overlap index, is a commonly used metric in validating medical image segmentation. For the binary ground truth images of each class, DICE can be written as:

$$DICE_t = \frac{2\sum_{i=1}^{N} p_{it}g_{it} + \epsilon}{\sum_{i=1}^{N} p_{it} + \sum_{i=1}^{N} g_{it} + \epsilon}. \tag{1}$$

In the above, $g_{it} \in \{0,1\}$ specifies the ground truth label of class t and pixel i, where N indicates the total number of pixels of the image. Similarly, $p_{it} \in [0,1]$ denotes the output probability. In practice, the ϵ term is adopted to guarantee the loss function stability by avoiding the numerical issue of dividing by 0.

A common method for class imbalance is introducing a weight $w_t \geq 0$ for each class t. Therefore, we write the Dice Loss (DL) as:

$$DL = \sum_t w_t\,(1 - DICE_t). \tag{2}$$

Focal Dice Loss. As mentioned by [3], the extreme class imbalance overwhelms the cross entropy loss during training. We propose to assign lower weights to the well-segmented classes, and focus on the hard classes with lower DICE.

Formally, a factor $1/\beta$ is applied as the power of $DICE_t$ for each class, where the exponent parameter $\beta \geq 1$. We define the Focal Dice Loss (FDL) as:

$$FDL = \sum_t w_t\,(1 - DICE_t^{1/\beta}). \tag{3}$$

Table 1. Average Class Frequencies. Average frequencies taken over the training set of HG images, approximate values. Classes are: background (0) necrosis (1), edema (2), non-enhancing tumor (3), and enhancing tumor (4).

Class	0	1	2	3	4
Frequency	0.9858	0.0006	0.0092	0.0015	0.0028

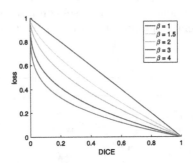

Fig. 3. Visualization of Focal Dice Loss. A factor $1/\beta$ is applied as the power of $DICE_t$, with the increase in β, the well-segmented classes are down-weighted.

The following are three properties of the FDL. (1) If a pixel is misclassified to class t with a large $DICE_t$ (i.e., the class is well segmented), then FDL is basically unaffected. On the contrary, if $DICE_t$ is small (i.e., the class is poorly segmented) and a pixel is misclassified, then the FDL will decrease significantly. (2) The exponent parameter β smoothly adjusts the rate where better-segmented classes are lower weighted. FDL is equal to DL when $\beta = 1$. With the increase in exponent factor β, the network focuses more on the poorly segmented classes than the others. (3) Different from focal loss [3], the overlap measurement FDL focus on the object of interest instead of the entire image, which meets the demand of brain tumor segmentation.

The FDL is visualized for several values of $\beta \in [1, 4]$ in Fig. 3. (we found $\beta = 2$ to work best in our experiments). We have validated the FDL in the BRATS2015 dataset, which shows an obvious improvement, especially for the small classes.

2.2   Dilation for Coarse-to-Fine Learning

Dilation. Dilation is one of the operators in the area of mathematical morphology. The effect of this operator on binary or grayscale images is enlarging the boundaries of foreground pixels using a structuring element. Mathematically, the dilation of A by B, denoted $A \oplus B$, is defined in terms of set operation:

$$A \oplus B = \{ z \,|\, (\hat{B})_z \cap A \neq \varnothing \}. \tag{4}$$

where $\varnothing$ is the empty set and B is the structuring element, $\hat{B}$ is the reflection of set B and $(B)_z$ is the translation of B by point $z = (z_1, z_2)$.

In image processing, one application of dilation is bridging the gaps of disconnected but close components, like broken characters. Similarly, we apply dilation to the ground truth to expanding the objects, and linking the disconnected parts. We aim at higher level feature extraction and therefore compromise on some low-level details in the early training stage.

Dilation on the Ground Truth. In our proposed method, dilation is applied to the binary ground truth images of each foreground class in the training set with a probability ratio α. Figure 4(f) to (j) show that the structuring element for dilation shrinks in size gradually during training, resulting in a coarse-to-fine learning process. Noted that eventually there is no dilation applied (dilation by structuring element in Fig. 4(j) remains no change to images). No dilation is applied to validation or test images in any of the experiments.

After dilation, it is possible that the dilated ground truth overlaps, and pixels (in the overlapping region) classified to all the intersected classes will result in a decrement of the loss function. Under this circumstance, the FDL is able to focus on the classes with lower DICE.

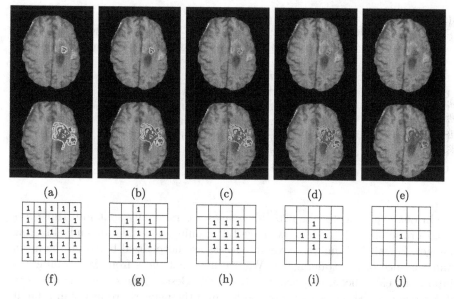

Fig. 4. Dilation on tumor sub-regions. (a) to (e): the dilated necrosis and nonenhancing tumor by structuring elements (f) to (j). The region in blue is the ground truth, and the region in yellow and blue is the dilated ground truth. (Color figure online)

In practice, the dilation has the following properties. (1) It expands the tiny regions and connects the close but separated pieces (Fig. 4(a) to (e)). Therefore, the ground truth of each foreground class shrinks from the dilated coarse features to the original fine labels. It also helps the network to focus on the higher level features. (2) Similar to Dropout that randomly discards units with its connections [9], the stochastic dilation on training labels prevents overfitting because of the dynamic changes during training. (3) The coarse-to-fine interface also boosts the learning speed as well as the training efficiency.

3 Evaluation

Our method has been evaluated on the BRATS2015 dataset. We use HG training set that contains MR images from 220 patients, and for each patient, there are 4 modalities (T1, T1-contrast (T1c), T2, and FLAIR) together with the ground truth. The label contains 5 classes: background, necrosis, edema, non-enhancing and enhancing tumor. The evaluation is performed on three different tumor sub-compartments: (1) the complete tumor (it contains all four tumor sub-regions); (2) the tumor core (it contains all tumor sub-regions except edema); (3) the enhancing tumor structure (it contains only the enhancing tumor sub-region).

Table 2. Performance on the BRATS 2015 44 test images.

Method	Dice				Sensitivity			Positive predictive value		
	Avg.	Comp.	Core	Enhan.	Comp.	Core	Enhan.	Comp.	Core	Enhan.
U-Net	77.38	86.15	72.77	73.23	85.62	70.00	73.76	89.03	81.21	79.18
U-Net+FDL	78.23	86.32	**73.71**	74.68	84.82	71.17	75.32	89.95	82.41	79.72
U-Net+Dilation	78.15	86.15	73.47	**74.85**	83.88	70.27	75.01	**90.61**	83.75	80.27
Proposed method	**78.38**	86.77	73.67	74.70	85.92	**74.98**	**79.88**	89.39	79.14	75.04
U-Net+Focal Loss	77.83	86.84	72.87	73.82	86.21	69.44	73.51	89.45	84.21	81.13
U-Net+CRF	77.04	86.55	70.97	73.60	**87.78**	71.17	75.32	89.94	82.41	79.72
Boundary-aware [7]	77.92	**87.31**	72.48	73.99	85.97	68.66	72.63	90.22	**84.71**	**81.20**

In our experiments, the 220 HG images are randomly split into three sets with a ratio of 6:2:2, therefore we have 132 training, 44 validation and 44 testing images. For all MR images, voxel intensities are normalized based on the mean and variance of the training set. We use 2D axial slices from MR volumes as input, and each slice is cropped into 192×200. Besides, the symmetric intensity difference map [8] of each slice is also fed into the network, resulting in 8 input channels. In our experiments, we use exponent factor $\beta = 2$ and dilation ration $\alpha = 0.6$. The duration of applying each structuring element in Fig. 4(g) to (j) for dilation is 15 epochs, the matrix in Fig. 4(f) is not used in our experiments. The model is implemented with Keras and Tensorflow backend, and trained for 60 epochs using Adam optimizer, with learning rate 8×10^{-5}.

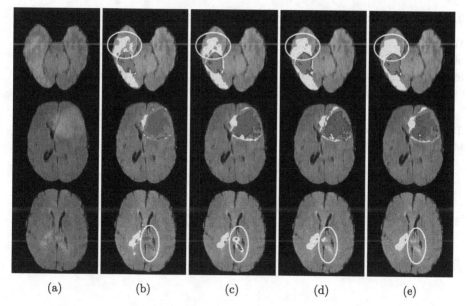

Fig. 5. Example results. Left to right: (a) Flair, (b) Flair with ground truth, (c) results of our method, (d) U-Net results, (e) Boundary-aware [7] results. Best viewed in color: necrosis (red), edema (yellow), non-enhancing tumor (blue), and enhancing tumor (green). (Color figure online)

The evaluation results of the 44 test images are shown in Table 2 on three tumor sub-regions. The hyper-parameters of mentioned models in Table 2 are identical to the proposed ones. Based on U-Net, the FDL and image dilation shows improvement especially on rather small regions like tumor core and enhancing tumor. It shows the capability of the FDL in improving the accuracy of classes with lower *Dice*. Our proposed method that combines the FDL and dilation outperforms the other methods in average *Dice* of three tumor regions. The example results are annotated in Fig. 5. Our method achieves better high-level understanding instead of misled by complex details. [7] generates smooth boundary of entire tumor but not for each tumor sug-regions, and our method also outperforms it on some disconnected components.

Besides the improvement in accuracy, one more advantage of our method is the low computational cost for new test images. Recent methods reported 8 min [6], 2 to 4 min [1], and 2 min [12] respectively for the prediction of each 3D volumes on the modern GPU. Our method just takes around 3 s on the NVIDIA Titan X Pascal, and including image normalization and computing symmetric difference maps.

3.1 Results on the Focal Dice Loss

We have tested the performance of the proposed method with different values of β in the FDL, as shown in Table 3. We plot the dice curves of 44 validation images during training. Noted that the *Dice* in Figs. 6 and 7 is the average DICE of 4 foreground classes, which differs from our evaluation matrix of 3 regions.

Table 3. Results on different values of exponent factor.

Exponent factor	Dice		
	Complete	Core	Enhancing
$\beta = 1$	86.15	73.47	74.85
$\beta = 1.5$	86.58	71.04	74.00
$\beta = 2$	86.77	73.67	74.70
$\beta = 3$	86.58	71.03	7.95

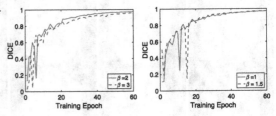

Fig. 6. *Dice* curves of different values of exponent factor.

3.2 Results on Dilation

We also conducted experiments to explore the properties of dilation on the ground truth. Table 4 shows that our model works best when $\alpha = 0.6$. It is worth noticing that the stability of the network is degraded when the dilation rate is 0.45 and 1 in Fig. 7. If the ground truth is dilated by a small ratio ($\alpha = 0.45$), the corresponding input images may be considered as noise during training as the occurrence of dilated images is limited. For large dilation rate, like $\alpha = 1$, it is likely that the network experiences great changes when the structuring element is switched to a smaller one and results in the oscillation of *Dice* curves.

Table 4. Results on different dilation ratios.

Dilation ratio	Dice		
	Complete	Core	Enhancing
$\alpha = 0.45$	86.49	72.93	74.41
$\alpha = 0.6$	86.77	73.67	74.70
$\alpha = 0.75$	86.40	73.09	75.10
$\alpha = 1$	86.32	73.71	74.68

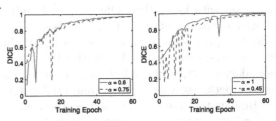

Fig. 7. *Dice* curves of different dilation ratios.

4 Conclusion

We introduced a FDL to address the data imbalance for multimodal brain tumor segmentation, which focuses on different objects of interest instead of the entire image (like focal loss). The experiments shows the capability of FDL in improving the class with lower accuracy. Dilation is also applied to training samples by a gradually downsized structuring elements to enlarge and connect the tiny regions for better high level feature extraction, which is a coarse-to-fine and incremental training approach with the structure of network unaffected. The performance of our method has been tested on the BRATS2015 dataset and achieves the state-of-the-art in Dice Coefficient with relatively low computational cost.

References

1. Kamnitsas, K., et al.: Efficient multi-scale 3D CNN with fully connected CRF for accurate brain lesion segmentation. Med. Image Anal. **36**, 61–78 (2017)
2. Krähenbühl, P., Koltun, V.: Efficient inference in fully connected CRFS with Gaussian edge potentials. In: Advances in Neural Information Processing Systems, pp. 109–117 (2011)
3. Lin, T.Y., Goyal, P., Girshick, R., He, K., Dollar, P.: Focal loss for dense object detection. In: Proceedings of the IEEE Conference on Computer Vision and Pattern Recognition, pp. 2980–2988 (2017)
4. Long, J., Shelhamer, E., Darrell, T.: Fully convolutional networks for semantic segmentation. In: Proceedings of the IEEE Conference on Computer Vision and Pattern Recognition, pp. 3431–3440 (2015)
5. Menze, B.H., et al.: The multimodal brain tumor image segmentation benchmark (BRATS). IEEE Trans. Med. Imaging **34**(10), 1993–2024 (2015)
6. Pereira, S., Pinto, A., Alves, V., Silva, C.A.: Brain tumor segmentation using convolutional neural networks in MRI images. IEEE Trans. Med. Imaging **35**(5), 1240–1251 (2016)
7. Shen, H., Wang, R., Zhang, J., McKenna, S.J.: Boundary-aware fully convolutional network for brain tumor segmentation. In: Descoteaux, M., Maier-Hein, L., Franz, A., Jannin, P., Collins, D.L., Duchesne, S. (eds.) MICCAI 2017. LNCS, vol. 10434, pp. 433–441. Springer, Cham (2017). https://doi.org/10.1007/978-3-319-66185-8_49
8. Shen, H., Zhang, J., Zheng, W.: Efficient symmetry-driven fully convolutional network for multimodal brain tumor segmentation. In: ICIP, pp. 3864–3868 (2017)
9. Srivastava, N., Hinton, G., Krizhevsky, A., Sutskever, I., Salakhutdinov, R.: Dropout: a simple way to prevent neural networks from overfitting. J. Mach. Learn. Res. **15**(1), 1929–1958 (2014)
10. Sudre, C.H., Li, W., Vercauteren, T., Ourselin, S., Jorge Cardoso, M.: Generalised dice overlap as a deep learning loss function for highly unbalanced segmentations. In: Cardoso, M.J., et al. (eds.) DLMIA/ML-CDS -2017. LNCS, vol. 10553, pp. 240–248. Springer, Cham (2017). https://doi.org/10.1007/978-3-319-67558-9_28
11. Yu, F., Koltun, V.: Multi-scale context aggregation by dilated convolutions. arXiv preprint arXiv:1511.07122 (2015)
12. Zhao, X., Wu, Y., Song, G., Li, Z., Zhang, Y., Fan, Y.: A deep learning model integrating FCNNs and CRFs for brain tumor segmentation. Med. Image Anal. **43**, 98–111 (2018)

Deep Particle Tracker: Automatic Tracking of Particles in Fluorescence Microscopy Images Using Deep Learning

Roman Spilger[1(✉)], Thomas Wollmann[1], Yu Qiang[1], Andrea Imle[2],
Ji Young Lee[3], Barbara Müller[4], Oliver T. Fackler[2], Ralf Bartenschlager[3],
and Karl Rohr[1]

[1] Division of Bioinformatics, Biomedical Computer Vision Group,
University of Heidelberg, BioQuant, IPMB, and DKFZ Heidelberg,
Im Neuenheimer Feld 267, 69120 Heidelberg, Germany
`roman.spilger@bioquant.uni-heidelberg.de`
[2] Department of Infectious Diseases, Integrative Virology,
University Hospital Heidelberg, Heidelberg, Germany
[3] Department of Infectious Diseases, Molecular Virology,
University Hospital Heidelberg, Heidelberg, Germany
[4] Department of Infectious Diseases, Virology, University Hospital Heidelberg,
Heidelberg, Germany

Abstract. Tracking of particles in fluorescence microscopy image sequences is essential for studying the dynamics of subcellular structures and virus structures. We introduce a novel particle tracking approach using an LSTM-based neural network. Our approach determines assignment probabilities jointly across multiple detections by exploiting both short and long-term temporal dependencies of individual object dynamics. Manually labeled data is not required. We evaluated the performance of our approach using image data of the ISBI Particle Tracking Challenge as well as real fluorescence microscopy image sequences of virus structures. It turned out that the proposed approach outperforms previous methods.

1 Introduction

Tracking of multiple particles in time-lapse fluorescence microscopy image sequences is an important task to quantify the dynamic behavior of subcellular and virus structures. Since a large number of particles needs to be tracked to draw statistically sound conclusions, accurate and robust automatic tracking approaches are indispensable.

Previous work on tracking biological particles can be subdivided into deterministic and probabilistic methods. Deterministic approaches follow a two step-paradigm comprising particle localization and motion correspondence (e.g., [13,14]). Probabilistic approaches are formulated within a Bayesian framework and take into account uncertainties to improve the robustness. The solution

© Springer Nature Switzerland AG 2018
D. Stoyanov et al. (Eds.): DLMIA 2018/ML-CDS 2018, LNCS 11045, pp. 128–136, 2018.
https://doi.org/10.1007/978-3-030-00889-5_15

is determined using Kalman filters or particle filters (e.g., $[1, 2, 4, 9, 11]$). A disadvantage of traditional tracking methods is that a handcrafted similarity measure is used to determine the degree of correspondence between detections in successive images. In addition, a suitable dynamic model needs to be selected, and often tedious manual tuning of (numerous) parameters is required. Often, these approaches have difficulties in cluttered environments with clustering objects. Deep learning methods have the potential to improve the performance. This has been demonstrated for different tasks such as segmentation and classification in the fields of computer vision and medical image analysis (e.g., [5]), however, much less work exists on tracking.

In the field of computer vision, Milan et al. [10] proposed a recurrent neural network (RNN) for tracking pedestrians in video images of natural scenes. However, tracking pedestrians is quite different from tracking biological particles since the motion and shape are very different, and appearance is not a reliable cue. Also, in [10] a handcrafted similarity measure is used for correspondence finding. In addition, two separate networks need to be trained for state prediction and data association. Sadeghian et al. [12] introduced an appearance-based RNN for tracking pedestrians in video images. However, there the similarity measure for correspondence finding is determined independently for each detection, and information on missing detections is not provided by the network. Also, a fixed input sequence length is used (last 6 time points). For training, manually labeled data was used. Yao et al. [17] used a similar approach as in [12] to track microtubules in synthetic data. However, the similarity measure for correspondence finding is not jointly computed across multiple detections, and a fixed input sequence length is used (as in [12]). In addition, objects are not automatically detected but ground truth positions are used, and real microscopy data was not considered. He et al. [6] introduced an approach based on convolutional neural networks (CNNs) for tracking of cells. However, this approach does not use an RNN, and tracking of particles was not considered.

In this contribution, we introduce a new approach for particle tracking in time-lapse fluorescence microscopy images based on an RNN. Both short- and long-term temporal dependencies of individual object dynamics are exploited for state prediction and correspondence finding using a long short-term memory (LSTM) [7]. The network automatically learns to determine assignment probabilities for correspondence finding, without requiring a handcrafted similarity measure. In contrast to [12, 17], our network computes assignment probabilities jointly across multiple detections, and also determines the probabilities of missing detections. In addition, the input sequence length is not limited but can be arbitrary long. Thus, we exploit more information and intrinsically cope with missing detections. Moreover our approach does not require manually labeled data (in contrast to [10, 12, 17]). Both state prediction and data association are trained within one network. Compared to traditional tracking methods, the dynamic model is automatically selected, and tuning of tracking parameters is not required. We performed a quantitative evaluation using data from the

ISBI Particle Tracking Challenge as well as using real live cell microscopy data of human immunodeficiency virus type 1 (HIV-1) particles and hepatitis C virus (HCV) proteins. It turned out that our approach yields better tracking results than previous methods.

2   Methods

Our approach, denoted as deep particle tracker (DPT), relies on a tracking-by-detection paradigm. For spot detection, we use the spot-enhancing filter (SEF) [13] yielding a set of detections. For correspondence finding, we introduce an LSTM-based recurrent neural network that determines assignment probabilities between tracked objects and particle detections. To establish one-to-one correspondences using the computed assignment probabilities of all objects and the probabilities of missing detections, the Hungarian algorithm is employed.

2.1   Network Architecture

In our DPT approach, for each object we use one neural network with the same network architecture. We employ both LSTM and fully-connected (FC) layers each consisting of K units (we used $K = 250$). We apply Gaussian dropout after each layer. Below, we describe the network architecture in more detail.

Let the vector $\mathbf{x}_t^i \in \mathbb{R}^D$ denote the state of an object i at time point t. In our work, we used $\mathbf{x}_t^i = (x_t^i, y_t^i, s_t^i, \alpha_t^i)$, i.e. $D = 4$. (x_t^i, y_t^i) is the object position. The speed and direction of the object motion is denoted by s_t^i and α_t^i (computed using the positions at two successive time points). The detections (positions as well as speed and direction for an assignment to object i) are represented by the vector $\mathbf{y}_t^i \in \mathbb{R}^{M \cdot D}$, where M is the overall number of detections. Note that M is often very high (in cluttered environments) and varies strongly between different images of a sequence. On the other hand, the neural network requires a fixed input vector size. To address this, in our approach we exploit the M-nearest detections (we used $M = 5$). For each time point $t - 1$, the network computes two output vectors for the next time point t: $\hat{\mathbf{x}}_t^i \in \mathbb{R}^D$ is the predicted object state, and $\mathbf{a}_t^i \in [0, 1]^{M+1}$ represents the assignment probabilities between object i and the M-nearest detections as well as probabilities for missing detections.

We use an LSTM to predict the state of an object i for the next time point t. The LSTM is composed of layers interacting which each other to determine the new hidden state $\mathbf{h}_t^i \in \mathbb{R}^K$ of dimension K which also represents the output. The main component of an LSTM is the cell state $\mathbf{c}_t^i \in \mathbb{R}^K$ which serves as long-term memory [7]. At each time point t, different types of gates determine which information is added to or removed from the previous cell state $\mathbf{c}_{t-1}^i$. Note that all gates compute their output based on the previous hidden state $\mathbf{h}_{t-1}^i$ and the current input. In our case, the input is the object state $\mathbf{x}_{t-1}^i$ mapped to the vector $\mathbf{z}_t^i \in \mathbb{R}^K$ by using a fully-connected (FC) layer and a hyperbolic tangent activation function. At time point t, the LSTM for an object i is updated as follows:

$$\mathbf{i}_t^i = \sigma(\mathbf{W}_{zi}\mathbf{z}_t^i + \mathbf{W}_{hi}\mathbf{h}_{t-1}^i + \mathbf{b}_i) \tag{1}$$

$$\mathbf{f}_t^i = \sigma(\mathbf{W}_{zf}\mathbf{z}_t^i + \mathbf{W}_{hf}\mathbf{h}_{t-1}^i + \mathbf{b}_f) \tag{2}$$

$$\mathbf{o}_t^i = \sigma(\mathbf{W}_{zo}\mathbf{z}_t^i + \mathbf{W}_{ho}\mathbf{h}_{t-1}^i + \mathbf{b}_o) \tag{3}$$

$$\mathbf{g}_t^i = \tanh(\mathbf{W}_{zg}\mathbf{z}_t^i + \mathbf{W}_{hg}\mathbf{h}_{t-1}^i + \mathbf{b}_g) \tag{4}$$

$$\mathbf{c}_t^i = \mathbf{f}_t^i \otimes \mathbf{c}_{t-1}^i + \mathbf{i}_t^i \otimes \mathbf{g}_t^i \tag{5}$$

$$\mathbf{h}_t^i = \mathbf{o}_t^i \otimes \tanh(\mathbf{c}_t^i) \tag{6}$$

where $\mathbf{i}_t^i$ is the input gate, $\mathbf{f}_t^i$ is the forget gate, $\mathbf{o}_t^i$ is the output gate, and $\mathbf{g}_t^i$ is the input modulation gate. Weight matrices $\mathbf{W} \in \mathbb{R}^{K \times K}$ and bias vectors $\mathbf{b} \in \mathbb{R}^K$ represent the parameters of a gate. σ is the logistic sigmoid activation function, and $\otimes$ denotes element-wise multiplication. We use the new hidden state $\mathbf{h}_t^i$ of the LSTM to compute the predicted object state $\hat{\mathbf{x}}_t^i$ by employing a FC layer and a hyperbolic tangent activation function. Since $\mathbf{h}_t^i$ is a function of all object states $\mathbf{x}_{1:t-1}^i$ from time point 1 to time point $t-1$, the network can exploit both short and long-term temporal dependencies for state prediction.

The vector $\mathbf{y}_t^i$ of the detections is passed to a FC layer with a hyperbolic tangent activation function for mapping it to a K-dimensional vector, which is then concatenated with the hidden state $\mathbf{h}_t^i$ of the LSTM. The resulting vector of dimension $2K$ is passed to another FC layer which maps it to a vector of dimension K. This vector is fed into a fully connected linear output layer with softmax normalization so that the final network output vector $\mathbf{a}_t^i$ can be interpreted as $M+1$ assignment probabilities, i.e. $\forall i : \sum_{j=1}^{M+1} a_t^{ij} = 1$, where a_t^{ij} denote the assignment probabilities between object i and detection j ($j = 1, ..., M$), and $a_t^{i(M+1)}$ are the probabilities of missing detections. The computed assignment probabilities and the probabilities for missing detections (dummy detections in the probability matrix) are used as input for the Hungarian algorithm. Note that a handcrafted similarity measure for the predicted state and the detections (e.g., Euclidean distance) is not required to compute the assignment probabilities.

The LSTM-based neural network is trained by minimizing the loss $\mathcal{L}$ over all trajectories defined by:

$$\mathcal{L} = \sum_{i=1}^{N} \mathcal{L}^i, \qquad \mathcal{L}^i = \sum_{t=1}^{T^i} \left(\frac{1}{D}\|\hat{\mathbf{x}}_t^i - \tilde{\mathbf{x}}_t^i\|^2 - \sum_{j=1}^{M+1} \tilde{a}_t^{ij} \log(a_t^{ij}) \right) \tag{7}$$

where N is the overall number of trajectories, $\mathcal{L}^i$ denotes the loss for the trajectory of object i, $\hat{\mathbf{x}}_t^i$ is the predicted state and $\tilde{\mathbf{x}}_t^i$ the true state at time point t. The deviation between the states is quantified by the mean squared error (MSE). The cross-entropy is used to measure the deviation between the computed assignment probabilities a_t^{ij} and the ground truth $\tilde{a}_t^{ij}$. T^i defines the total number of time points for a trajectory.

2.2 Training

Since deep learning architectures involve a large number of parameters, vast amounts of training data are generally required. However, ground truth for microscopy image sequences of biological particles is hardly available and manual annotation is very tedious. Therefore, in our approach we do not use manually labeled data but rely on synthetic data for training. We generated a large number of simulated trajectories of particles, which perform Brownian motion or directed motion. The diffusion coefficients and velocities of individual particles were sampled from a uniform distribution and the initial positions were chosen randomly. In addition, we randomly removed particle positions which enables the network to learn coping with missing detections.

For training our network, we used the RMSprop optimizer [15] with an initial learning rate of 3×10^{-5}, which was decreased by 5% when the validation loss stopped improving. To avoid overfitting, we employed early stopping and set the Gaussian dropout rate to $p = 0.2$. We used a dataset with 85,000 synthetically generated trajectories with variable track length. The dataset was split into 82% for training and 18% for validation. We used a mini-batch size of 10 trajectories.

3   Experimental Results

3.1   Particle Tracking Challenge Data

We evaluated our DPT approach based on data of the ISBI Particle Tracking Challenge [2] and compared the performance with the overall top-three approaches (Methods 5, 1, and 2). Method 5 uses the spot-enhancing filter (SEF) [13] for particle localization and probabilistic data association [4]. Method 1 employs intensity-weighted centroids for particle localization and combinatorial optimization [14]. Method 2 localizes particles by local maxima selection and performs linking by multiple hypothesis tracking [3]. In addition, we compared the performance of DPT with a recent approach employing a piecewise-stationary motion model smoother (PMMS) [11]. This approach uses SEF for particle localization and linear programming for linking (extension of u-track [8]).

To study the performance in cluttered environments, we used data of the vesicle scenario for signal-to-noise ratios of SNR = 4 and SNR = 7 as well as medium and high particle densities (medium: 500 particles/frame, high: 1000 particles/frame). The data is challenging due to conflicting correspondences (in total 15,682 trajectories). The image sequences consist of 100 images (512×512 pixels) with random appearance and disappearance of particles. To quantitatively assess the performance of the tracking methods, we computed the metrics α, β, JSC, JSC_θ, and $RMSE$ as described in [2]. $\alpha \in [0, 1]$ indicates the overall degree of matching of ground truth and estimated tracks excluding spurious tracks. $\beta \in [0, \alpha]$ includes an additional penalization for spurious tracks compared to α. The Jaccard similarity coefficient $JSC \in [0, 1]$ represents the overall particle detection performance, and $JSC_\theta \in [0,1]$ is the rate of correctly estimated tracks. The overall localization accuracy is indicated by the root mean square error $(RMSE)$.

The quantitative results are presented in Table 1 (bold values indicate the best performance). It can be seen that DPT performs best for all metrics and cases. Note that for PMMS the results in [11] are given only up to two decimal places and $RMSE$ is not provided. Note that for our DPT approach, we did not use the Particle Tracking Challenge data for training, but used our own generated synthetic data as described in Sect. 2.2 above.

Table 1. Tracking performance of different approaches for data of the vesicle scenario from the Particle Tracking Challenge. Bold indicates best performance.

Density	Meth	SNR = 4					SNR = 7				
		α	β	JSC	JSC_θ	$RMSE$	α	β	JSC	JSC_θ	$RMSE$
Med	Meth 5	0.658	0.588	0.641	0.776	0.754	0.677	0.605	0.646	0.783	0.667
	Meth 1	0.687	0.609	0.652	0.767	0.607	0.700	0.619	0.650	0.758	0.544
	Meth 2	0.582	0.514	0.590	0.757	0.970	0.611	0.547	0.606	0.775	0.828
	PMMS	0.67	0.60	0.64	0.77	-	0.68	0.61	0.64	0.78	-
	DPT	**0.695**	**0.624**	**0.658**	**0.790**	**0.545**	**0.711**	**0.631**	**0.651**	**0.790**	**0.525**
High	Meth 5	0.488	0.408	0.466	0.671	1.004	0.533	0.453	0.503	0.698	0.931
	Meth 1	0.531	0.442	0.487	0.641	0.801	0.582	0.494	0.526	0.683	0.683
	Meth 2	0.430	0.356	0.429	0.649	1.208	0.466	0.395	0.458	0.665	1.027
	PMMS	0.51	0.44	0.48	0.67	-	0.55	0.48	0.51	0.69	-
	DPT	**0.547**	**0.462**	**0.505**	**0.680**	**0.746**	**0.590**	**0.507**	**0.535**	**0.702**	**0.677**

3.2   Real Fluorescence Microscopy Images of Virus Structures

We also evaluated the performance of the DPT approach using real fluorescence microscopy image sequences displaying human immunodeficiency virus type 1 (HIV-1) particles and hepatitis C virus (HCV) proteins. The fluorescence labeled HIV-1 particles were imaged by a confocal spinning disk microscope and an EM-CCD camera. For our evaluation we used two image sequences (each 50 time points, 1000 × 1000 pixels, 16-bit) denoted by Seq. A and Seq. B. We also used one image sequence showing the HCV nonstructural protein 5A (30 time points, 1000 × 1000 pixels, 16-bit) denoted by Seq. C (an example section with 115 × 115 pixels is shown in Fig. 1). The images were acquired by a confocal spinning disk microscope and a CMOS camera. This dataset is challenging due to relatively low SNRs and clutter (high particle density, often crossing of trajectories). Ground truth trajectories for regions with clutter and large motion were determined by manual annotation. Seq. A, Seq. B, and Seq. C comprise 117, 125, and 55 ground truth trajectories, respectively (with up to 30 time points).

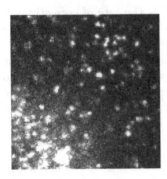

Fig. 1. Section of image sequence Seq. C (HCV). The image contrast was enhanced.

Table 2. Tracking performance of different approaches for real fluorescence microscopy images. Bold indicates best performance.

Sequence	Meth	α	β	JSC	JSC_θ	$RMSE$
Seq. A (HIV-1)	PT	0.312	0.255	0.348	0.442	2.701
	KF	0.388	0.317	0.421	0.456	2.775
	MHT	0.367	0.304	0.454	0.440	3.393
	DPT	**0.413**	**0.360**	**0.462**	**0.497**	**2.673**
Seq. B (HIV-1)	PT	0.328	0.261	0.338	0.399	2.559
	KF	0.352	0.312	0.396	0.373	**2.121**
	MHT	0.366	0.303	0.429	0.416	2.991
	DPT	**0.435**	**0.331**	**0.444**	**0.527**	2.717
Seq. C (HCV)	PT	0.590	0.496	0.629	0.557	1.064
	KF	0.559	0.481	0.564	0.550	1.088
	MHT	0.540	0.480	0.588	0.611	1.237
	DPT	**0.647**	**0.571**	**0.669**	**0.625**	**1.024**

We compared the performance of DPT with the ParticleTracker (PT) [14], a Kalman filter based approach (KF) [16], and multiple-hypothesis tracking (MHT) using multiple motion models [1]. PT uses intensity-weighted centroids for particle localization and combinatorial optimization [14]. KF uses SEF for particle localization and particle linking is based on a linear assignment method used in u-track [8]. MHT employs a wavelet-based detection scheme for particle localization. For PT, KF, and MHT we performed a grid search to determine optimal parameter settings. Note that for DPT, adaption of tracking parameters was not necessary (except the two detection parameters for SEF), i.e. we directly applied our tracking approach to the real data while training was performed only on synthetic data (see Sect. 2.2 above). Table 2 shows the tracking performance for all three image sequences. It turns out that DPT outperforms the other methods for all metrics and sequences (except $RMSE$ for Seq. B). Sample results for Seq. C are shown in Fig. 2. It can be seen that DPT yields the best result and maintains the correct identity for all three particles. KF causes an identity switch (between the blue and green trajectory). MHT yields a broken trajectory (yellow).

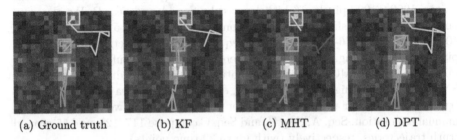

(a) Ground truth   (b) KF   (c) MHT   (d) DPT

Fig. 2. Ground truth and results of different tracking approaches for image sequence Seq. C (HCV). The image contrast was enhanced for better visualization. (Color figure online)

4   Conclusion

We presented a novel approach for tracking particles in time-lapse microscopy images using an LSTM-based recurrent neural network which computes assignment probabilities jointly across multiple detections and also determines probabilities for missing detections. Manually labeled data is not required. In addition, a handcrafted similarity measure is not needed. We evaluated our approach based on synthetic and real image sequences. It turned out that our approach yields better results than previous methods.

Acknowledgment. Support of the DFG (German Research Foundation) within the SFB 1129 is gratefully acknowledged.

References

1. Chenouard, N., Bloch, I., Olivo-Marin, J.C.: Multiple hypothesis tracking for cluttered biological image sequences. IEEE Trans. Pattern Anal. Mach. Intell. **35**(11), 2736–3750 (2013)
2. Chenouard, N., et al.: Objective comparison of particle tracking methods. Nat. Methods **11**(3), 281–289 (2014)
3. Coraluppi, S., Carthel, C.: Multi-stage multiple-hypothesis tracking. J. Adv. Inf. Fusion **6**, 57–67 (2011)
4. Godinez, W.J., Rohr, K.: Tracking multiple particles in fluorescence time-lapse microscopy images via probabilistic data association. IEEE Trans. Med. Imag. **34**(2), 415–432 (2015)
5. Greenspan, H., van Ginneken, B., Summers, R.M.: Deep learning in medical imaging: overview and future promise of an exciting new technique. IEEE Trans. Med. Imag. **35**(5), 1153–1159 (2016)
6. He, T., Mao, H., Guo, J., Yi, Z.: Cell tracking using deep neural networks with multi-task learning. Image Vis. Comput. **60**, 142–153 (2017)
7. Hochreiter, S., Schmidhuber, J.: Long short-term memory. Neural Comput. **9**(8), 1735–1780 (1997)
8. Jaqaman, K., et al.: Robust single-particle tracking in live-cell time-lapse sequences. Nat. Methods **5**(8), 695–702 (2008)
9. Liang, L., Shen, H., Camilli, P.D., Duncan, J.S.: A novel multiple hypothesis based particle tracking method for clathrin mediated endocytosis analysis using fluorescence microscopy. IEEE Trans. Image Process. **23**(4), 1844–1857 (2014)
10. Milan, A., Rezatofighi, S.H., Dick, A., Reid, I., Schindler, K.: Online multi-target tracking using recurrent neural networks. In: Proceedings of 2017 Conference on Artificial Intelligence (AAAI), San Francisco, CA, USA, pp. 4225–4232, February 2017
11. Roudot, P., Ding, L., Jaqaman, K., Kervrann, C., Danuser, G.: Piecewise-stationary motion modeling and iterative smoothing to track heterogeneous particle motions in dense environments. IEEE Trans. Image Process. **26**(11), 5395–5410 (2017)
12. Sadeghian, A., Alahi, A., Savarese, S.: Tracking the untrackable: learning to track multiple cues with long-term dependencies. In: Proceedings of 2017 IEEE International Conference on Computer Vision (ICCV), Venice, Italy, pp. 300–311, October 2017

13. Sage, D., Neumann, F.R., Hediger, F., Gasser, S.M., Unser, M.: Automatic tracking of individual fluorescence particles: application to the study of chromosome dynamics. IEEE Trans. Image Process. **14**(9), 1372–1383 (2005)
14. Sbalzarini, I., Koumoutsakos, P.: Feature point tracking and trajectory analysis for video imaging in cell biology. J. Struct. Biol. **151**(2), 182–195 (2005)
15. Tieleman, T., Hinton, G.: Lecture 6.5-RMSPROP: divide the gradient by a running average of its recent magnitude. COURSERA Neural Netw. Mach. Learn. **4**(2), 26–31 (2012)
16. Tinevez, J.Y., et al.: TrackMate: an open and extensible platform for single-particle tracking. Methods **115**, 80–90 (2017)
17. Yao, Y., Smal, I., Meijering, E.: Deep neural networks for data association in particle tracking. In: Proceedings of 2018 IEEE 15th International Symposium on Biomedical Imaging (ISBI 2018), Washington, D.C., USA, pp. 458–461, April 2018

3D Convolutional Neural Networks for Classification of Functional Connectomes

Meenakshi Khosla[1], Keith Jamison[2,3], Amy Kuceyeski[2,3],
and Mert R. Sabuncu[1,4(✉)]

[1] School of Electrical and Computer Engineering, Cornell University, Ithaca, USA
msabuncu@cornell.edu
[2] Radiology, Weill Cornell Medical College, New York City, USA
[3] Brain and Mind Research Institute, Weill Cornell Medical College,
New York City, USA
[4] Nancy E. and Peter C. Meinig School of Biomedical Engineering,
Cornell University, Ithaca, USA

Abstract. Resting-state functional MRI (rs-fMRI) scans hold the potential to serve as a diagnostic or prognostic tool for a wide variety of conditions, such as autism, Alzheimer's disease, and stroke. While a growing number of studies have demonstrated the promise of machine learning algorithms for rs-fMRI based clinical or behavioral prediction, most prior models have been limited in their capacity to exploit the richness of the data. For example, classification techniques applied to rs-fMRI often rely on region-based summary statistics and/or linear models. In this work, we propose a novel volumetric Convolutional Neural Network (CNN) framework that takes advantage of the full-resolution 3D spatial structure of rs-fMRI data and fits non-linear predictive models. We showcase our approach on a challenging large-scale dataset (ABIDE, with $N > 2,000$) and report state-of-the-art accuracy results on rs-fMRI-based discrimination of autism patients and healthy controls.

Keywords: Functional connectivity · fMRI
Convolutional neural networks · Autism · ABIDE

1 Introduction

The connectome, which can be captured via neuroimaging techniques such as diffusion and resting-state functional MRI, is a research area of intense focus, as it has delivered and continues to promise novel neuroscientific insights and clinical tools. In recent years, machine learning algorithms have been increasingly applied to connectome data [14,18,22]. These models often employ hand-engineered features such as pairwise correlations between regions of interest (ROIs) and network topological measures of clustering, small-worldness, integration, or segregation [2,10]. Furthermore, a vast majority of these models collapse the data into a feature vector for use in standard classification algorithms. Vectorization, however, discards the spatial structure of the connectome, which is an important

© Springer Nature Switzerland AG 2018
D. Stoyanov et al. (Eds.): DLMIA 2018/ML-CDS 2018, LNCS 11045, pp. 137–145, 2018.
https://doi.org/10.1007/978-3-030-00889-5_16

source of predictive information [12]. Finally, many machine learning techniques used with connectome data rely on linear or "shallow" models, which are limited in their capacity to capture relationships between connectomic features and clinical/behavioral variables.

In related work, deep neural networks exploiting the topological properties of brain networks have been recently explored. For example, the BrainNetCNN architecture of [11] extends convolutional neural networks (CNNs) to handle graph-structured data. While CNNs are motivated via the translation-invariance property of image-based classification problems and thus have achieved tremendous success, the neuroscientific basis of the invariance property exploited by BrainNetCNN remains elusive. Furthermore, this approach works directly with an adjacency matrix derived from the connectome data, while disregarding spatial information. Graph convolution networks [16], while increasingly popular, also seem sub-optimal to use with connectome data, since they rely on a common graph and the variation of interest is in the node properties. In the connectome, however, the main variation is the adjacency matrix, i.e., edge properties.

Our core contribution is an easy-to-implement 3D CNN framework for connectome-based classification. Our key insight is to use the connectivity "fingerprint", or functional coupling of each voxel to distinct target ROIs, as input features for a traditional volumetric CNN, represented as a multi-channel image volume. This allows us to characterize connectivity at a much finer scale than previously used with machine learning techniques, and without losing the spatial relationship between voxels. We are agnostic to the exact definition of target ROIs, yet as we demonstrate empirically this choice can impact final accuracy. In our experiments, we present an ensemble learning strategy that averages models obtained with different ROI definitions (called "atlases"), which yields robust and accurate results.

The proposed approach establishes a new benchmark model for autism classification on ABIDE, which is a particularly difficult dataset because of its heterogeneity, comprising subjects across a wide age range (5–64 years), and from sites that used different imaging protocols. Previous studies have reported cross-validated classification accuracies up to 67% on ABIDE-I, the first phase of the ABIDE study [1]. The proposed CNN approach improves this accuracy to above 73%. We also report, for the first time, independent test performance for benchmark and proposed models on the recently released second phase of ABIDE.

2   Materials and Methods

2.1   Proposed 3D CNN Approach

Here, we present our strategy to adopt a CNN architecture for use with connectomic data. The input to the CNN is formed by concatenating voxel-level maps of "connectivity fingerprints", which are represented as a multi-channel 3D volume. Each channel is a connectivity feature, such as the (Pearson) correlation between each voxel's time series and the average signal within a target ROI. In our implementation, we use atlas-based brain parcellation schemes to

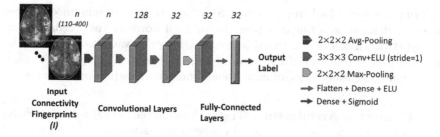

Fig. 1. Implemented CNN architecture. Number of channels denoted above.

define the target ROIs. The total number of input channels thus represents the number of ROIs used for creating voxel-level fingerprints. We used a variety of so-called atlases, which define a specific parcellation of the brain into ROIs (see below for details). Each atlas consisted of between 110 and 400 ROIs, where a larger number of regions corresponded to a finer scale parcellation. For each atlas, we trained a separate model, which we report performance values for. We also implemented an ensemble learning strategy, where the prediction was computed by taking a majority vote of the models corresponding to the different atlases.

In our experiments, we employed a simple CNN architecture, illustrated in Fig. 1. Our architecture has several convolutional layers, interspersed with max-pooling based down-sampling layers, followed by a couple of densely connected layers. The models were trained for 50 epochs with a batch size of 64. The learning rate and momentum for Stochastic Gradient Descent (SGD) were set to 0.001 and 0.9 respectively. The same architecture and settings were used for all atlases. We note that each atlas is defined on a unique grey matter mask. To ensure that all classifiers (baseline and proposed) use information from the same voxels while computing mean ROI signals or connectivity patterns, respective gray matter masks of these atlas were used for masking the input image of connectivity fingerprints before feeding into the proposed convolutional architecture.

2.2   Baseline Methods

Proposed CNN was compared against following baselines.

Ridge Classifier: A linear regression model was trained with a loss function equal to the sum of squared differences between prediction and ground truth values and α times the squared norm of the weight vector. The ground truth labels were encoded as ±1 for the two output categories. We test 10 linearly spaced values for the hyper-parameter α in the range $[0.1, 10]$ and report the highest cross-validation accuracy. Thus this baseline result reflects an *optimistic* estimate of performance.

Support Vector Machine: A linear SVM was trained to minimize β times the squared hinge loss function plus the squared norm of the weight vector. The hyper-parameter β was tuned by maximizing cross-validation accuracy by searching over two orders of magnitude ($[0.5, 50]$). As with the ridge classifier, this should be considered as an upper bound on generalization performance.

Fully Connected Architecture: The fully-connected neural network (FCN) architecture takes as input functional connectivity estimates between pairs of ROIs, which is vectorized and processed by a feed-forward network. We implemented following architecture: 4 fully connected hidden layers, with 800, 500, 100 and 20 numbers of features and each linear layer followed by an elementwise Exponential Linear Unit (ELU) activation. The output node was a sigmoid and computes disease probability, which is subsequently used for classification. The models were trained for 30 epochs with a batch size of 64. We monitored training curves to ensure that all trained models had converged before terminating the optimization. Stochastic Gradient Descent was used as the optimizer with learning rate and momentum set to 0.01 and 0.9 respectively. Dropout regularization parameter was set to 0.2 and applied to each layer during training.

2.3   Experiments

Data: Autism Brain Imaging Data Exchange (ABIDE) is a multi-site open-access MRI study [6]. The first phase of ABIDE (ABIDE-I) compiled data from 1112 individuals, comprising 539 individuals diagnosed with Autism Spectrum Disorder (ASD) and 573 typical controls, from 17 sites. The second phase (ABIDE-II) was recently released, and consists of an additional 521 individuals with ASD and 593 healthy controls, from 19 sites.

In our experiments, we used ABIDE-I subject data that passed manual quality assessments (QA) by all the functional raters. This yielded a final sample size of 774 ABIDE-I subjects, comprising 379 subjects with ASD and 395 typical controls. As an independent test dataset, we employed ABIDE-II subjects from sites that participated in ABIDE-I and used the same MRI sequence parameters for data collection. Since manual QA was not yet available for ABIDE-II, we performed an automatic quality control by selecting those subjects that retained at least 100 frames or 4 min of fMRI scans after motion scrubbing [19]. Motion scrubbing was performed based on Framewise Displacement (FD), discarding one volume before and two volumes after the frame with FD exceeding 0.5 mm [15]. This step yielded a final ABIDE-II sample size of 163 individuals with ASD and 230 healthy controls.

Data Preprocessing: ABIDE-I: The Preprocessed Connectomes Project (PCP) released preprocessed versions of ABIDE using several pipelines [4]. We used the data processed through Configurable Pipeline for Analysis of Connectomes (CPAC). This pipeline includes slice timing correction, motion correction, global mean intensity normalization and standardization of functional data to

MNI space ($3 \times 3 \times 3$ mm resolution) before the extraction of ROI time series. Among the different versions of the release, data extracted with global signal regression and band-pass filtering (0.01–10 Hz) was used in our analysis.

ABIDE-II: We preprocessed the ABIDE-II dataset following the same sequence of steps listed for ABIDE-I in CPAC (v1.0.2a). Connectivity between distinct brain regions was estimated using Pearson's correlation coefficient.

Table 1. 10-fold cross-validation on ABIDE-I/independent test on ABIDE-II accuracy of baseline models and proposed CNN approach. Best results are **bolded**.

Parcellation	Ridge classifier	SVC (l2 penalty)	SVC (l1 penalty)	Deep network	3D-CNN
HO	66.7/63.3	66.7/63.1	67.9/62.8	69.4/**67.7**	**70.5/67.7**
CC200	69.7/67.4	69.5/68.7	68.8/66.4	70.5/71.5	**71.2/72.8**
EZ	66.4/63.3	66.9/63.3	65.9/61.0	68.6/63.8	**69.3/66.4**
TT	64.4/66.1	65.3/66.7	64.3/61.3	67.1/65.9	**69.4/70.0**
CC400	70.2/69.4	70.5/69.7	67.5/68.1	71.0/69.9	**71.7/70.5**
AAL	65.4/63.3	65.7/62.3	68.1/62.6	66.7/65.4	**71.4/69.5**
DOS160	66.2/66.7	66.7/66.1	65.3/61.6	67.2/66.1	**68.6/67.0**
Ensemble	69.8/66.7	69.6/67.1	70.1/64.2	71.5/69.9	**73.3/71.7**

Atlases: In our experiments, we considered all atlases that were used for ROI time series extraction in PCP. These include the following seven atlases: Harvard-Oxford (HO), Craddock 200 (CC200), Eickhoff-Zilles (EZ), Talaraich and Tournox (TT), Dosenbach 160 (DOS160), Automated Anatomical Labelling (AAL) and Craddock 400 (CC400) [3,5,7,8,13,21].

For the baseline methods, each atlas was used to define a corresponding connectivity matrix which was fed as input to each model. For the proposed model, the atlas ROIs were used as target ROIs to derive the input connectivity features at the voxel-level. We also report results for an ensemble learning strategy, where we combined the predictions of models corresponding to individual atlases through majority voting to obtain improved and robust predictions.

Evaluation: We evaluated our model on the challenging task of autism classification using the two schemes. First, we implemented a 10-fold cross-validation scheme for ABIDE-I to be consistent with previously reported classification results [1,18]. Second, we trained each model on all of ABIDE-I and computed test performance on an independent held-out set from ABIDE-II. This is used for assessing the generalization behavior of different classifiers. We report accuracy and the receiver operating curves (ROC), along with corresponding area under the curves (AUC) for each of these scenarios.

3 Results

Table 1 shows cross-validation and independent test accuracy values for different models. Proposed 3D CNN model consistently outperforms baselines. The ensemble CNN approach yields a classification accuracy of **73.3** % on ABIDE-I, significantly exceeding the state of the art [9]. Further, with an accuracy of **71.7** % on independent test data, the model also achieves good generalization. Figure 2 shows ROC curve obtained of individual atlases and their ensemble on ABIDE-II. The ensemble achieves an AUC of **75.8%**.

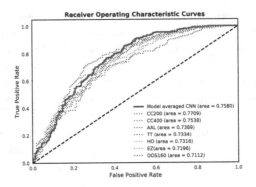

Fig. 2. ROC on independent ABIDE-II

3.1 Visualization of CNN Model

Visualization techniques for CNNs can help reveal salient features used by the model for discriminating between output classes. We employed the saliency map of [20], which is a gradient-based technique. Essentially, this visualization approach computes the gradient of the output score with respect to the input image, i.e., the 3D volume, using a single backward pass through the trained neural network. We then computed voxel-level saliency as the maximum absolute gradient value across all input channels corresponding to different target ROIs. Figure 3 shows these saliency maps averaged across all ABIDE-II cases for different atlases.

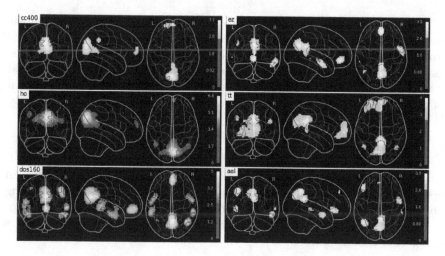

Fig. 3. CNN saliency maps averaged over ABIDE-II cases for different atlases.

4   Discussion

In this paper, we presented a novel strategy to use 3D-CNN architectures for connectome classification. We conducted detailed empirical evaluations of the proposed model on a large dataset, which yielded significant improvements over state-of-the-art accuracy. In almost all cases, the performance of the proposed approach exceeded that of the baseline models, although the differences were modest for higher resolution parcellations.

Another contribution of our paper is to highlight the advantage of ensemble learning, for example by majority voting over models corresponding to different atlases. Atlases, or more generally ROIs, are often selected arbitrarily in the rs-fMRI community and our experiments demonstrate that averaging across these decisions can yield more robust and accurate predictions.

The interpretation of classification models is invaluable for biomedical applications, for example by offering biological insights or understanding the information that was used to make the prediction. Several previous studies have attempted to visualize abnormal connectivity patterns in disease. In this work, we present a strategy that allows us to interrogate the trained CNN models. Our approach allows for visualizing the saliency map for a given individual, yet we leave the analysis of this for future work. Instead we presented group-averaged maps for the different atlases. As shown in Fig. 3, the saliency maps for the different atlases are rather consistent and highlight the so-called default mode network, which has been implicated in autism in prior studies [17]. We also note some differences between the atlas saliency maps, which suggests that the different models are utilizing slightly different information content and thus can be complementary, explaining why model averaging can improve accuracy.

While the proposed CNN approach achieves promising accuracy on autism detection, there is room for further improvement. We have not yet conducted a comprehensive optimization of the convolutional architecture. Furthermore, there is likely more optimal choices than atlas-based target ROI correlations that are used as input to the model. We envision an end-to-end learning strategy that can enable the optimization of these connectomic features.

5   Conclusion

Our experiments highlight the potential of deep neural network algorithms in the classification of functional connectomes and in expanding our understanding of brain disorders. When tailored for connectomes, modern DNN architectures like Convolutional Neural Networks offer an unparalleled opportunity to probe brain networks in disease.

Acknowledgements. This work was supported by NIH grants R01LM012719 & R01AG053949 (MS), R21NS10463401 & R01NS10264601A1 (AK), NSF NeuroNex grant 1707312 (MS) & Anna-Maria & Stephen Kellen Foundation Junior Faculty Fellowship (AK).

References

1. Abraham, A., et al.: Deriving reproducible biomarkers from multi-site resting-state data: an autism-based example. NeuroImage **147**, 736–745 (2017)
2. Brown, C.J., Hamarneh, G.: Machine learning on human connectome data from MRI. CoRR, 1611.08699 (2016)
3. Cameron, C.R., et al.: A whole brain fMRI atlas generated via spatially constrained spectral clustering. Hum. Brain Mapp. **33**(8), 1914–1928 (2012)
4. Craddock, C., et al.: The neuro bureau preprocessing initiative: open sharing of preprocessed neuroimaging data and derivatives. Front. Neuroinformatics (2013)
5. Desikan, R.S., et al.: An automated labeling system for subdividing the human cerebral cortex on MRI scans into gyral based regions of interest. NeuroImage **31**(3), 968–980 (2006)
6. Di Martino, A., et al.: Enhancing studies of the connectome in autism using the autism brain imaging data exchange II. Sci. Data **4**, 170010 (2017)
7. Dosenbach, N.U.F., Nardos, B., Cohen, A.L., et al.: Prediction of individual brain maturity using fMRI. Science **329**(5997), 1358–1361 (2010)
8. Eickhoff, S.B., et al.: A new spm toolbox for combining probabilistic cytoarchitectonic maps and functional imaging data. NeuroImage **25**(4), 1325–1335 (2005)
9. Heinsfeld, A.S., et al.: Identification of autism spectrum disorder using deep learning and the abide dataset. NeuroImage Clin. **17**, 16–23 (2018)
10. Kaiser, M.: A Tutorial in Connectome Analysis: Topological and Spatial Features of Brain Networks. ArXiv e-prints, May 2011
11. Kawahara, J., et al.: BrainNetCNN: convolutional neural networks for brain networks; towards predicting neurodevelopment. NeuroImage **146**, 1038–1049 (2017)
12. Kong, R., et al.: Spatial topography of individual-specific cortical networks predicts human cognition, personality, and emotion. Cereb. Cortex (2018)

13. Lancaster, J.L., Woldorff, M.G., et al.: Automated talairach atlas labels for functional brain mapping. Hum. Brain Mapp. **10**(3), 120–131 (2000)
14. Mennes, M., et al.: Resting state functional connectivity correlates of inhibitory control in children with ADHD. Front Psychiatry (2012)
15. Muschelli, J., Nebel, M.B., et al.: Reduction of motion-related artifacts in resting state fMRI using aCompCor. NeuroImage **96**, 22–35 (2014)
16. Niepert, M., et al.: Learning convolutional neural networks for graphs. In: Proceedings of Machine Learning Research, New York, USA, June 2016
17. Padmanabhan, A., et al.: The default mode network in autism. Biol. Psychiatry Cogn. Neurosci. Neuroimaging **2**(6), 476–486 (2017)
18. Plitt, M., et al.: Functional connectivity classification of autism identifies highly predictive brain features but falls short of biomarker standards. NeuroImage Clin. **7**, 359–366 (2015)
19. Power, J.D., Mitra, A., et al.: Methods to detect, characterize, and remove motion artifact in resting state fMRI. NeuroImage **84**, 320–341 (2014)
20. Simonyan, K., et al.: Deep inside convolutional networks: visualising image classification models and saliency maps. CoRR, 1312.6034 (2013)
21. Tzourio-Mazoyer, N., et al.: Automated anatomical labeling of activations in SPM using a macroscopic anatomical parcellation of the MNI MRI single-subject brain. NeuroImage **15**(1), 273–289 (2002)
22. Varoquaux, G., Baronnet, F., Kleinschmidt, A., Fillard, P., Thirion, B.: Detection of brain functional-connectivity difference in post-stroke patients using group-level covariance modeling. In: Jiang, T., Navab, N., Pluim, J.P.W., Viergever, M.A. (eds.) MICCAI 2010. LNCS, vol. 6361, pp. 200–208. Springer, Heidelberg (2010). https://doi.org/10.1007/978-3-642-15705-9_25

Segmentation of Head and Neck Organs-At-Risk in Longitudinal CT Scans Combining Deformable Registrations and Convolutional Neural Networks

Liesbeth Vandewinckele[1,3], David Robben[1,3], Wouter Crijns[2,4], and Frederik Maes[1,3(✉)]

[1] KU Leuven, Department of ESAT/PSI, Kasteelpark Arenberg 10 bus 2441, 3001 Leuven, Belgium
frederik.maes@kuleuven.be
[2] KU Leuven, Department of Oncology - Laboratory of Experimental Radiotherapy, Herestraat 49 bus 7003 40, 3000 Leuven, Belgium
[3] UZ Leuven, Medical Imaging Research Center, Herestraat 49 bus 7003, 3000 Leuven, Belgium
[4] UZ Leuven, Radiation Oncology, Herestraat 49 bus 7003 40, 3000 Leuven, Belgium

Abstract. Automated segmentation of organs-at-risk (OAR) in follow-up images of the patient acquired during the course of treatment could greatly facilitate adaptive treatment planning in radiotherapy. Instead of segmenting each image separately, the segmentation could be improved by making use of the additional information provided by longitudinal data of previously segmented images of the same patient. We propose a tool for automated segmentation of longitudinal data that combines deformable image registration (DIR) and convolutional neural networks (CNN). The segmentation propagated by DIR from a previous image onto the current image and the segmentation obtained by a separately trained cross-sectional CNN applied to the current image, are given as input to a longitudinal CNN, together with the images itself, that is trained to optimally predict the manual ground truth segmentation using all available information. Despite the fairly limited amount of training data available in this study, a significant improvement of the segmentations of four different OAR in head and neck CT scans was found compared to both the results of DIR and the cross-sectional CNN separately.

1 Introduction

Delineation of Organs-At-Risk (OAR) in a pre-treatment CT scan of the patient is an essential step in radiotherapy (RT) planning to be able to deliver the required dose to the target volume while at the same time minimizing the dose to the surrounding normal tissues in order to reduce the risk of complications. However, since the treatment is fractionated over multiple RT sessions during

© Springer Nature Switzerland AG 2018
D. Stoyanov et al. (Eds.): DLMIA 2018/ML-CDS 2018, LNCS 11045, pp. 146–154, 2018.
https://doi.org/10.1007/978-3-030-00889-5_17

the course of several weeks, anatomical changes may occur that invalidate the initial treatment plan. Hence, it can be useful to acquire a new CT scan during the course of treatment and adapt the treatment to the new anatomy if needed, which requires delineation of each of these longitudinal CT scans [1]. Manual segmentation by a clinical expert of OAR in the head and neck (H&N) region is time consuming and takes about 45 min up to two hours in clinical practice, since there are on average 13 3D structures to be delineated. Moreover, the manual delineations are prone to intra- and interobserver variations.

Automatic segmentation of OAR in longitudinal CT scans in the context of RT planning is usually solved by using deformable image registration (DIR) [2]. An already segmented image (a so called atlas) is deformed to fit the new image to be segmented and the delineations in the atlas are deformed in the same way to yield a segmentation of the new image. Several choices for the atlas can be made, but the best results are obtained with a previous CT scan from the same patient, as the similarity between the atlas and the new CT image to be segmented is then likely very high [2]. This strategy was applied by Zhang et al. [3], Veiga et al. [4] and Castadot et al. [5]. Unfortunately, manual adaptation may still be necessary, but the time needed for the adaptation is usually small compared to manual segmentation [6]. The purpose of this work is to replace this manual correction by a neural network that can do the needed corrections.

Convolutional neural networks (CNN) are currently the state-of-the-art neural network architectures for medical image segmentation. The segmentation is formulated as a voxel-wise classification problem, whereby each voxel is individually classified as belonging to a particular organ of interest based on the intensity values within a certain neighborhood (the receptive field). A CNN for segmentation of OAR in the H&N-region is proposed by Ibragimov et al. [7]. The network gives state-of-the-art results for organs with recognizable boundaries in CT-images. However, organs without recognizable boundaries are more difficult to segment, which suggests that additional information is required.

Longitudinal data are not frequently used yet in CNN based segmentation, although such data could provide relevant additional information. Examples of neural networks that incorporate longitudinal data are Birenbaum et al. [8], who used a CNN on longitudinal data for MS lesion segmentation, and Vivanti et al. [9], who proposed an algorithm for liver tumor segmentation in follow-up CT scans. Vivanti et al. [9] did not train their network on longitudinal data, but only used the previous scans to define a region of interest (ROI) to give as input to the neural network for segmenting the tumor. The benefit of defining a ROI is that the amount of false positives will be reduced. In contrast to Vivanti et al. [9], we propose to include the previous segmentations registered to the new CT scan as additional features for CNN-based classification.

2 Methods

2.1 Available Data and Preprocessing

The dataset consists of 17 sets of longitudinal H&N data. Each such set consists of five types of images:

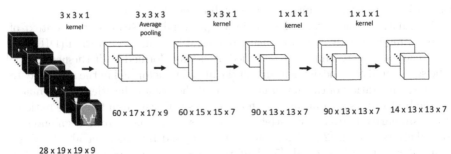

Fig. 1. The proposed CNN architecture for segmentation using longitudinal data. The size of each layer is given by # feature maps × 3D segment size.

- I_0: a previous CT scan acquired before or in week two of the RT treatment;
- I_1: the current CT scan acquired in week two or four of the RT treatment;
- $S_{0,m}$: the clinically approved binary segmentation maps of OAR in I_0;
- $S_{1,m}$: the clinically approved binary segmentation maps of OAR in I_1;
- $S_{1,c}$: the automatically generated binary segmentation maps of OAR in I_1 using the state-of-the-art cross-sectional CNN defined in [10], trained on a separate non-longitudinal dataset (acquired on the same scanner and delineated by the same observer as the longitudinal dataset).

The 17 sets of longitudinal data originate from 9 different patients. All CT scans were acquired in our institute on the same Siemens Sensation Open CT scanner using the same clinical protocol at 120kV. Clinically approved OAR segmentations are available for 13 H&N structures: the brainstem, the cochlea (left and right), the upper esophagus, the glottic area, the mandible, the extended oral cavity, the parotid glands (left and right), the pharyngeal constrictor muscles (PCM inferior, medial and superior), the spinal cord, the submandibular glands (left and right) and the supraglottic larynx. All images are preprocessed to have the same voxel size of $1 \times 1 \times 3$ mm^3 and the intensities of the CT scans are normalized to have zero mean and unit variance over all CT scans together.

2.2 Deformable Image Registration

The first step is to align the previous image I_0 and its segmentation $S_{0,m}$ onto the current image I_1 using DIR, yielding the deformed image $I_{0,r}$ and a DIR-based segmentation $S_{0,r}$ of the OAR in I_1. The registration process consists of two steps: first rigid and then non-rigid B-spline registration. The hyperparameters for each step are optimized in terms of a volume-weighted average of the Dice similarity coefficients (DSC) of $S_{0,r}$ compared to $S_{1,m}$ over all OAR. The most important DIR hyperparameters are the similarity metric used, the number of histogram bins in case mutual information is used, and the final spacing of the B-spline control point grid. Optimal performance was obtained with mutual information as similarity metric, with 64 bins for rigid and 32 bins for non-rigid registration, and a final B-spline grid spacing of 16 mm. All registrations were performed using Elastix [11].

2.3   Neural Network Architecture

The registered longitudinal images $I_{0,r}$ and I_1 and both segmentations $S_{0,r}$ and $S_{1,c}$ are given as input to the neural network, which generates the segmentation $S_{1,l}$ as a prediction of the true segmentation $S_{1,m}$ for image I_1. The longitudinal neural network is built by taking into account two different considerations. Firstly, a certain size of the receptive field is required. Secondly, the amount of parameters must be kept as low as possible to reduce overfitting since the amount of training data is small. The network has four convolutional layers. The first two layers are the feature extraction part with a kernel size of $(3, 3, 1)$ and a stride of 1 and the last two layers are fully connected layers implemented as convolutional layers with a kernel size of $(1, 1, 1)$ to make the network fully convolutional. A scheme of the architecture can be found in Fig. 1. An average pooling layer is inserted since this increases the receptive field without increasing the amount of parameters. It has a pooling size of $(3, 3, 3)$ with a stride of 1. The amount of feature maps cannot be made too low since we expect a lot of interactions between the inputs (and OAR) and the amount of redundant information is not high. The amount of feature maps is set to 60 in the first layer, 90 in the subsequent layers and 14 in the output layer, one for each class (13 OAR and background). The size of the receptive field thus becomes $7 \times 7 \times 3$ voxels or $7 \times 7 \times 9$ mm^3, which is small, implying that the neural network has not much contextual information to base its predictions on. It only makes uses of the intensities of both images and the available segmentations within a small neighborhood around each voxel.

2.4   Neural Network Training

The neural network is trained in a supervised way using the training scheme from Kamnitsas et al. [12], which was implemented by [13]. The training scheme does fully-convolutional predictions on image segments, since the memory requirements for full 3D images and 3D networks are high. In this way, several consecutive segments must be given as input to the network to obtain a segmentation of the complete image. The used evaluation metric is categorical cross-entropy. To prevent class imbalance, the image segments are sampled from the training images with an equal probability to be centered at a voxel of any of the different classes. The Adam optimizer is used with the originally proposed parameters [14]. The initial learning rate is set to 0.008 and is divided by four when a convergence plateau of the cost function is reached. This is done two times. The weights are initialized using He's initialization and PReLU activation functions are used in the hidden layers. Furthermore, batch normalization is applied to all hidden layers. A softmax function is used at the output layer. As the amount of data available to train the network was low, regularization is quite important in this work. Dropout is used in the last layers of the network with a dropout probability of 0.5. The weight against L_2-regularization is equal to 0.001. Data augmentation is done on the samples by flipping them around the sagittal plane.

2.5   Postprocessing

Postprocessing is a standard approach in literature to improve the resulting segmentations of the neural network. Voxels are classified individually to belong to the object of interest or not, without explicitly considering connectivity constraints. Postprocessing can be used to impose such constraints, which causes single pixels or holes to be removed [7,8,12,15]. However, in this work, no postprocessing is used in order to be able to evaluate the intrinsic segmentation performance of the network itself.

3   Results and Discussion

DIR took on average 15 min per dataset on an Intel Xeon E5645. After registration, the segmentation of the OAR by the longitudinal CNN took on average 2–3 min on a Nvidia GTX 1080 Ti.

A 6-fold cross-validation is performed on the longitudinal dataset to obtain segmentations for all patients with the longitudinal CNN. The results of the three segmentation approaches $S_{0,r}$ (DIR), $S_{1,c}$ (cross-sectional CNN), and $S_{1,l}$ (the proposed longitudinal CNN) are summarized in Table 1 by their average DSC compared to the manual ground truth segmentation $S_{1,m}$. Statistical significance between different approaches based on differences in DSC is assessed with a one-sided, paired Wilcoxon signed-rank test with a significance level of 0.05.

DIR ($S_{0,r}$) performs better than the cross-sectional CNN of [10] ($S_{1,c}$) in terms of DSC for five different organs (brainstem, upper esophagus, oral cavity, parotid glands and spinal cord), while the opposite is true for the mandible, which is a bony structure that is clearly defined on a CT scan.

The longitudinal CNN ($S_{1,l}$) performs at least as good as its both input segmentations (except for the spinal cord). It performs better than the cross-sectional CNN for 7 structures and better than DIR for 5 structures, including also the mandible. Moreover, the longitudinal CNN improves the results of both input segmentations for 4 structures: the oral cavity, the parotid glands, the submandibular glands and the supraglottic larynx. Hence, the longitudinal CNN not just selects the best of both segmentations, but succeeds at improving segmentation quality by combining the results of both inputs. An exception is the segmentation of the spinal cord. This can be explained by an inconsistency in the lower border of the spinal cord in the training data for the cross-sectional CNN of [10] and for the longitudinal CNN, which makes it impossible for the longitudinal CNN to learn a consensus.

Table 1. DSC (mean ± SD) for OAR segmentation in image I_1 based on DIR of the previous image I_0 onto the current image I_1 ($S_{0,r}$), the cross-sectional CNN of [10] applied to I_1 ($S_{1,c}$) and the proposed longitudinal CNN ($S_{1,l}$) w.r.t. the manual expert segmentation of I_1 ($S_{1,m}$), averaged over all performed predictions on N datasets. Statistical significant results are indicated by ($> r, c, l$) if the result is better than $S_{0,r}$, $S_{1,c}$ or $S_{1,l}$ respectively. Significance was assessed using a one-sided, paired Wilcoxon signed-rank test ($\alpha = 0.05$).

OAR	N	$S_{0,r}$	$S_{1,c}$	$S_{1,l}$
Brainstem	17	0.88 ± 0.01 ($> c$)	0.84 ± 0.03	0.88 ± 0.02 ($> c$)
Cochlea	5	0.60 ± 0.11	0.55 ± 0.12	0.67 ± 0.09
Upper Esophagus	16	0.64 ± 0.13 ($> c$)	0.58 ± 0.12	0.62 ± 0.12 ($> c$)
Glottic Area	15	0.57 ± 0.18	0.58 ± 0.22	0.56 ± 0.23
Mandible	17	0.87 ± 0.02	0.91 ± 0.02 ($> r$)	0.91 ± 0.02 ($> r$)
Oral Cavity	15	0.88 ± 0.02 ($> c$)	0.87 ± 0.04	0.89 ± 0.02 ($> r, c$)
Parotid Glands	17	0.82 ± 0.03 ($> c$)	0.79 ± 0.06	0.84 ± 0.04 ($> r, c$)
PCM inferior	13	0.59 ± 0.10	0.53 ± 0.18	0.51 ± 0.24
PCM medial	15	0.48 ± 0.16	0.52 ± 0.17	0.50 ± 0.12
PCM superior	10	0.42 ± 0.12	0.38 ± 0.08	0.45 ± 0.11
Spinal Cord	17	0.75 ± 0.10 ($> c, l$)	0.73 ± 0.10	0.73 ± 0.09 ($> c$)
Submandibular Glands	17	0.75 ± 0.05	0.71 ± 0.11	0.78 ± 0.09 ($> r, c$)
Supraglottic Larynx	13	0.71 ± 0.08	0.64 ± 0.13	0.76 ± 0.07 ($> r, c$)

Some example delineations are shown in Fig. 2. We observed that the delineations obtained with the longitudinal CNN mostly lie between the delineations obtained with DIR and the cross-sectional CNN, unless a clear boundary can be perceived in the CT scan. The longitudinal CNN can thus improve the input segmentations if one systematically constitutes an oversegmentation and the other an undersegmentation. This appears to be the case for the parotid glands segmentations. Another possibility is that inaccuracies in both input segmentations occur at different positions in the object. An example are the submandibular glands, for which the cross-sectional CNN performs well for segmenting the upper part, while DIR performs well for the lower part. At the moment, little can be concluded about the other organs, for which segmentation performance is not significantly improved by the longitudinal CNN. Since the receptive field of the proposed longitudinal CNN is limited, it has only limited ability to differentiate between different positions in the structures to be segmented, and therefore has only limited ability to adapt its prediction depending on the position. Improvements can occur if the longitudinal CNN would be able to recognize typical errors of both types of input segmentations at different positions in the organ. Therefore, extra hidden layers or additional pathways should be added to the network. Since this increases the amount of parameters, extra training data would be required.

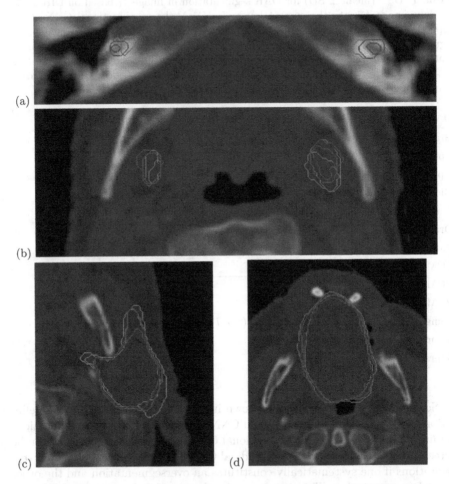

Fig. 2. Examples of OAR segmentations obtained with DIR ($S_{0,r}$, orange), the cross-sectional CNN ($S_{1,c}$, purple), and the longitudinal CNN ($S_{1,l}$, blue), compared to the manual ground truth segmentations ($S_{1,m}$, green), for: (a) cochlea; (b) submandibular glands; (c) right parotid gland; (d) oral cavity. (Color figure online)

4 Conclusion

We propose a manner to combine two different segmentation methods for OAR in H&N CT scans: longitudinal DIR and a CNN trained on cross-sectional data. Both techniques base their predictions on a different type of information: longitudinal data similarity for DIR versus learned intensity features for CNN. Combining both methods using the proposed longitudinal CCN effectively combines both sources of information. This hybrid approach was shown not only to be able to choose the best segmentation obtained with both methods, but also to improve the segmentation performance as achieved with either method separately.

References

1. Castadot, P., Lee, J., Geets, X., Gregoire, V.: Adaptive radiotherapy for head and neck cancer. Semin. Radiat. Oncol. **20**(2), 84–93 (2010)
2. Han, X., et al.: Atlas-based auto-segmentation of head and neck CT images. In: Metaxas, D., Axel, L., Fichtinger, G., Székely, G. (eds.) MICCAI 2008. LNCS, vol. 5242, pp. 434–441. Springer, Heidelberg (2008). https://doi.org/10.1007/978-3-540-85990-1_52
3. Zhang, T., Chi, Y., Meldolesi, E., Yan, D.: Automatic delineation of on-line head-and-neck computed tomography images: toward on-line adaptive radiotherapy. Int. J. Radiat. Oncol. Biol. Phys. **68**(2), 522–530 (2007)
4. Veiga, C., McClelland, J., Ricketts, K., D'Souza, D., Royle, G.: Deformable registrations for head and neck cancer adaptive radiotherapy. In: Proceedings of the First MICCAI Workshop on Image-Guidance and Multimodal Dose Planning in Radiation Therapy, pp. 66–73 (2012)
5. Castadot, P., Lee, J., Parraga, A., Geets, X., Macq, B., Gregoire, V.: Comparison of 12 deformable registration strategies in adaptive radiation therapy for the treatment of head and neck tumors. Radiother. Oncol. **89**(1), 1–12 (2008)
6. Daisne, J.F., Blumhofer, A.: Atlas-based automatic segmentation of head and neck organs at risk and nodal target volumes: a clinical validation. Radiat. Oncol. **8**, 154 (2013)
7. Ibragimov, B., Xing, L.: Segmentation of organs-at-risk in head and neck CT images using convolutional neural networks. Med. Phys. **44**(2), 547–557 (2017)
8. Birenbaum, A., Greenspan, H.: Multi-view longitudinal CNN for multiple sclerosis lesion segmentation. Eng. Appl. Artif. Intell. **65**, 111–118 (2017)
9. Vivanti, R., Ephrat, A., Joskowicz, L., Lev-Cohain, N., Karaaslan, O.A., Sosna, J.: Automatic liver tumor segmentation in follow-up CT scans: preliminary method and results. In: Wu, G., Coupé, P., Zhan, Y., Munsell, B., Rueckert, D. (eds.) Patch-MI 2015. LNCS, vol. 9467, pp. 54–61. Springer, Cham (2015). https://doi.org/10.1007/978-3-319-28194-0_7
10. La Greca Saint-Esteven, A.: Deep convolutional neural networks for automated segmentation of organs-at-risk in radiotherapy. Master's thesis, KU Leuven (2018)
11. Klein, S., Staring, M., Murphy, K., Viergever, M.A., Pluim, J.P.W.: elastix: a toolbox for intensity based medical image registration. IEEE Trans. Med. Imaging **29**(1), 196–205 (2010)
12. Kamnitsas, K., et al.: Efficient multi-scale 3D CNN with fully connected CRF for accurate brain lesion segmentation. Med. Image Anal. **36**, 61–78 (2017)

13. Robben, D., Bertels, J., Willems, S., Vandermeulen, D., Maes, F., Suetens, P.: DeepVoxNet: voxel-wise prediction for 3D images. Technical report: KUL/ESAT/PSI/1801 (2018)
14. Kingma, D.P., Ba, J.: Adam: a method for stochastic optimization. In: Proceedings of the 3rd International Conference on Learning Representations (ICLR) (2014)
15. Hu, P., Wu, F., Peng, J., Bao, Y., Chen, F., Kong, D.: Automatic abdominal multi-organ segmentation using deep convolutional neural network and time-implicit level sets. Int. J. Comput. Assist. Radiol. Surg. **12**(3), 399–411 (2017)

Unpaired Deep Cross-Modality Synthesis with Fast Training

Lei Xiang[1], Yang Li[2,3], Weili Lin[3], Qian Wang[1(✉)],
and Dinggang Shen[3(✉)]

[1] Institute for Medical Imaging Technology, School of Biomedical Engineering,
Shanghai Jiao Tong University, Shanghai, China
wang.qian@sjtu.edu.cn
[2] Department of Computer Science, University of North Carolina at Chapel Hill,
Chapel Hill, NC, USA
[3] Department of Radiology and BRIC, University of North Carolina at Chapel
Hill, Chapel Hill, NC, USA
dgshen@med.unc.edu

Abstract. Cross-modality synthesis can convert the input image of one modality to the output of another modality. It is thus very valuable for both scientific research and clinical applications. Most existing cross-modality synthesis methods require large dataset of paired data for training, while it is often non-trivial to acquire perfectly aligned images of different modalities for the same subject. Even tiny misalignment (i.e., due patient/organ motion) between the cross-modality paired images may place adverse impact to training and corrupt the synthesized images. In this paper, we present a novel method for cross-modality image synthesis by training with the unpaired data. Specifically, we adopt the generative adversarial networks and conduct the fast training in cyclic way. A new structural dissimilarity loss, which captures the detailed anatomies, is introduced to enhance the quality of the synthesized images. We validate our proposed algorithm on three popular image synthesis tasks, including brain MR-to-CT, prostate MR-to-CT, and brain 3T-to-7T. The experimental results demonstrate that our proposed method can achieve good synthesis performance by using the unpaired data only.

1 Introduction

Due to the complementary information contained in different imaging modalities (e.g., CT images, T1- and T2-weighted MR images), multi-modal images are usually captured and fused for disease diagnosis, treatment planning, etc. However, acquisition of multimodal images can be time-consuming and costly. Furthermore, the fusion often requires accurate cross-modality registration and can be degraded by the deformation of the organs.

L. Xiang and Y. Li—Contributed equally to this work.

The original version of this chapter was revised: an Acknowledgements section has been added. The correction to this chapter is available at https://doi.org/10.1007/978-3-030-00889-5_44

Cross-modality synthesis is thus valuable for both scientific research and clinical application. Although each modality presents different characteristic of the underlying anatomy, individual modalities are highly correlated when scanning the same anatomical structure and revealing the tissue appearance from different perspectives. Thus, synthesizing images of one modality based on the images of another modality is theoretically possible. However, the mapping between the two different modalities are highly nonlinear, which makes the synthesis task difficult to accomplish.

Over the past few years, various methods have been proposed for cross-modality medical image synthesis. Typical works include coupled sparse representation [1] and deep convolutional neural networks [2–4]. These methods usually require paired data for training, i.e., well-aligned source and target modalities from the same subject. However, it is not always easy to get the perfectly paired data, which thus strongly limits the application of cross-modality synthesis. Moreover, misalignment within the paired source/target data is sometimes inevitable (though tiny), and it could cause ambiguity or even devastate current synthesis methods.

Unsupervised synthesis has already been explored in [5], which only requires unpaired data for training. They used cross-modality nearest neighbor search to produce the candidate for each target voxel, then simultaneously maximized the global mutual information between candidate and source images. Local spatial consistency was enforced to generate the final target image. The performance of the method is highly dependent on the accuracy of the nearest neighbor searching.

Recently, unsupervised deep learning models have been applied for image synthesis. Cycle-GAN [6], for example, has been used to synthesize CT from MR [7]. However, it is insufficient to simply borrow the Cycle-GAN model while many properties of the medical images are ignored. We argue that the synthesis of medical images is quite different from natural images due to the 3D nature of many medical image modalities. Thus, in this work, we train the deep network in a quasi-3D way and design a 3D structural dissimilarity loss for several popular medical tasks. Particularly, inspired by the structural similarity metric (SSIM), we introduce a new structural dissimilarity loss to improve the boundary contrast of the synthesized image.

We also simplify the generator in GAN to decrease the number of the parameters, which leads to faster training yet better synthesis quality. Our generator combines the advantages of Unet [8] and deep residual net [9], and is termed as Res-Unet. Our simplified model can then be well trained within 3 h. We conduct abundant experiments to verify the promising performances of our method. Specifically, we perform brain MR-to-CT synthesis, prostate MR-to-CT synthesis and brain 3T-to-7T MR synthesis, respectively. Several examples of our datasets are shown in Fig. 1, where the differences between the paired and the unpaired data are clear. Note that in this paper we use the unpaired data only for all the experiments.

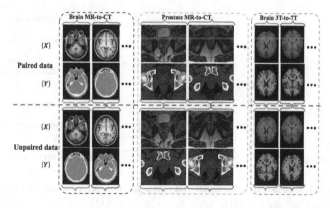

Fig. 1. Examples of the paired (top) and unpaired training data (bottom) for threes tasks: brain MR-to-CT, prostate MR-to-CT, and brain 3T-to-7T MR. In the paired data, the input images (X and Y) belong to the same subject and registered. In the unpaired data, the inputs images are clearly misaligned.

2 Method

2.1 Loss Design

We aim to accomplish the cross-modality synthesis by the Cycle-Consistent Adversarial Networks. Suppose we have two modality images X and Y. Then, the goal of our method is to learn the mapping function between these two modalities. We define the training samples as $\{x_i\}_{i=1}^{N} \in X$ and $\{y_j\}_{j=1}^{M} \in Y$. As illustrated in Fig. 2(a), there are two mapping functions, i.e., $G : X \rightarrow Y$ and $F : Y \rightarrow X$ in this cross-modality synthesis task. The two mapping functions can be modeled by deep neural networks. Besides, two adversarial discriminators D_X and D_Y are trained, such that D_X tries to distinguish real images $\{x_i\}$ and the synthesized images $\{F(y_j)\}$. Similarly, D_Y tries to distinguish $\{y_j\}$ and $\{G(x_i)\}$. In order to quantify the variation of the anatomical structures between the real images and the synthesized images, we also introduce the new structural dissimilarity loss. Therefore, the objective of the network as shown in Fig. 2 (a) mainly contains three terms: the adversarial loss ($\mathcal{L}_{GAN}$), the cycle consistency loss ($\mathcal{L}_{CYC}$) and the structural dissimilarity loss ($\mathcal{L}_{DSSIM}$):

$$\mathcal{L}(G, F, D_X, D_Y) = \mathcal{L}_{GAN}(G, D_Y, X, Y) + \mathcal{L}_{GAN}(F, D_X, Y, X) \\ + \lambda \mathcal{L}_{CYC}(G, F) + \beta \mathcal{L}_{DSSIM}(G, F), \tag{1}$$

where λ and β control the relative importance of individual loss terms. We set $\lambda = 10$ and set $\beta = 1$ in this work.

Adversarial Loss. Adversarial loss is applied to both mapping functions G and F. For the mapping function $G : X \rightarrow Y$ and its corresponding discriminator D_Y, the objective function is expressed as:

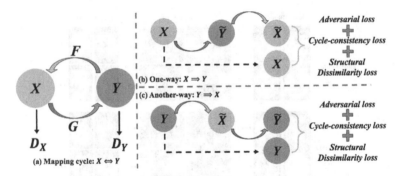

Fig. 2. The Cycle-Consistent Adversarial Networks (a) used for cross-modality synthesis are illustrated in (a). There are two cycle mappings as in (b) and (c).

$$\mathcal{L}_{GAN}(G, D_Y, X, Y) = E_{y \sim P_{data}(y)}[logD_Y(y)] + E_{x \sim P_{data}(x)}[log(1 - D_Y(x))] \quad (2)$$

G intends to generate the target modality image $G(x)$ that appears to be similar to real target image (Y), while D_Y aims to distinguish whether the input to the discriminator is the synthesized image $G(x)$ or a real image $y \in Y$. Therefore, G tries to minimize this objective function while the adversarial D tries to maximize it, i.e. $G^* = \arg \min_G \max_{D_Y} \mathcal{L}_{GAN}(G, D_Y, X, Y)$. Similar adversarial loss is also applied for the mapping function $F : Y \rightarrow X$: i.e. $F^* = \arg \min_F \max_{D_X} \mathcal{L}_{GAN}(F, D_X, Y, X)$.

Cycle Consistency Loss. To further reduce the ambiguity in solving the mapping functions, we enforce the cycle-consistency constraint, which means the difference between the input modality image and the cyclically synthesized image should be minimized. The illustration for the cycle consistency loss is shown in Fig. 2(b) and (c) for both synthesis direction, i.e., $x \rightarrow G(x) \rightarrow F(G(x))$ should be similar with x and $y \rightarrow G(y) \rightarrow F(G(y))$ should be similar with y. This cycle-consistency loss can thus be defined as:

$$\mathcal{L}_{cyc}(G, F) = E_{x \sim P_{data}(x)}[\|F(G(x)) - x\|_1] + E_{y \sim P_{data}(y)}[\|F(G(y)) - y\|_1]. \quad (3)$$

Structural Dissimilarity Loss. As the global L1 loss focuses on the entire image space, it ignores many local structural details. Structural information is usually critical in medical images as they are closely related to delineating the boundaries of tissues and organs. In order to further improve the quality of the synthesized images regarding anatomical details, we propose to take advantage of SSIM to restore the local structures in the synthesized image. This leads to the new structural dissimilarity loss (DSSIM), which is a distance metric extended from SSIM:

$$\mathcal{L}_{DSSIM}(G,F) = \mathrm{E}_{x \sim P_{data}(x)} \left[\frac{1 - SSIM(x, F(G(x)))}{2} \right]$$
$$+ \mathrm{E}_{y \sim P_{data}(y)} \left[\frac{1 - SSIM(y, F(G(y)))}{2} \right]. \tag{4}$$

2.2   Architecture of the Generator/Discriminator

There are two networks in the Cycle-Consistent Adversarial Networks, i.e., the generator and the discriminator. The generator, which is critical to the quality of the generated images, has many layers with abundant parameters, making the training process very slow. In order to design a more efficient network, we intend to take advantages from two popular architectures, i.e., Unet [8] and deep residual network [9].

Unet is widely used in many medical image analysis researches, as it has shown promising results on various tasks, including image segmentation and image synthesis. Unet consists of an encoding path and a decoding path, with skip connection in each corresponding level. This design ensures the network to have a large receptive field to capture both local and global image appearances. Salient high-level features can thus be extracted, which is essential to the cross-modality mapping trained with unpaired samples. Deep residual network, is also adopted in many research tasks, such as image classification and image super-resolution. The most important component of deep residual network is the residual block, which consists of two convolutional layers with an identity mapping, as shown in Fig. 3. The residual block is designed to alleviate the gradient vanishing issue; in the meantime, it can also boost information exchange across different layers. Inspired by the two networks, we design a deep network called Res-Unet in this work. Our network fuses advantages of Unet and the residual block, as its architecture is illustrated in Fig. 3. There are 2 pooling stages, 2 deconvolution stages and 5 residual blocks in our generator.

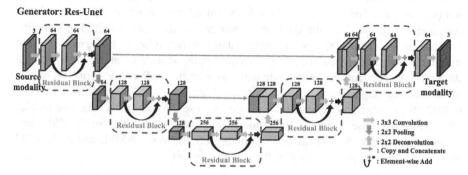

Fig. 3. Illustration of the proposed Res-Unet architecture as the generator.

3   Experimental Results

3.1   Datasets and Tasks

We utilize three real datasets to evaluate our cross-modality synthesis method. The datasets and the relative synthesis tasks are introduced below.

(1) **Brain MR-to-CT dataset.** This dataset consists of 16 subjects, each of whom comes with an MR and a CT scan. The voxel sizes of the CT and MR images are $0.59 \times 0.59 \times 0.59$ mm^3 and $1.2 \times 1.2 \times 1$ mm^3, respectively. We separate the 16 subjects into a training set containing 10 subjects and a testing set containing 6 subjects.

(2) **Prostate MR-to-CT dataset.** The prostate dataset consists of 22 subjects. The voxel sizes of the CT and MR images are $1.17 \times 1.17 \times 1$ mm^3 and $1 \times 1 \times 1$ mm^3, respectively. We also separate the 22 subjects into two parts: a training set containing 14 subjects and a testing set containing 8 subjects.

(3) **Brain 3T-to-7T dataset.** This dataset consists of 15 subjects. The voxel sizes of the 3T MR and 7T MR are $1 \times 1 \times 1$ mm^3 and $0.65 \times 0.65 \times 0.65$ mm^3, respectively. These 15 subjects are separated into a training set containing 10 subjects and a testing set containing 5 subjects.

For both brain and prostate MR-to-CT tasks, the CT images are linearly aligned (by FLIRT in FSL) to the corresponding MR images and resampled to the same size of the MR images. For brain 3T-to-7T dataset, corresponding 3T and 7T images are also linearly aligned. The nonlinear deformations between images in the same subject are left there. The intensities are normalized to $[0, 1]$ in each image.

3.2   Implementation Details

In this paper, PyTorch implementation for the basic Cycle-GAN [6] is used in all the experiments[1]. The generator is replaced by the proposed Res-Unet in our method. In the training phase, we extract consecutive 2D axial slices from the 3D image as the training samples. The training samples from two different input modalities are drawn separately, such that the samples in each pair are totally independent. The sampling process results in the ***unpaired*** training dataset, which allows no alignment of the training images in practical usage. Horizontal flipping is used to augment the training datasets. We apply Adam optimization with momentum of 0.9 and perform 100 epochs in the training stage. The batch size is set to 1 and the initial learning rate is set to 0.0002. To quantitatively evaluate the results, we use the commonly accepted metrics of peak signal-noise ratio (PSNR), normalized mean squared error (NMSE) and structural similarity (SSIM). In general, higher PSNR, lower NMSE and high SSIM indicate better perceptive quality of the synthesis result.

---

[1] https://github.com/junyanz/pytorch-CycleGAN-and-pix2pix.

3.3   Quantitative and Visual Comparisons

In this section, we compare the cross-modality synthesis results by our proposed method and the previously reported Cycle-GAN model. Comparisons are conducted on all three tasks: brain MR-to-CT, prostate MR-to-CT, and brain 3T-to-7T. First, we show the effectiveness of the proposed new generator Res-Unet. Comparisons between 'Basic Cycle-GAN' and 'Res-Unet' have been summarized in Table 1. We can see that with the new generator the synthesis results are improved on all three datasets, which demonstrates the superiority of the proposed generator. Moreover, with the new DSSIM loss added, the synthesis performance is further improved. In general, the quantitative results in Table 1 show that our proposed method ('Res-Unet + DSSIM') achieves best results on all three tasks, in terms of all evaluation metrics of PSNR, NMSE and SSIM.

Table 1. Comparisons of the synthesis results by different methods.

	Brain MR-to-CT			Prostate MR-to-CT			Brain 3T-to-7T		
	PSNR	NMSE	SSIM	PSNR	NMSE	SSIM	PSNR	NMSE	SSIM
Basic cycle-GAN	24.89	0.0569	0.896	30.27	0.0306	0.931	26.71	0.0461	0.918
Res-Unet	25.41	0.0532	0.904	30.58	0.0303	0.929	27.21	0.0436	0.922
Res-Unet + DSSIM (Proposed method)	**25.62**	**0.0525**	**0.909**	**31.23**	**0.0277**	**0.937**	**27.52**	**0.0421**	**0.926**

To give an intuitive view, visualization of the synthesized results using 'Basic Cycle-GAN' and the proposed 'Res-Unet + DSSIM' are presented in Figs. 4, 5 and 6 for prostate MR-to-CT, brain MR-to-CT, and brain 3T-to-7T, respectively. Compared to 'Basic Cycle-GAN', 'Res-Unet + DSSIM' can obtain better synthesis results with clearer tissue/organ boundaries. For example, in the coronal view of the prostate MR-to-CT task in Fig. 4, the two bones in the hip joint are successfully separated and synthesized by 'Res-Unet + DSSIM', while the boundaries of the bones appear blur in the synthesized result by 'Basic Cycle-GAN' (orange box in the figure). Also we could observe that the anatomical details pointed by the red and green boxes are clearer in 'Res-Unet + DSSIM'. Similar observations can be found on brain MR-to-CT and brain 3T-to-7T dataset in Figs. 5 and 6.

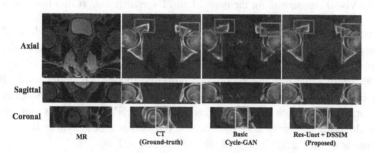

Fig. 4. Visual comparison for the prostate MR-to-CT synthesis task. (Color figure online)

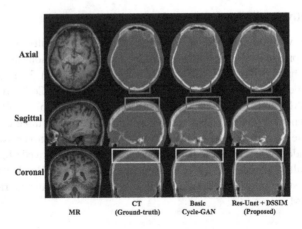

Fig. 5. Visual comparison for the brain MR-to-CT synthesis task. (Color figure online)

Meanwhile, note that our training is based on 3 consecutive axial slices, while the synthesized results are consistent on all three views. That is, our method can well handle the synthesis task of 3D medical images, even though only 3 consecutive slices are used in training. In the testing stage, we process every 3 axial slices each time, while the final output of the 3D volume can be obtained by averaging all synthesis results.

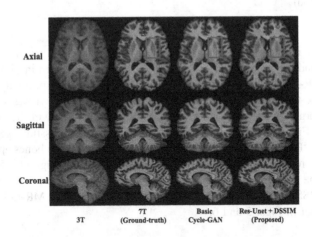

Fig. 6. Visual comparison for the brain 3T-to-7T synthesis task. (Color figure online)

We conduct another experiment on brain MR-to-CT dataset to show the fast convergence of our 'Res-Unet + DSSIM' compared to 'Basic Cycle-GAN'. We show the synthesis result by training with same epoch. The results are shown in Fig. 7. We can see that with same training epoch, our proposed model gets better result. It takes 3 h to train our model, while Basic Cycle-GAN takes 17 h. And our model contains 13.3 M parameters, which is 1/4 of 'Basic Cycle-GAN'. That means our proposed model could train fast with less parameters, but achieve best synthesis result. The testing time is 6 s for a 3D image of size $181 \times 234 \times 149$.

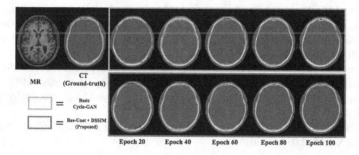

Fig. 7. Visual comparison for Basic Cycle-GAN and proposed method during training.

4   Conclusion

We proposed a novel Res-Unet architecture as the generator and solve cross-modality image synthesis by GAN. In particular, we accomplish the synthesis tasks on three different scenarios by training with the unpaired data, which indicates that our method has great potentials to many real clinical applications. This Res-Unet generator, which benefits from the novel loss design, has shown its superior performances by mapping between different images modalities with large appearance variation. In our future work, we will conduct large-scale evaluation in clinical applications, and demonstrate that the proposed image synthesis technique can be used as a new tool to reshape multimodal image fusion and subsequent analysis.

Acknowledgement. This work was supported in part by NIH grant **EB006733**.

References

1. Cao, T., Zach, C., Modla, S., Powell, D., Czymmek, K., Niethammer, M.: Multi-modal registration for correlative microscopy using image analogies. Med. Image Anal. **18**, 914–926 (2014)
2. Xiang, L., et al.: Deep embedding convolutional neural network for synthesizing CT image from T1-Weighted MR image. Med. Image Anal. **47**, 31–44 (2018)
3. Nie, D., et al.: Medical image synthesis with context-aware generative adversarial networks. In: Descoteaux, M., Maier-Hein, L., Franz, A., Jannin, P., Collins, D.L., Duchesne, S. (eds.) MICCAI 2017. LNCS, vol. 10435, pp. 417–425. Springer, Cham (2017). https://doi.org/10. 1007/978-3-319-66179-7_48
4. Xiang, L., et al.: Deep auto-context convolutional neural networks for standard-dose PET image estimation from low-dose PET/MRI. Neurocomputing **267**, 406–416 (2017)
5. Vemulapalli, R., Van Nguyen, H., Kevin Zhou, S.: Unsupervised cross-modal synthesis of subject-specific scans. In: Proceedings of the IEEE International Conference on Computer Vision, pp. 630–638 (2015)
6. Zhu, J.-Y., Park, T., Isola, P., Efros, A.A.: Unpaired image-to-image translation using cycle-consistent adversarial networks. arXiv preprint arXiv:1703.10593 (2017)

7. Wolterink, J.M., Dinkla, A.M., Savenije, M.H.F., Seevinck, P.R., van den Berg, C.A.T., Išgum, I.: Deep MR to CT synthesis using unpaired data. In: Tsaftaris, S.A., Gooya, A., Frangi, A.F., Prince, J.L. (eds.) SASHIMI 2017. LNCS, vol. 10557, pp. 14–23. Springer, Cham (2017). https://doi.org/10.1007/978-3-319-68127-6_2
8. Ronneberger, O., Fischer, P., Brox, T.: U-Net: convolutional networks for biomedical image segmentation. In: Navab, N., Hornegger, J., Wells, W.M., Frangi, A.F. (eds.) MICCAI 2015. LNCS, vol. 9351, pp. 234–241. Springer, Cham (2015). https://doi.org/10.1007/978-3-319-24574-4_28
9. He, K., Zhang, X., Ren, S., Sun, J.: Deep Residual Learning for Image Recognition. arXiv preprint arXiv:1512.03385 (2015)

UOLO - Automatic Object Detection and Segmentation in Biomedical Images

Teresa Araújo[1,2(✉)], Guilherme Aresta[1,2(✉)], Adrian Galdran[1], Pedro Costa[1], Ana Maria Mendonça[1,2], and Aurélio Campilho[1,2]

[1] INESC TEC - Institute for Systems and Computer Engineering, Technology and Science, Porto, Portugal
{tfaraujo,guilherme.m.aresta,adrian.galdran,pvcosta}@inesctec.pt
[2] Faculdade de Engenharia da Universidade do Porto, Porto, Portugal
{amendon,campilho}@fe.up.pt

Abstract. We propose UOLO, a novel framework for the simultaneous detection and segmentation of structures of interest in medical images. UOLO consists of an object segmentation module which intermediate abstract representations are processed and used as input for object detection. The resulting system is optimized simultaneously for detecting a class of objects and segmenting an optionally different class of structures. UOLO is trained on a set of bounding boxes enclosing the objects to detect, as well as pixel-wise segmentation information, when available. A new loss function is devised, taking into account whether a reference segmentation is accessible for each training image, in order to suitably backpropagate the error. We validate UOLO on the task of simultaneous optic disc (OD) detection, fovea detection, and OD segmentation from retinal images, achieving state-of-the-art performance on public datasets.

Keywords: Detection · Segmentation · Biomedical images
Eye fundus images · Convolutional neural networks

1 Introduction

Detection and segmentation of anatomical structures are central medical image analysis tasks since they allow to delimit Regions-Of-Interest (ROI), create landmarks and improve feature collection. In terms of segmentation, Deep Fully-Convolutional (FC) Neural Networks (NNs) achieve the highest performance on a variety of images and problems. Namely, U-Net [1] has become a reference model – its autoencoder structure with skip connections enables the propagation from the encoding to the decoding part of the network, allowing a more robust multi-scale analysis while reducing the need for training data.

Similarly, Deep Neural Networks (DNNs) have become the technique of choice in many medical imaging detection problems. The standard approach is to use

---

T. Araújo and G. Aresta—Authors contributed equally to this work.

© Springer Nature Switzerland AG 2018
D. Stoyanov et al. (Eds.): DLMIA 2018/ML-CDS 2018, LNCS 11045, pp. 165–173, 2018.
https://doi.org/10.1007/978-3-030-00889-5_19

networks pre-trained on large datasets of natural images as feature extractors of a detection module. For instance, Faster-R CNN [2] uses these features to identify ROIs via a specialized layer. ROIs are then pooled, rescaled and supplied to a pair of Fully-Connected NNs responsible for adjusting the size and label the bounding boxes. Alternatively, YOLOv2 [3] avoids the use of an auxiliary ROI proposal model by directly using region-wise activations from pre-trained weights to predict coordinates and labels of ROIs.

When a ROI has been identified, the segmentation of an object contained on it becomes much easier. For this reason, the combination of detection and segmentation models into a single method is being explored. For instance, Mask-R CNN [4] extends Faster-R CNN with the addition of FC layers after its final pooling, enabling a fine segmentation without a significant computational overhead. In this architecture, the segmentation and detection modules are decoupled, *i.e.* the segmentation part is only responsible for predicting a mask, which is then labeled class-wise by the detection module. However, despite the high performance achieved by Mask-R CNN in computer vision, its application to medical image analysis problems remains limited. This is due to the large requirement of data annotated at a pixel level, which is usually not available in medical applications.

In this paper we propose UOLO (Fig. 1), a novel architecture that performs simultaneous detection and segmentation of structures of interest in biomedical images. UOLO harvests the best of its individual detection and segmentation modules to allow robust and efficient predictions even when few training data is available. Moreover, training UOLO is simple since the entire network can be updated during back-propagation. We experimentally validate UOLO on eye fundus images for the joint task of fovea (FV) detection, optic disc (OD) detection, and OD segmentation, where we achieve state-of-the-art performance.

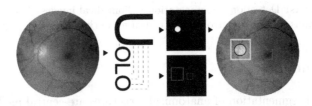

Fig. 1. Using UOLO for fovea detection and optic disc detection and segmentation.

2   UOLO Framework

2.1   Object Segmentation Module

For object segmentation we consider an adapted version of the U-Net network presented in [1]. U-Net is composed of FC layers organized on an auto-encoder scheme, which allows to obtain an output of the same size of the input, thus enabling pixel-wise predictions. Skip connections between the encoding and decoding parts are used for avoiding the information loss inherent to encoding. The model's upsampling path includes a large number of feature channels with the aim of propagating the multi-scale context information to higher resolution layers. Ultimately, the segmentation prediction results from the analysis of abstract representations of the images from multiple scales, with the majority of the relevant classification information being available on the decoder portion of the network due to the skip connections. We modify the network by adding batch normalization after each convolutional layer, and replacing the pooling layers by convolutions with stride. The soft intersection over union (IoU) is used as loss:

$$\mathcal{L}_{\text{U-Net}} = 1 - \text{IoU} = 1 - \frac{\sum I_t \circ I_p}{\sum (I_t + I_p) - \sum I_t \circ I_p}, \tag{1}$$

where I_t and I_p are the ground truth mask and the soft prediction mask, respectively, and $\circ$ is the Hadamard product.

2.2   Object Detection Module

For object detection we take inspiration from YOLOv2 [3], a network composed of: (1) a DNN that extracts features from an image (F_{YOLO}); (2) a feature interpretation block that predicts both labels and bounding boxes for the objects of interest (D_{YOLO}). YOLOv2 assumes that every image's patch can contain an object of size similar to one of various template bounding boxes (or *anchors*) computed *a priori* from the objects' shape distribution in the training data.

Let the output of F_{YOLO} be a tensor F of shape $S \times S \times N$, where S is the dimension of the spatial grid and N is the number of maps. F_{YOLO} convolves and reshapes F into Y, a tensor of shape $S \times S \times A \times (C + 5)$, where A is the number of anchors, C is the number of object classes, and 5 is the number of variables to be optimized: center coordinates x and y, width w, height h, and the confidence c (how likely is the bounding box to be an object) of the bounding boxes. For each anchor A_k in Y, the value of each feature map element $m_{i,j}$ is responsible for adjusting a property of the predicted bounding box $\hat{b}$,

$$(\hat{b}_x, \hat{b}_y) = (\sigma(\hat{x}) + x_{i,j,k}, \sigma(\hat{y}) + y_{i,j,k})$$
$$(\hat{b}_w, \hat{b}_h) = (w_{i,j,k}e^{\hat{w}}, h_{i,j,k}e^{\hat{h}}) \tag{2}$$
$$\text{confidence} = \sigma(\hat{c})$$

where σ is a sigmoid function. YOLOv2 is trained by optimizing the loss function:

$$\mathcal{L}_{\text{YOLO}} = \lambda_1 \mathcal{L}_{\text{centers}} + \lambda_2 \mathcal{L}_{\text{dimensions}} + \lambda_3 \mathcal{L}_{\text{confidence}} + \lambda_4 \mathcal{L}_{\text{classes}} \tag{3}$$

where λ_i are predefined weighting factors, $\mathcal{L}_{\text{centers}}$, $\mathcal{L}_{\text{dimensions}}$ and $\mathcal{L}_{\text{confidence}}$ are mean squared errors, and $\mathcal{L}_{\text{classes}}$ is the cross-entropy loss. Each loss term penalizes a different error: (1) $\mathcal{L}_{\text{centers}}$ penalizes the error in the center position of the cells; (2) $\mathcal{L}_{\text{dimensions}}$ penalizes the incorrect size, *i.e.* height and width, of the bounding box; (3) $\mathcal{L}_{\text{confidence}}$ penalizes the incorrect prediction of a box presence; (4) $\mathcal{L}_{\text{classes}}$ penalizes the misclassification of the objects.

2.3   UOLO for Joint Object Detection and Segmentation

UOLO framework for object detection and segmentation is depicted in Fig. 2, where the segmentation module itself is used as a feature extraction module, adopting the role of F_{YOLO}, and serving as input for the localization module D_{YOLO}. The intuition behind this design is that the abstract representation learned by the decoding part of U-Net contains multi-scale information that can be useful not only to segment objects, but also to detect them. In addition, the class of objects that UOLO can detect is not limited to those for which segmentation ground-truth is available.

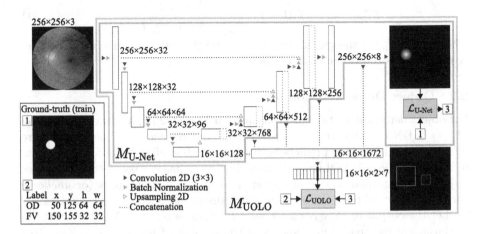

Fig. 2. UOLO framework, nesting an U-Net responsible for segmentation and feature extraction for an YOLOv2-based detector. $M_{U\text{-}Net}$: U-net part; M_{UOLO}: full UOLO.

Let $M_{U\text{-}Net}$ be an U-Net-like network that, given pairs of images and binary masks, can be trained for performing segmentation by minimizing $\mathcal{L}_{U\text{-}Net}$ (Eq. 1). $M_{U\text{-}Net}$ has a second output corresponding to the concatenation of the down-sampled decoding maps with its bottle neck (last encoder layer). The resulting tensor corresponds to a set of multi-scale representations of the original image that are supplied to the object detection block D_{YOLO}, which, by its turn, can be optimized via $\mathcal{L}_{YOLO}$, defined in Eq. 3. D_{YOLO} and $M_{U\text{-}Net}$ are then merged by concatenation into M_{UOLO}, a single model that can be optimized by minimizing the addition of the corresponding loss functions:

$$\mathcal{L}_{UOLO} = \mathcal{L}_{YOLO} + \mathcal{L}_{U\text{-}Net} \tag{4}$$

Thanks to the straightforward definition of the loss function in Eq. (4), M_{UOLO} can be trained with a simple iterative scheme detailed in Algorithm 1. In essence, $\mathcal{L}_{U\text{-}Net}$ is updated only when segmentation information is available. However, a global weight update is performed at every step based on the prediction error backpropagation. Furthermore, the outlined training scheme allows

Algorithm 1. Loss computation scheme of UOLO. $M_{\text{U-Net}}$: U-net part from the UOLO model; M_{UOLO}: full UOLO model; b_{det}: batches of images with objects' bounding boxes ground truth; b_{seg}: batches of images with segmentation ground truth.

$\mathcal{L}_{\text{U-Net}} \leftarrow 1$
for each training step **do**
　$M_{\text{UOLO}} \leftarrow \textbf{train}(M_{\text{UOLO}}, b_{\text{det}}, \mathcal{L}_{\text{UOLO}})$ {train on n_{det} batches from b_{det}, back-propagating $\mathcal{L}_{\text{UOLO}}$};
　$\textbf{update}(\mathcal{L}_{\text{YOLO}})$

　$M_{\text{U-Net}} \leftarrow \textbf{train}(M_{\text{U-Net}}, b_{\text{seg}}, \mathcal{L}_{\text{U-Net}})$ {train on n_{seg} batches from b_{seg}, backpropagating $\mathcal{L}_{\text{U-Net}}$}
　$\textbf{update}(\mathcal{L}_{\text{U-Net}})$
　$\mathcal{L}_{\text{UOLO}} \leftarrow \mathcal{L}_{\text{YOLO}} + \mathcal{L}_{\text{U-Net}}$

for a different number of strong (pixel-wise) and weak (bounding boxes) annotations, easing its application to medical images.

3 Experiments and Results

3.1 Datasets and Experimental Details

We test UOLO on 3 public eye fundus datasets with healthy and pathological images: (1) Messidor [5] has 1200 images (1440×960, 2240×1488 and 2304×1536 pixels, $45°$ field-of-view (FOV)), 1136 having ground truth (GT) for OD segmentation and FV centers[1]; (2) IDRID[2] training set has 413 images (4288×2848 pixels, $50°$ FOV) with OD and FV centers and 54 with OD segmentation; (3) DRIVE [6] has 40 images (768×584 pixels, $45°$ FOV) with OD segmentation[3].

All images are cropped around the FOV (determined via Otsu's thresholding) and resized to 256×256 pixels. The side of the square GT bounding boxes is set to 32 and 64 for the FV and OD following their relative size in the image. For training, n_{det} and n_{seg} (Algorithm 1) are set to 256 and 32, respectively. Online data augmentation, a mini-batch size of 8, and the Adam optimizer (learning rate of 1e–4) were used for training, while 25% of the data was kept for validation. The bounding box with highest confidence for each class is kept. The predicted soft segmentations are binarized using a threshold of 0.5.

The OD segmentation is evaluated with IoU and Sorensen-Dice coefficient overlap metrics. The detection is evaluated in terms of mean euclidean distance (ED) between the prediction and the GT. We also evaluate ED relatively to the OD radius, $\bar{D}$ [7,8]. Finally, detection success, S_{1R}, is assessed using the maximum distance criteria of 1 OD radius.

---

[1] http://www.uhu.es/retinopathy.

[2] https://idrid.grand-challenge.org/, available since January 20, 2018.

[3] https://sites.google.com/a/uw.edu/src/useful-links.

3.2   Results and Discussion

We evaluate UOLO both inter and intra-dataset-wise. For inter-dataset experiments, UOLO was trained on Messidor and tested in the other datasets whereas for intra-dataset studies stratified 5-fold cross-validation was used. We do not extensively optimize the training parameters to verify how robust UOLO is when dealing with segmentation and detection simultaneously. Table 1 shows the results of UOLO for the OD detection and segmentation and FV detection tasks, Table 2 compares our performance with state-of-the-art methods and Fig. 3 shows two prediction examples in complex detection and segmentation cases.

UOLO achieves equal or better performance in comparison to the state-of-the-art on both detection and segmentation tasks (IoU 0.88 ± 0.09 on Messidor) in a single step prediction. Furthermore, the proposed network is robust even in inter-dataset scenarios, maintaining both segmentation and detection performances. This indicates that the abstract representations learned by UOLO are

Table 1. UOLO performance on optic disc (OD) detection and segmentation and fovea (FV) detection. n: number of training images for detection and segmentation.

Datasets		n		OD seg.		OD det.		FV det.	
Train	Test	seg.	det.	IoU	Dice	$\bar{D}$	S_{1R}	$\bar{D}$	S_{1R}
Messidor		680	680	0.88	0.93	0.111	99.74	0.121	99.38
Messidor		100	680	0.87	0.93	0.114	99.74	0.114	97.89
IDRID		30	280	0.88	0.93	0.095	99.79	0.288	93.78
Messidor	IDRID	852	852	0.84	0.91	0.138	99.78	0.403	89.06
Messidor	DRIVE	852	852	0.82	0.89	0.171	97.50	-	-

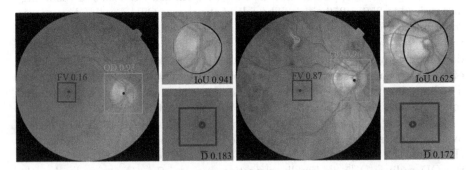

Fig. 3. Examples of results of UOLO on Messidor images. Green curve: segmented optic disc (OD), green and blue boxes: predicted OD and FV locations, respectively; black curve: ground truth OD segmentation; black and blue dots: ground truth OD and FV locations, respectively. The object detection confidence is shown next to each box. IoU (intersection over union) and normalized distance ($\bar{D}$) values are also shown. (Color figure online)

highly effective for solving the task at hands. It is worth noting that our segmentation and detection performances do not alter significantly even when UOLO is trained with only 15% of the pixel-wise annotated images. This means that UOLO does not require a significant amount of pixel-wise annotations, easing its application on the medical field, where these are expensive to obtain.

Our results also suggest that UOLO is capable of using multi-scale information (*eg.* relative position to the OD or vessel tree) to perform predictions. For instance, Fig. 3 shows UOLO's output for two Messidor images, illustrating that the network is capable of detecting the FV in a low contrast scenario. On the other hand, the segmentation and detection processes are not completely interdependent, as expected from the proposed training scheme, since the network segments OD confounders outside the detected OD region. Another advantage of UOLO is that these segmentation errors are easily correctable by limiting the pixel-wise predictions to the found OD region. Unlike hand-crafted feature-based methods, UOLO does not require an extensive parameter tunning and it is simple to extend to different applications.

We also evaluate U-Net ($\mathcal{M}_{\text{U-Net}}$, Fig. 2) for OD segmentation and YOLOv2 (with a pretrained Inceptionv3 as feature extractor) for OD and FV detection (Table 2). The training conditions were set as in UOLO. UOLO segmentation performance is practically the same as U-Net, whereas the detection drops slightly when comparing with YOLOv2, mainly for OD detection. However, one has to consider the trade-off between computational burden and performance, since UOLO network has 23 347 063 parameters, whereas U-Net has 15 063 985 and YOLOv2 has 21 831 470, being that for training U-Net and YOLO a total of 36 895 455 parameters have to be optimized (60% increase).

Table 2. State-of-the-art for OD detection and segmentation and FV detection.

(a) OD segmentation

Dataset	Messidor		DRIVE	
Method	IoU	Dice	IoU	Dice
UOLO	0.88	0.93	0.82	0.89
U-Net	0.88	0.93	0.81	0.88
[9]	0.91	-	-	-
[10]	0.89	0.94	-	-
[11]	0.84	-	0.81	-
[12]	0.82	-	0.72	-
[13]	-	-	0.82	-

(b) OD and FV detection

Task	OD det.				FV detection	
Dataset	Messidor		DRIVE		Messidor	
Method	ED	S_{1R}	ED	S_{1R}	ED	S_{1R}
UOLO	9.40	99.74	8.13	97.5	10.44	99.38
YOLOv2	6.86	100	7.20	97.5	9.01	100
[14]	-	97	-	-	-	96.6
[8]	-	-	-	-	16.09	98.24
[7]	-	-	-	-	20.17	98.24
[15]	-	98.83	-	-	-	-
[16]	23.17	99.75	15.57	100	34.88	99.40
[10]		99.75	-	-	-	-

4   Conclusions

We presented UOLO, a novel network that performs joint detection and segmentation of objects of interest in medical images by using the abstract representations learned by U-Net. Furthermore, UOLO can detect objects from a different class for which segmentation ground-truth is available.

We tested UOLO for simultaneous fovea detection and optic disk detection and segmentation, achieving state-of-the-art results. This network can be trained with relatively few images with segmentation ground-truth and still maintain a high performance. UOLO is also robust to inter-dataset settings, thus showing great potential for applications in the medical image analysis field.

Acknowledgements. T. Araújo is funded by the FCT grant SFRH/BD/122365/2016. G. Aresta is funded by the FCT grant SFRH/BD/120435/2016. This work is funded by the ERDF European Regional Development Fund, Operational Programme for Competitiveness and Internationalisation - COMPETE 2020, and by National Funds through the FCT - project CMUP-ERI/TIC/0028/2014.

References

1. Ronneberger, O., Fischer, P., Brox, T.: U-Net: convolutional networks for biomedical image segmentation. In: Navab, N., Hornegger, J., Wells, W.M., Frangi, A.F. (eds.) MICCAI 2015. LNCS, vol. 9351, pp. 234–241. Springer, Cham (2015). https://doi.org/10.1007/978-3-319-24574-4_28
2. Ren, S., He, K., Girshick, R., Sun, J.: Faster R-CNN: towards real-time object detection with region proposal networks. IEEE Trans. Patt. Anal. Mach. Intell. **39**(6), 1137–1149 (2017)
3. Redmon, J., Farhadi, A.: YOLO9000: Better, Faster, Stronger. arXiv (2016)
4. He, K., Gkioxari, G., Dollár, P., Girshick, R.: Mask R-CNN. arXiv (2017)
5. Decenciere, E., Zhang, X., Cazuguel, G.: Feedback on a publicly distributed image database: the Messidor database. Image Anal. Stereol. **33**(3), 231–234 (2014)
6. Staal, J., Niemeijer, M., Viergever, M.A., Ginneken, B.V.: Ridge-based vessel segmentation in color images of the retina. IEEE Trans. Med. Imaging **23**(4), 501–509 (2004)
7. Gegundez-Arias, M.E., Marin, D., Bravo, J.M., Suero, A.: Locating the fovea center position in digital fundus images using thresholding and feature extraction techniques. Comput. Med. Imaging Graph. **37**(5–6), 386–393 (2013)
8. Aquino, A.: Establishing the macular grading grid by means of fovea centre detection using anatomical-based and visual-based features. Comput. Biol. Med. **55**, 61–73 (2014)
9. Dai, B., Wu, X., Bu, W.: Optic disc segmentation based on variational model with multiple energies. Patt. Recogn. **64**, 226–235 (2017)
10. Dashtbozorg, B., Mendonça, A., Campilho, A.: Optic disc segmentation using the sliding band filter. Comput. Biol. Med. **56**, 1–12 (2015)
11. Roychowdhury, S., Koozekanani, D.D., Kuchinka, S.N., Parhi, K.K.: Optic disc boundary and vessel origin segmentation of fundus images. IEEE J. Biomed. Health Inform. **20**(6), 1562–1574 (2016)

12. Morales, S., Naranjo, V., Angulo, U., Alcaniz, M.: Automatic detection of optic disc based on PCA and mathematical morphology. IEEE Trans. Med. Imaging **32**(4), 786–796 (2013)
13. Salazar-Gonzalez, A., Kaba, D., Li, Y., Liu, X.: Segmentation of blood vessels and optic disc in retinal images. IEEE J. Biomed. Health Inform. **18**(6), 1874–1886 (2014)
14. Al-Bander, B., Al-Nuaimy, W., Williams, B.M., Zheng, Y.: Multiscale sequential convolutional neural networks for simultaneous detection of fovea and optic disc. Biomed. Sig. Process. Control **40**, 91–101 (2018)
15. Aquino, A., Gegúndez-arias, M.E., Marín, D.: Detecting the optic disc boundary in digital fundus feature extraction techniques. IEEE Trans. Med. Imaging **29**(11), 1860–1869 (2010)
16. Kamble, R., Kokare, M., Deshmukh, G., Hussin, F.A., Mériaudeau, F.: Localization of optic disc and fovea in retinal images using intensity based line scanning analysis. Comput. Biol. Med. **87**, 382–396 (2017)

Unpaired Brain MR-to-CT Synthesis Using a Structure-Constrained CycleGAN

Heran Yang[1,2(✉)], Jian Sun[1], Aaron Carass[2], Can Zhao[2], Junghoon Lee[3], Zongben Xu[1], and Jerry Prince[2]

[1] School of Mathematics and Statistics, Xi'an Jiaotong University, Xi'an, China
yhr.7017@stu.xjtu.edu.cn
[2] Department of Electrical and Computer Engineering, Johns Hopkins University, Baltimore, USA
[3] Department of Radiation Oncology and Molecular Radiation Sciences, Johns Hopkins University, Baltimore, USA

Abstract. The cycleGAN is becoming an influential method in medical image synthesis. However, due to a lack of direct constraints between input and synthetic images, the cycleGAN cannot guarantee structural consistency between these two images, and such consistency is of extreme importance in medical imaging. To overcome this, we propose a structure-constrained cycleGAN for brain MR-to-CT synthesis using unpaired data that defines an extra structure-consistency loss based on the modality independent neighborhood descriptor to constrain structural consistency. Additionally, we use a position-based selection strategy for selecting training images instead of a completely random selection scheme. Experimental results on synthesizing CT images from brain MR images demonstrate that our method is better than the conventional cycleGAN and approximates the cycleGAN trained with paired data.

Keywords: MR-to-CT synthesis · CycleGAN · Deep learning · MIND

1 Introduction

Magnetic resonance (MR) imaging has been widely utilized to diagnose patients, as it is non-ionizing, non-invasive, and has a range of contrast mechanisms. However, MR images do not directly provide electron density information, which is essential for some applications such as MR-based radiotherapy treatment planning or attenuation correction in hybrid PET/MR scanners. A straightforward solution is to separately scan a computed tomography (CT) image, but this is time-consuming, costly, potentially harmful to patients, and requires accurate MR/CT registrations. Therefore, to avoid the CT scan, a variety of approaches have been proposed to synthesize CT images from available MR images [1,4–7]. For example, by using paired MR and CT atlases, atlas-based methods [4] first register multiple atlas MR images to a subject MR image, and then the warped

© Springer Nature Switzerland AG 2018
D. Stoyanov et al. (Eds.): DLMIA 2018/ML-CDS 2018, LNCS 11045, pp. 174–182, 2018.
https://doi.org/10.1007/978-3-030-00889-5_20

atlas CT images are combined to synthesize a subject CT image. Deep learning-based methods [5] have designed different convolutional neural network (CNN) structures to directly learn the MR-to-CT mapping.

Although these methods can produce good synthetic images, they rely on a large number of paired CT and MR images, which are hard to obtain in practice, especially for specific MR tissue contrasts. To relax the requirement of paired data, Wolterink et al. [6] and Chartsias et al. [1] used a cycleGAN [8] for MR-to-CT synthesis on unpaired data with promising results. They used a CNN to learn the MR-to-CT mapping with the help of an adversarial loss, which forces synthetic CT images to be indistinguishable from real CT images. To ensure the synthetic CT image correctly corresponds to an input MR image, another CNN is utilized to map synthetic CT back to the MR domain and the reconstructed image should be identical to the input MR image (i.e., cycle-consistency loss).

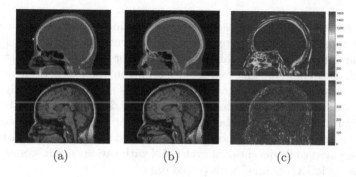

(a)   (b)   (c)

Fig. 1. Visual example of a cycleGAN result. We show (a) ground-truth CT image and input MR image, (b) synthetic CT image and reconstructed MR image, and (c) the relative errors between the ground-truth/synthetic CT images (upper) and the input/reconstructed MR images (lower).

However, due to a lack of direct constraints between the synthetic and input images, the cycleGAN cannot guarantee structural consistency between these two images. As shown in Fig. 1, the reconstructed MR image is almost identical to the input MR image, indicating the cycle consistency is well kept, but the synthetic CT image is quite different from the ground-truth, especially for the skull region, which illustrates that the structure of the synthetic CT image is not consistent with that of the input MR image. To overcome this, Zhang et al. [7] trained two auxiliary CNNs respectively for segmenting MR and CT images and also defined a loss to force the segmentation of the synthetic image to be the same as the ground-truth segmentation of the input image. This requires a training dataset with ground-truth segmentations of MR and CT images, which further complicates the training data requirements.

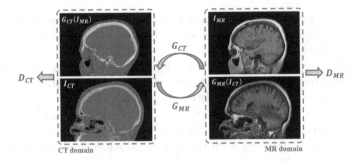

Fig. 2. Illustration of our proposed structure-constrained cycleGAN. Two generators (i.e., G_{CT} and G_{MR}) learn cross-domain mappings between CT and MR domains. The training of these mappings is supervised by adversarial, cycle-consistency, and structure-consistency losses.

In this work, we propose a structure-constrained cycleGAN to constrain structural consistency without requiring ground-truth segmentations. By using the modality independent neighborhood descriptor [3], we define a structure-consistency loss enforcing the extracted features in the synthetic image to be voxel-wise close to the ones extracted in the input image. Additionally, we use a position-based selection strategy for selecting training images instead of a completely random selection scheme. Experimental results on synthesizing CT images from brain MR images show that our method achieves significantly better results compared to a conventional cycleGAN with various metrics, and approximates the cycleGAN trained with paired data.

2   Method

In this section, we introduce our proposed structure-constrained cycleGAN. As shown in Fig. 2, our method contains two generators G_{CT} and G_{MR}, which provide the MR-to-CT and CT-to-MR mappings, respectively. In addition, discriminator D_{CT} is used to distinguish between real and synthetic CT images, and discriminator D_{MR} is for MR images. Our training loss includes three types of terms: an adversarial loss [2] for matching the distribution of synthetic images to target CT or MR domain; a cycle-consistency loss [8] to prevent generators from producing synthetic images that are irrelevant to the inputs; and a structure-consistency loss to constrain structural consistency between input and synthetic images.

2.1   Adversarial Loss

The adversarial loss [2] is applied to both generators. For the generator G_{CT} and its discriminator D_{CT}, the adversarial loss is defined as

$$\mathcal{L}_{GAN}(G_{CT}, D_{CT}) = D_{CT}(G_{CT}(I_{MR}))^2 + (1 - D_{CT}(I_{CT}))^2 , \quad (1)$$

where I_{CT} and I_{MR} denote the unpaired input CT and MR images. During the training phase, G_{CT} tries to generate a synthetic CT image $G_{\mathrm{CT}}(I_{\mathrm{MR}})$ close to a real CT image, i.e., $\max_{G_{\mathrm{CT}}} \mathcal{L}_{\mathrm{GAN}}(G_{\mathrm{CT}}, D_{\mathrm{CT}})$, while D_{CT} is to distinguish between a synthetic CT image $G_{\mathrm{CT}}(I_{\mathrm{MR}})$ and a real image I_{CT}, i.e., $\min_{D_{\mathrm{CT}}} \mathcal{L}_{\mathrm{GAN}}(G_{\mathrm{CT}}, D_{\mathrm{CT}})$. Similarly, the adversarial loss for G_{MR} and D_{MR} is defined as

$$\mathcal{L}_{\mathrm{GAN}}(G_{\mathrm{MR}}, D_{\mathrm{MR}}) = D_{\mathrm{MR}}(G_{\mathrm{MR}}(I_{\mathrm{CT}}))^2 + (1 - D_{\mathrm{MR}}(I_{\mathrm{MR}}))^2 \; . \tag{2}$$

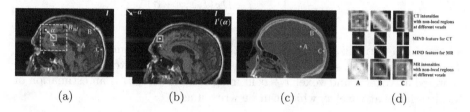

(a)   (b)   (c)   (d)

Fig. 3. Illustration of the MIND feature. (a) To extract the MIND feature at x, a patch around $x + \alpha$ is compared with a patch around x for each $x + \alpha \in R_{nl}$; (b) comparison between x and $x + \alpha$ of I in (a) equals a comparison of I and $I'(\alpha)$ at x; (c) the CT image paired with MR image in (a); (d) visual examples of MIND features extracted at voxels A, B, C within paired MR and CT images in (a) and (c).

2.2 Cycle-Consistency Loss

To prevent the generators from producing synthetic images that are irrelevant to the inputs, a cycle-consistency loss [8] is utilized for G_{CT} and G_{MR} forcing the reconstructed images $G_{\mathrm{CT}}(G_{\mathrm{MR}}(I_{\mathrm{CT}}))$ and $G_{\mathrm{MR}}(G_{\mathrm{CT}}(I_{\mathrm{MR}}))$ to be identical to their inputs I_{CT} and I_{MR}. This loss is written as

$$\mathcal{L}_{cycle}(G_{\mathrm{CT}}, G_{\mathrm{MR}}) = \|G_{\mathrm{CT}}(G_{\mathrm{MR}}(I_{\mathrm{CT}})) - I_{\mathrm{CT}}\|_1 \\ + \|G_{\mathrm{MR}}(G_{\mathrm{CT}}(I_{\mathrm{MR}})) - I_{\mathrm{MR}}\|_1 \; . \tag{3}$$

2.3 Structure-Consistency Loss

Since the cycle-consistency loss does not necessarily ensure structural consistency (as discussed in Sect. 1), our method uses an extra structure-consistency loss between the synthetic and input images. However, as these two images are respectively in MR and CT domains, we first map these images into a common feature domain by using a modal-independent structural feature, and then the structural consistency between the synthetic and input images is measured in this feature domain. In this work, we use the modality independent neighborhood descriptor (MIND) [3] as the structural feature. MIND is defined using a non-local patch-based self-similarity and depends on image local structure instead of intensity values. It has been previously applied to MR/CT image registration as a similarity metric. Figure 3(d) shows visual examples of MIND features extracted at different voxels in MR and CT images. In the following paragraphs, we introduce the MIND feature and our structure-consistency loss in detail.

The MIND feature extracts distinctive image structure by comparing each patch with all its neighbors in a non-local region. As shown in Fig. 3(a), for voxel x in image I, the MIND feature F_x is an $|R_{nl}|$-length vector, where R_{nl} denotes a non-local region around voxel x, and each component $F_x^{(\alpha)}$ for a voxel $x + \alpha \in R_{nl}$ is defined as

$$F_x^{(\alpha)}(I) = \frac{1}{Z} \exp \left(-\frac{D_{\mathcal{P}}(I, x, x + \alpha)}{V(I, x)} \right) , \tag{4}$$

where Z is a normalization constant so that the maximal component of F_x is 1. $D_{\mathcal{P}}(I, x, x+\alpha)$ denotes the L_2 distance between two image patches $\mathcal{P}$ respectively centered at voxel x and voxel $x + \alpha$ in image I, and $V(I, x)$ is an estimation of local variance at voxel x, which can be written as

$$D_{\mathcal{P}}(I, x, x + \alpha) = \sum_{p \in \mathcal{P}} (I(x + p) - I(x + \alpha + p))^2 , \tag{5}$$

$$V(I, x) = \frac{1}{4} \sum_{n \in \mathcal{N}} D_{\mathcal{P}}(I, x, x + n) , \tag{6}$$

where $\mathcal{N}$ is the 4-neighborhood of voxel x.

It is difficult to directly compute the operation $D_{\mathcal{P}}$ and its gradient using Eq. 5 in a deep network. Instead, as shown in Fig. 3(b), $D_{\mathcal{P}}$ can be equivalently computed by using a convolutional operation as

$$D_{\mathcal{P}}(I, x, x + \alpha) = C * (I - I'(\alpha))^2 , \tag{7}$$

where C is an all-one kernel of the same size as patch $\mathcal{P}$, and $I'(\alpha)$ denotes I translated by α. By doing this, the structural feature can be extracted via several simple operations and the gradients of these operations can be easily computed.

Based on the MIND feature introduced above, the structure-consistency loss in our method is defined to enforce the extracted MIND features in the synthetic images $G_{CT}(I_{MR})$ or $G_{MR}(I_{CT})$ to be voxel-wise close to the ones extracted in their inputs I_{MR} or I_{CT}, which can be written as

$$\mathcal{L}_{\text{structure}}(G_{CT}, G_{MR}) = \frac{1}{N_{MR}|R_{nl}|} \sum_x \|F_x(G_{CT}(I_{MR})) - F_x(I_{MR})\|_1$$
$$+ \frac{1}{N_{CT}|R_{nl}|} \sum_x \|F_x(G_{MR}(I_{CT})) - F_x(I_{CT})\|_1 , \tag{8}$$

where N_{MR} and N_{CT} respectively denote the number of voxels in input images I_{MR} and I_{CT}, and $\| \cdot \|_1$ is the L_1 norm. In this work, we use a 9×9 non-local region and a 7×7 patch for computing structure-consistency loss. Furthermore, instead of an all-one kernel C, we utilize a Gaussian kernel C_σ with standard deviation $\sigma = 2$ to reweight the importance of voxels within patch $\mathcal{P}$ in Eq. 7. In preliminary experiments, we tried different non-local regions, patch sizes, and σ values, but did not observe improved performance.

2.4   Training Loss

Given the definitions of adversarial, cycle-consistency, and structure-consistency losses above, the training loss of our proposed method is defined as:

$$\mathcal{L}(G_{\mathrm{CT}}, G_{\mathrm{MR}}, D_{\mathrm{CT}}, D_{\mathrm{MR}}) = \mathcal{L}_{\mathrm{GAN}}(G_{\mathrm{CT}}, D_{\mathrm{CT}}) + \mathcal{L}_{\mathrm{GAN}}(G_{\mathrm{MR}}, D_{\mathrm{MR}})$$
$$+ \lambda_1 \mathcal{L}_{cycle}(G_{\mathrm{CT}}, G_{\mathrm{MR}}) + \lambda_2 \mathcal{L}_{structure}(G_{\mathrm{CT}}, G_{\mathrm{MR}}) , \quad (9)$$

where λ_1 and λ_2 control the relative importance of the loss terms. During training, λ_1 is set to 10 as per [6,8] and λ_2 is set to 5. To optimize $\mathcal{L}$, we alternatively update $D_{\mathrm{MR/CT}}$ (with $G_{\mathrm{MR/CT}}$ fixed) and $G_{\mathrm{MR/CT}}$ (with $D_{\mathrm{MR/CT}}$ fixed).

2.5   Network Structure

Our method is composed of four trainable neural networks, i.e., two generators, G_{CT} and G_{MR}, and two discriminators, D_{CT} and D_{MR}, and we use the same network structures as [6,8] in this work. That is, two generators, G_{CT} and G_{MR}, are 2D fully convolutional networks (FCNs) with two stride-2 convolutional layers, nine residual blocks, and two fractionally-strided convolutional layers with stride $\frac{1}{2}$. The two discriminators, D_{CT} and D_{MR}, are 2D FCNs consisting of five convolutional layers to classify whether 70×70 overlapping image patches are real or synthetic. For further details, please refer to [8].

2.6   Position-Based Selection Strategy

Although our input MR and CT slices are unpaired, we can get the positions of their slices within the volumes. Slices in the middle of the volume necessarily have more brain tissue than peripheral slices. Thus, instead of feeding in slices at extremely different positions of the brain, e.g., a peripheral CT slice and a medial MR slice, we input training slices at similar positions; this is referred to as a position-based selection (PBS) strategy. That is, the MR and CT slices are linearly aligned considering their respective numbers of slices within the volumes, and given the i-th MR slice in its volume, the index $T(i)$ of corresponding CT slice selected by our method is determined by

$$T(i) = \begin{cases} \left[i \cdot \frac{K_{\mathrm{CT}}-1}{K_{\mathrm{MR}}-1} \right] + m , & \text{if } 5 \leq \left[i \cdot \frac{K_{\mathrm{CT}}-1}{K_{\mathrm{MR}}-1} \right] < K_{\mathrm{CT}} - 5, \\ \left[i \cdot \frac{K_{\mathrm{CT}}-1}{K_{\mathrm{MR}}-1} \right] , & \text{otherwise,} \end{cases} \quad (10)$$

where K_{MR} and K_{CT} respectively denote the number of slices in unpaired MR and CT volumes. $[\cdot]$ denotes the rounding function, and m is a random integer within the range of $[-5, 5]$. This strategy forces the discriminators to be stronger at distinguishing synthetic images from real ones, thus avoiding mode collapse. This in turn forces our generators to be better in order to *trick* our discriminators. We evaluate this position-based selection strategy in Sect. 3.

3 Experiments

3.1 Data Set

The MR and CT volumes are respectively obtained using a Siemens Magnetom Espree 1.5T scanner (Siemens Medical Solutions, Malvern, PA) and a Philips Brilliance Big Bore scanner (Philips Medical Systems, Netherlands) under a routine clinical protocol for brain cancer patients. Geometric distortions in MR volumes are corrected using a 3D correction algorithm in the Siemens Syngo console workstation. All MR volumes are N4 corrected and normalized by aligning the white matter peak identified by fuzzy C-means.

The data set contains the brain MR and CT volumes of 45 patients, which were divided into a training set containing MR and CT volumes of 27 patients, a validation set of 3 patients for model and epoch selection, and a test set of 15 patients for performance evaluation. As in [6], the experiments were performed on 2D sagittal image slices. Each MR or CT volume contains about 270 sagittal images, which are resized and padded to 384×256 while maintaining the aspect ratio, and the intensity ranges are respectively $[-1000, 3500]$ HU for CT and $[0, 3500]$ for MR. To augment the training set, each image is padded to 400×284 and then randomly cropped to 384×256 as training samples.

3.2 Experimental Results

We compare the proposed method to the conventional cycleGAN [6,8] (denoted as "cycleGAN") and a cycleGAN trained with paired data (denoted as "cycle-GAN (paired)"), which represents the best that a cycleGAN can achieve.

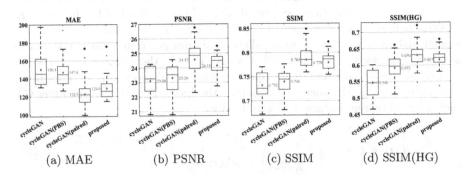

(a) MAE   (b) PSNR   (c) SSIM   (d) SSIM(HG)

Fig. 4. Comparison of different methods on synthesizing CT images in boxplots, where the diamond and number in blue denote the respective mean and * denotes $p < 0.001$ compared to the conventional cycleGAN using a paired sample t-test.

To evaluate the position-based selection strategy in Sect. 2.6, a cycleGAN using this strategy during training, denoted as "cycleGAN (PBS)", is also included in comparison. As in [6,8], the learning rate is set to 0.0002 for all compared methods.

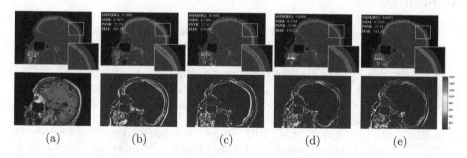

(a)   (b)   (c)   (d)   (e)

Fig. 5. Visual comparison of synthetic CT images using different methods. For one test subject, we show (a) the ground-truth CT image and input MR image; the synthetic CT image and its difference image (compared to ground-truth CT image) generated by (b) cycleGAN, (c) cycleGAN (PBS), (d) cycleGAN (paired), and (e) proposed method. The small text in each sub-image is the corresponding accuracy on this test subject.

To quantitatively compare these methods, we use mean absolute error (MAE), peak signal-to-noise ratio (PSNR), and structural similarity (SSIM) between the ground-truth CT volume and the synthetic one, which are computed within the head region mask and averaged over 15 test subjects. Furthermore, SSIM over regions with high gradient magnitudes (denoted as "SSIM(HG)") is also computed to measure the quality of bone regions in synthetic images. The maximum value in PSNR and the dynamic range in SSIM are set to 4500, as the range of our CT data is $[-1000, 3500]$ HU.

As shown in Fig. 4, our proposed method achieves significantly better performance than conventional cycleGAN in all the metrics ($p < 0.001$) and produces similar results compared to the cycleGAN trained with paired data. Compared to randomly selecting training slices at any position, our proposed position-based selection strategy produces significantly higher SSIM(HG) score ($p < 0.001$) with marginal improvement in the other three metrics. Figure 5 shows visual examples of synthetic CT images by different methods from a test subject.

4   Conclusion

We propose a structure-constrained cycleGAN for brain MR-to-CT synthesis using unpaired data. Compared to the conventional cycleGAN [6,8], we define an extra structure-consistency loss based on the modality independent neighborhood descriptor to constrain structural consistency and also introduce a position-based selection strategy for selecting training images. The experiments show that our method generates better synthetic CT images than the conventional cycleGAN and produces results similar to a cycleGAN trained with paired data.

Acknowledgments. This work is supported by the NSFC (11622106, 11690011, 61721002) and the China Scholarship Council.

References

1. Chartsias, A., Joyce, T., Dharmakumar, R., Tsaftaris, S.A.: Adversarial image synthesis for unpaired multi-modal cardiac data. In: Tsaftaris, S.A., Gooya, A., Frangi, A.F., Prince, J.L. (eds.) SASHIMI 2017. LNCS, vol. 10557, pp. 3–13. Springer, Cham (2017). https://doi.org/10.1007/978-3-319-68127-6_1
2. Goodfellow, I., et al.: Generative adversarial nets. In: NIPS, pp. 2672–2680 (2014)
3. Heinrich, M.P., et al.: MIND: modality independent neighbourhood descriptor for multi-modal deformable registration. Med. Image Anal. **16**(7), 1423–1435 (2012)
4. Hofmann, M., Bezrukov, I., et al.: MRI-based attenuation correction for whole-body PET/MRI: quantitative evaluation of segmentation- and atlas-based methods. J. Nucl. Med. **52**(9), 1392–1399 (2011)
5. Roy, S., Butman, J.A., Pham, D.L.: Synthesizing CT from ultrashort echo-time MR images via convolutional neural networks. In: Tsaftaris, S.A., Gooya, A., Frangi, A.F., Prince, J.L. (eds.) SASHIMI 2017. LNCS, vol. 10557, pp. 24–32. Springer, Cham (2017). https://doi.org/10.1007/978-3-319-68127-6_3
6. Wolterink, J.M., Dinkla, A.M., Savenije, M.H.F., Seevinck, P.R., van den Berg, C.A.T., Išgum, I.: Deep MR to CT synthesis using unpaired data. In: Tsaftaris, S.A., Gooya, A., Frangi, A.F., Prince, J.L. (eds.) SASHIMI 2017. LNCS, vol. 10557, pp. 14–23. Springer, Cham (2017). https://doi.org/10.1007/978-3-319-68127-6_2
7. Zhang, Z., et al.: Translating and segmenting multimodal medical volumes with cycle- and shape-consistency generative adversarial network. In: CVPR (2018)
8. Zhu, J.Y., Park, T., et al.: Unpaired image-to-image translation using cycle-consistent adversarial networks. In: ICCV, pp. 2242–2251 (2017)

Active Learning for Segmentation by Optimizing Content Information for Maximal Entropy

Firat Ozdemir[1(✉)], Zixuan Peng[1], Christine Tanner[1], Philipp Fuernstahl[2], and Orcun Goksel[1]

[1] Computer-assisted Applications in Medicine, ETH Zurich, Zurich, Switzerland
ozdemirf@vision.ee.ethz.ch
[2] CARD, University Hospital Balgrist, University of Zurich, Zurich, Switzerland

Abstract. Segmentation is essential for medical image analysis tasks such as intervention planning, therapy guidance, diagnosis, treatment decisions. Deep learning is becoming increasingly prominent for segmentation, where the lack of annotations, however, often becomes the main limitation. Due to privacy concerns and ethical considerations, most medical datasets are created, curated, and allow access only locally. Furthermore, current deep learning methods are often suboptimal in translating anatomical knowledge between different medical imaging modalities. Active learning can be used to select an informed set of image samples to request for manual annotation, in order to best utilize the limited annotation time of clinical experts for optimal outcomes, which we focus on in this work. Our contributions herein are two fold: (1) we enforce domain-representativeness of selected samples using a proposed penalization scheme to maximize information at the network *abstraction layer*, and (2) we propose a Borda-count based sample querying scheme for selecting samples for segmentation. Comparative experiments with baseline approaches show that the samples queried with our proposed method, where both above contributions are combined, result in significantly improved segmentation performance for this active learning task.

1 Introduction

Segmentation has several medical applications, such as patient-specific surgical planning. Due to limited resources of expert physicians, detailed manual annotations are often not possible, even when desired anatomy may be visible with sufficient contrast using non-invasive imaging modalities such as MRI and ultrasound. Deep learning has shown encouraging performance for segmentation [1,2], but often only when sufficient amount of labeled data for a target anatomy is available. Medical image data across different medical centers is often not uniform, for instance with respect to machine manufacturer, imaging settings, and cohort demographics. Thus, studies and corresponding annotations are only carried out in isolated datasets, with difficulties in merging information with data

© Springer Nature Switzerland AG 2018
D. Stoyanov et al. (Eds.): DLMIA 2018/ML-CDS 2018, LNCS 11045, pp. 183–191, 2018.
https://doi.org/10.1007/978-3-030-00889-5_21

sharing, patient rights, and confidentiality concerns. Hence, a sufficiently large dataset for a given task needs to be labeled. *Active learning* aims at maximizing the prediction performance through an intelligent sample querying system so that the limited expert annotation resources can be properly managed as opposed to training on a randomly selected next batch of samples which would contain a lot of redundancy. In a clinical environment, one can imagine that expert(s) will allocate a fixed amount of annotation time per time interval (i.e., week), hence the correct use of this time (i.e., on most valuable samples) is essential. Therefore, the segmentation framework would be initially provided a very limited labeled dataset, which will be extended with a certain batch size of samples intelligently selected at each iteration of the active learning.

Intuitively, the prediction confidence of a learned model can be used as a surrogate metric for its potential accuracy, in order to propose the most *uncertain* predictions for future manual annotation. In [3], *MC dropout* is proposed to sample from the approximate trained model posterior, which can be used to quantify an *uncertainty* metric through variations in the model predictions for a given input. Based on this, several approaches of querying the next batch of data are studied and compared with uniform random sampling in [4]. Unfortunately, it is intractable to assess conditional uncertainty of multiple samples; e.g. would i^{th} sample be still as uncertain as before once j^{th} sample is queried and trained for. Thus, it is intuitive to select a *representative* subset of these uncertain samples to reduce redundancy. Using a simplified version of DCAN [2] architecture (which has won the first place in the 2015 MICCAI Gland Segmentation Challenge [5]) for the purpose of faster training, a state-of-the-art method was proposed in [6] to select optimal sample images to annotate. First, a batch of *uncertain* samples is chosen based on the mean variance of multiple network predictions, followed by picking a subset of these using *maximum set coverage* [7] over the *image descriptors* of these samples. Recently in [8], a *content distance* [9] concept was proposed to quantify the similarity between two images, for selecting representative samples in class-incremental learning.

Herein we propose two main novelties for querying samples at an active learning step: (1) we add an additional constraint on the *abstraction layer* [8] activations during training to maximize information content at this level. We show that this additional constraint improves sample suitability that boosts segmentation performance from active learning. (2) Instead of the two step sample querying procedure (i.e., first select based on *uncertainty*, then cull using *representativeness*), we propose a Borda-count based method. This alone provides improvement over the state-of-the-art [6]; and when used in conjunction with our novel constraint above, it yields even further segmentation improvement.

2 Estimating Surrogate Metrics for Representativeness

Background. In [6], multiple FCNs were trained to estimate uncertainty for a given image through variation in their inferences. To make the FCN predictions diverse, the annotated dataset was also bootstrapped when training each model.

However, training several models is a costly operation and with larger number of models, one should bootstrap a smaller portion of the already-minimal dataset available in the early stages of typical active learning scenarios.

In our work, as a baseline, we implemented an improved version of the *Suggestive Annotation* framework [6]. We added dropout layers (c.f. Fig. 1) to allow for MC dropout [3], through which one can compute the voxel-wise variance across n_i inferences, and average it over all input voxels. The first step in querying samples is to pick the most uncertain n_{unc} samples S_{unc} from the set of non-annotated data D_{pool}. For representativeness, "image descriptor" I_i^c of every image $I_i \in D_{pool}$ is computed as described in [6] at the abstraction layer, l_{abst} (c.f. Fig. 1). Using cosine similarity $d_{sim}(I_i, I_j) = \cos(I_i^c, I_j^c)$ between the descriptors of images I_i and I_j, the maximum set-cover [7] over D_{pool} is computed using descriptors from S_{unc} for the top n_{rep} images. We call this method of using uncertainty and the above image descriptor (ID) as UNC-ID hereafter.

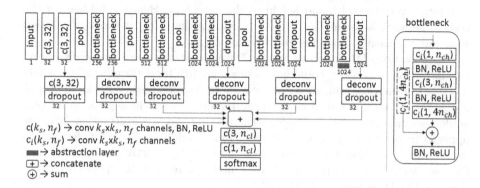

Fig. 1. DCAN network for *Suggestive Annotation* with additional spatial dropout layers. n_{ch} is the number of filters in respective block, BN is batch normalization, and n_{cl} is the number of classes. In consecutive bottlenecks, the first uses convolution filter in shortcuts to match tensor size while the second does not.

Content Distance. The image descriptor I_i^c averages the spatial information at the corresponding layer activations. While this allows for a spatially invariant means of representing a given image at a very abstract level, higher order features extracted at this stage would be blurred by this process. Alternatively, layer activation responses $R^l(I_i)$ of a pretrained classification network at a layer l can be used to describe the content of an image I_i [9]. Then, content distance (d_{cont}) between images I_i and I_j is defined as the mean squared error between their responses at layer l:

$$d_{cont}(I_i, I_j) = \frac{1}{N} \sum^N (R^l(I_i) - R^l(I_j))^2 \qquad (1)$$

A similar notion can be applied to active learning problems, where input images are described by the activation response at the l_{abst} of the currently trained network (c.f. Fig. 1).

Encoding Representativeness by Maximizing Entropy. Content distance defined in Eq. (1) allows for finer content discrimination than image descriptors [6]. However, it has been suggested that activations at a single layer may not be sufficient for accurate content description [8]. This is likely to particularly apply to segmentation networks, since network weights until l_{abst} are not optimized to describe the input image. Therefore, it has been proposed to stack activations from multiple layers. For a typical segmentation network, storing all layer activations of D_{pool} can quickly diverge to an unfeasible size. Alternatively, one can try to increase information content at the l_{abst} through maximizing its activation entropy [10] along the feature channels. Entropy loss can then be defined as:

$$L_{ent} = -\sum_x H(R^{(l_{abst},x)}) \tag{2}$$

where $R^{(l_{abst},x)}$ are the input activations of all channels for spatial location x, and x iterates over the width and height of the layer l_{abst}. Hence, total loss for the trained network becomes $L_{total} = L_{seg} + \lambda L_{ent}$, where L_{seg} is the segmentation loss, and λ is used to scale the entropy loss L_{ent}.

Optimization of the network weights through entropy maximization is a novel regularization. L_{ent} alone would have a tendency to alter network weights to only increase information, which may also encourage randomness. With an appropriate λ, the network is forced to optimize parameters for the segmentation task while also increasing "useful" information content at the abstraction layer; as opposed to producing just noise at l_{abst}. Hence, additional content description for a given image can be retrieved from a single layer activation, making it a feasible alternative. We refer to this method, where an entropy-based content distance (**ECD**) is used, as UNC-ECD.

3   Sample Selection Strategy

For active learning, one should emphasize that the initial data size can be very small. Until the model parameters are optimized for a sufficient coverage of the data distribution, the defined "uncertainty" metric might be misleading. As a result, one can explore different ways to combine multiple metrics when querying samples instead of the conventional 2-step process. An intuitive way to combine two metrics m_k and m_l would be to use $w_k m_k + w_l m_l$, where w_k, w_l are weights. However, *uncertainty* and *representativeness* metrics defined in Sect. 2 are not linearly combinable, even if normalized, due to non-linear unit increments. Therefore, we propose to use Borda count, where samples are ranked for each metric, and the next query sample I_{i^*} is picked based on the best combined rank:

$$i^* = \arg\min_i \left(\sum_{m_k \in S_m} f_{rank}(m_k(I_i)) \right) \tag{3}$$

where S_m is the set of metrics m_k to combine, and the f_{rank} function sorts the images based on the metric m_k. When we use the ranking in Eq. (3) for samples selection, we denote this in our results with "+", e.g. content distance with uncertainty is named UNC+ECD. In an active learning framework, the methods mentioned until now can be denoted as UNC+ID, UNC+ECD for ranking based sample selection and UNC-ID, UNC-ECD for uncertainty selection followed by representativeness selection.

Table 1. Dataset configuration

Config	#volumes	Left/Right	vox res. [mm]	image size [px]	TR [s]	TE [s]	FA [°]
1	20	9/11	0.91 × 0.91 × 3.0	192 × 192 × 64	20	1.70	10
2	16	8/8	0.83 × 0.83 × 3.0	144 × 144 × 56	20	2.39	10

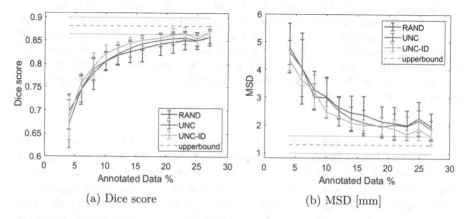

(a) Dice score   (b) MSD [mm]

Fig. 2. Comparison between our implementation of the baseline method (UNC-ID) with random sampling (RAND) and only uncertainty-based (UNC) active learning methods. Training on 100% of the data (D_{pool}) is shown as upperbound. (a) Mean Dice score and (b) mean surface distance (MSD) with error bars covering the standard deviation of 5 hold-out experiments at every evaluation point.

4   Experiments and Results

We have conducted experiments on an MR dataset of 36 patients diagnosed with rotator cuff tear (shoulders) according to specifications shown on Table 1. In an effort to regularize the dataset, Config2 images have been resized to match the voxel resolution of Config1, and then zero padded to match the in-plane image size of Config1. The data has expert annotations of two bones (humerus & scapula) and two muscle groups (supraspinatus & infraspinatus + teres minor). Experiments have been conducted using NVIDIA Titan X GPU and Tensorflow library [11].

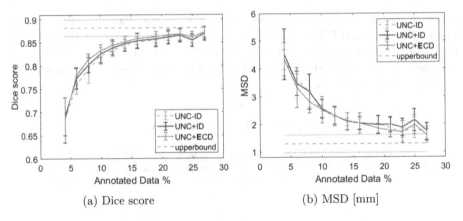

(a) Dice score   (b) MSD [mm]

Fig. 3. Comparison of the baseline method (UNC-ID) with ranking based sample selection (UNC+ID) and the combination of our proposed extensions (UNC+ECD). Training on 100% of the data (D_{pool}) is shown as upperbound. (a) Mean Dice score and (b) mean surface distance (MSD) with error bars covering the standard deviation of 5 hold-out experiments at every evaluation point. The mean Dice score of UNC+ECD was statistically significantly higher than the baseline in 4 of 5 experiments (one-sided paired t-test at the 0.05 level).

For all compared methods, we have used the modified DCAN architecture shown in Fig. 1, training it on 2D in-plane slices with the parameters $n_{ch} = 32$ and Adam optimizer. When training the networks, learning rate of 5×10^{-4}, dropout rate of 0.5, $n_i = 17$, and minibatch size of 8 images were applied. At each active learning stage, including the initial training, models were trained for 8000 steps, which took about 48 mins. Uncertainty metric is aggregated over the foreground classes to represent their mean uncertainty. We used cross-entropy loss at the softmax layer (c.f. Fig. 1) for the L_{seg}. Weight λ for scaling L_{ent} in methods UNC-ECD and UNC+ECD is empirically set to $\lambda = 1/(360 \times |R^{l_{abst}}|)$.

To provide quantitative results, we have evaluated Dice score coefficient and mean surface distance (MSD). In an effort to efficiently utilize the available dataset, we have generated 5 hold-out experiments where the initial training set D_{an}, the non-annotated set D_{pool}, the validation set (all slices from 2 patients) and the test set (all slices from 9 patients) are randomly picked. All experiments are initially trained on 64 slices. For every active learning step, $n_{rep} = 32$ and $n_{unc} = 64$ is used. In Figs. 2 and 3, we show the Dice score and MSD of different methods evaluated for the test set at 11 stages of active learning ranging from 4% up to 27% of the D_{pool}. Conducted experiments are shown in two groups to increase clarity: (1) Comparison of our implementation of the baseline (UNC-ID) to uniform random sample querying (RAND) and sample querying based only on uncertainty (UNC) as seen in Fig. 2; (2) Building on top of (1), improvements of ranking (UNC+ID) and the gain from L_{ent} during training and representativeness capabilities of d_{cont} for sample querying, UNC+ECD (c.f. Fig. 3).

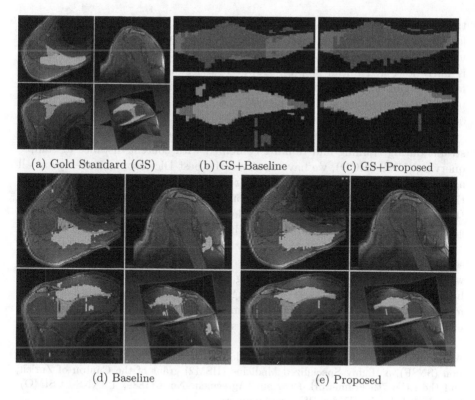

(a) Gold Standard (GS)   (b) GS+Baseline   (c) GS+Proposed

(d) Baseline   (e) Proposed

Fig. 4. Segmentation of a test volume comparing baseline (UNC-ID) with proposed method (UNC+ECD) after the first active learning step. Segmentation of two muscles overlaid on GS annotation (red) for (b) baseline and (c) proposed method. (d) Some of the substantial differences are pointed out by red arrows. (Color figure online)

In Fig. 4, we show an example cross-section from a test volume, where segmentation superiority of our proposed method (UNC+ECD) when compared to baseline is already visible after a single active learning step.

We conducted one-sided paired-sample t-tests at the 5% significance level on the mean Dice scores over all active learning steps for each hold-out experiment for UNC+ECD being superior to UNC-ID. Performance of UNC+ECD was statistically significantly better in 4 of 5 experiments.

5 Discussions and Conclusions

At early steps of active learning, one can see that the only uncertainty-based query sampling method (UNC) performs similar to random sample querying (RAND), with UNC only improving soon after $\approx 12\%$ of D_{pool} is used in training (c.f. Fig. 2). While UNC-ID already yields better segmentation performance than just uncertainty-based sampling, by simply using ranking, one can see that the baseline method achieves a more substantial boost at early stages of active learning (see UNC+ID in Fig. 3). This behavior suggests that the surrogate uncertainty metric can give a bad approximation when the trained data size is fairly low; i.e., initial step(s). However, the suboptimal segmentation performance gain can be compensated with representativeness, and even further improved when given a higher priority; i.e., ranking instead of 2-step sample querying.

Upon combination of the proposed additional information maximization constraint during training and ranking combined with content distance at sample querying (UNC+ECD), we have observed the best Dice score on average at all active learning steps among the compared baseline and ranking extensions of the baseline methods. Other possible combinations of our proposed extensions (UNC-CD, UNC+CD, UNC-ECD) yielded inferior performance to UNC+ECD, and hence are not included in the quantitative comparisons to reduce clutter.

In this paper, we have comparatively studied the impact of different sample selection methods in active learning for segmentation. We have proposed 2 novel ways to query samples for active learning, which also can be combined to further boost performance during active learning steps. Compared to a state-of-the-art method, we have shown our proposed method to yield statistically significant improvement of segmentation Dice scores.

Acknowledgements. This work was funded by the Swiss National Science Foundation (SNSF), a Highly Specialized Medicine (HSM2) grant of the Canton of Zurich, and the EU's 7th Framework Program (Agreement No. 611889, TRANS-FUSIMO). We acknowledge NVIDIA GPU Grant support.

References

1. Baumgartner, C.F., Koch, L.M., Pollefeys, M., Konukoglu, E.: An Exploration of 2D and 3D Deep Learning Techniques for Cardiac MR Image Segmentation. In: Pop, M., et al. (eds.) STACOM 2017. LNCS, vol. 10663, pp. 111–119. Springer, Cham (2018). https://doi.org/10.1007/978-3-319-75541-0_12
2. Chen, H., Qi, X., Yu, L., Dou, Q., Qin, J., Heng, P.A.: DCAN: deep contour-aware networks for object instance segmentation from histology images. Med. Image Anal. **36**, 135–146 (2016)
3. Gal, Y., Ghahramani, Z.: Dropout as a Bayesian approximation: representing model uncertainty in deep learning. In: International Conference on Machine Learning (ICML), pp. 1050–1059 (2016)
4. Gal, Y., Islam, R., Ghahramani, Z.: Deep Bayesian active learning with image data. In: Proceedings of the 34th International Conference on Machine Learning (ICML) (2017)
5. Sirinukunwattana, K., Pluim, J.P., Chen, H., et al.: Gland segmentation in colon histology images: the GlaS challenge contest. Med. Imag Anal. **35**, 489–502 (2017)
6. Yang, L., Zhang, Y., Chen, J., Zhang, S., Chen, D.Z.: Suggestive annotation: a deep active learning framework for biomedical image segmentation. In: Descoteaux, M., Maier-Hein, L., Franz, A., Jannin, P., Collins, D.L., Duchesne, S. (eds.) MICCAI 2017. LNCS, vol. 10435, pp. 399–407. Springer, Cham (2017). https://doi.org/10.1007/978-3-319-66179-7_46

7. Feige, U.: A threshold of ln n for approximating set cover. ACM **45**, 634–652 (1998)
8. Ozdemir, F., Fuernstahl, P., Goksel, O.: Learn the new, keep the old: extending pretrained models with new anatomy and images. In: Frangi, A.F., Schnabel, J.A., Davatzikos, C., Alberola-López, C., Fichtinger, G. (eds.) Medical Image Computing and Computer Assisted Intervention (MICCAI), pp. 361–369. Springer International Publishing, Cham (2018). https://doi.org/10.1007/978-3-030-00937-3_42. ISBN: 978-3-030-00937-3
9. Gatys, L.A., Ecker, A.S., Bethge, M.: Image style transfer using convolutional neural networks. In: IEEE CVPR, pp. 2414–2423 (2016)
10. Shannon, C.E.: A mathematical theory of communication. ACM SIGMOBILE Mob. Comput. Commun. Rev. **5**, 3–55 (2001)
11. Abadi, M., Agarwal, A., Barham, P., Brevdo, E., et al.: TensorFlow: large-scale machine learning on heterogeneous systems (2015). www.tensorflow.org

Weakly Supervised Localisation for Fetal Ultrasound Images

Nicolas Toussaint[1(✉)], Bishesh Khanal[1,2], Matthew Sinclair[2], Alberto Gomez[1], Emily Skelton[1], Jacqueline Matthew[1], and Julia A. Schnabel[1]

[1] School of Biomedical Engineering and Imaging Sciences, King's College, London, UK
`nicolas.a.toussaint@kcl.ac.uk`
[2] Department of Computing, Imperial College, London, UK

Abstract. This paper addresses the task of detecting and localising fetal anatomical regions in 2D ultrasound images, where only image-level labels are present at training, i.e. without any localisation or segmentation information. We examine the use of convolutional neural network architectures coupled with soft proposal layers. The resulting network simultaneously performs anatomical region detection (classification) and localisation tasks. We generate a proposal map describing the attention of the network for a particular class. The network is trained on 85,500 2D fetal Ultrasound images and their associated labels. Labels correspond to six anatomical regions: head, spine, thorax, abdomen, limbs, and placenta. Detection achieves an average accuracy of 90% on individual regions, and show that the proposal maps correlate well with relevant anatomical structures. This work presents itself as a powerful and essential step towards subsequent tasks such as fetal position and pose estimation, organ-specific segmentation, or image-guided navigation.

Keywords: Deep learning · Weakly supervised learning · Object localisation · Ultrasound · Fetal imaging · Image-guided navigation

1 Introduction

Ultrasound (US) is the most popular obstetric imaging modality for antenatal detection of fetal abnormalities. A routine US screening examination consists of manually scanning the fetal anatomy, mainly using 2D imaging, selecting a series of standard planes, and measuring biometric data to assess fetal normality. The plane selection process depends on the local/departmental protocol (e.g. FASP [2] in the UK). Steering the US transducer to obtain these anatomical planes of interest is a challenging task due to the large variability in image orientation and appearance, within an anatomical region as well as within a standard plane [7]. Recent years have seen significant efforts to detect such planes in US video sequences [1,9]. While these methods are extremely valuable, they disregard more than 95% of the examination images that do not fall into a

© Springer Nature Switzerland AG 2018
D. Stoyanov et al. (Eds.): DLMIA 2018/ML-CDS 2018, LNCS 11045, pp. 192–200, 2018.
https://doi.org/10.1007/978-3-030-00889-5_22

standard plane category. The remaining images do however contain valuable information about the global fetal anatomy. With that in mind, categorisation of any generic fetal US image in global anatomical regions is of great clinical interest. Such categorisation could for instance provide anatomical context to a subsequent organ specific task. Furthermore, localising general fetal structures could play an important role in the development of navigation systems, and could also be used to better understand and learn the patterns of steering towards specific planes of interests.

Related Work: Weakly supervised object localisation is a relatively active field of research in Neural Network literature [5]. Recently, Zhu et al. proposed a their Soft Proposal Networks (SPN) [11], consisting of a dedicated extra layer attached to any CNN architecture, specifically designed for this task. It was initially inspired by the class activation map (CAM) approach in [10]. One of the main advantages of SPNs over conventional Region Proposal Networks [6] for instance is that the proposal itself is an objectness confidence, and does not necessitate back propagation at inference time to retrieve saliency. As a consequence, it can be used directly in an end-to-end learning manner: the proposal couples with convolutional activation and evolves with the deep feature learning.

In the context of US images and fetal screening in particular, recent papers focused on classification or detection [1] of standard planes in US video sequences. In [1], the authors detected a standard plane within a real screening session video. They used saliency maps to infer the regions of interest attached to the detected standard plane using back propagation. They however discard the vast majority of acquired images (~95%) as background. In contrast, our work provides semantic level of labels for any arbitrary image. Thus, during scanning, the proposed method provides useful information and context from all images captured in a fetal US examination.

Contribution: We propose a method to detect and localise fetal anatomical regions applicable to any arbitrary 2D US fetal image within 22–32 week gestational age. The system is based on Convolutional Neural Networks (CNNs) and soft proposal layers [11] for weakly supervised localisation. It is to our knowledge the first attempt to transfer this technology to free hand 2D US fetal anatomical region localisation. The network is able to detect six separate anatomical regions of the fetal body with high accuracy (~90%), and localise key anatomical structures within an image in real time (~20 Hz).

2   Data

Image Data: The image data used in this work consists of a set of 20 free-hand fetal US examinations from patients, with gestational age of 27±5 weeks from free-hand ultrasound. The system used was a Philips EPIQ 7G machine. Each examination generated a stream of approximately 40,000 frames. Example of images are shown in Fig. 2(left). Each frame was stored on disk at acquisition time at full resolution and full frame rate. Acquisition parameters were provided from the manufacturer in real time.

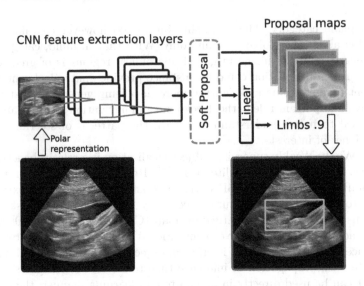

Fig. 1. Overview of our framework: A fetal ultrasound image is processed in real-time via a Convolutional Neural Network coupled with a Soft Proposal layer. The anatomical region is detected and localised using weakly supervised learning.

Image Labels: Each examination dataset was uploaded into a custom-made browser, which enabled the entire batch to be split into six different categories (+ background), or labels, forming an anatomical parcellation of the gestational sac. Regions are shown in Fig. 2(right), and defined as follows (number of labelled frames in brackets):

- **Head:** [25,249 fr.] Should contain the skull, full or in part.
- **Thorax:** [32,254 fr.] Should contain the cardiac chambers, full or in part.
- **Abdomen:** [16,220 fr.] Should contain the abdomen (diaphragm to pelvis).
- **Spine:** [5,980 fr.] Should contain part of the spine.
- **Limbs:** [11,617 fr.] Should contain one or more extremity(ies).
- **Placenta:** [6,081 fr.] Should contain part of the placenta.
- **Background:** [12,687 fr.] No distinguishable structure in image.

Categories were chosen such that they cover the entirety of the fetal body, ensuring that any image containing fetal tissue will fall into one of them. The following heuristics were followed for categorisation:

- An image is categorised as label **X** if **X** is the only category visible.
- If more than one category is visible, an image can be categorised as label **X** if **X** occupies the majority of the image.
- Images disagreeing with those rules (indistinguishable objects(s), no prominent category, strong blur, etc) are discarded.

Labelling of the 20 datasets was performed by 3 clinical experts. The total time spent per dataset was approximately 1.5h. The labelled data was then split between training and test sets using an 80% − 20% ratio, resulting in 85,500 images for training and 24,500 for testing. The split was performed at the subject level to ensure that we were testing the generality of the network.

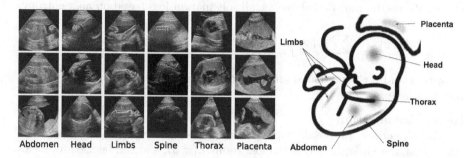

Fig. 2. Left: Selection of images from a fetal US examination, each column corresponds to an anatomical region. Right: Description of the anatomical regions detected and localised by our network.

3 Methods

Preprocessing

1. Polar projection: Unlike most other imaging modalities, fetal ultrasound images are sampled in polar cordinates, yielding the characteristic frustum-shaped images. The geometric properties of the frustum vary drastically at acquisition time, depending on the organ of interest, the fetal lie or the gestational age. To prevent our network from inadvertently learning the shape of the frustum as a feature associated with a specific class (i.e. to be invariant to sector width and depth), we transformed each image into its associated polar coordinate representation. We used acquisition parameters from the frame's header in order to retrieve the intrinsic polar coordinate system (Depth of Scan, Voxel Size, Sector Width, Zoom Level).

2. Crop and resize: In order to prevent our algorithm from focusing on acoustic reverberations artefacts, we cut 10% off the polar projected image on either side in the depth direction. The resulting image was resized to a standard 224 × 224 pixel size.

Network

We examined different architectures for the base feature extraction layers: VGG [8] and ResNets [3]. We used batch normalisation to accelerate convergence [4]. We adapted the tail of the networks to incorporate the Soft Proposal block. As suggested in [11], the soft proposal layer (SP) is inserted after the latest convolutional layer of the network. It is followed by a spatial pooling layer, and a fully connected linear classifier.

At training, our images were associated with a unique label corresponding to the prominent anatomical region present in the image. However, it is often the case in practice that multiple anatomical regions are visible in a single image. It is therefore important to consider that in the loss function used for our optimisation. We used a multi-label one *vs.* all soft margin loss based on max-entropy:

$$L(x, y) = - \sum_i y_i \log \frac{1}{1 + \exp(-x_i)} + (1 - y_i) \log \frac{\exp(-x_i)}{1 + \exp(-x_i)} \qquad (1)$$

with x and y the predicted and target class score vectors respectively, and i the class index.

Region Localisation

The objectness proposal maps from the SP-layer highlight regions of the image that were informative to the loss result $L(x, y)$, and can be used for localisation purposes. To quantify localisation accuracy, we computed a bounding box on the soft proposal map corresponding to the highest score. First the map is thresholded to 30% above the median pixel value, and the enclosing bounding box is extracted. We compared the predicted bounding box against the one annotated by a clinical expert, using the intersection over union (IoU) metric.

Implementation: The labelling tool was built using C++ and Qt software. Preprocessing was performed using the Insight ToolKit. We used pyTorch for the implementation of the network architecture. We trained our networks using CUDA 8.0 on an Nvidia GeForce GTX 960M GPU.

4   Experiments and Results

Training: We trained four different feature extraction networks with batch normalisation coupled with a soft proposal layer: VGG13-SP, VGG16-SP, ResNet18-SP, and ResNet34-SP, in an end-to-end manner. We used $K = 512$ feature channels in the SP layer (see [11]). Mini-batch Nesterov gradient descent was chosen with a momentum of 0.8. L2 regularisation was used with a weight decay of 5×10^{-4}. The initial learning rate was 0.05 and was divided by a factor 10 every 5 epochs until convergence. Since the training data contained large variability in size and orientation, the only data augmentation used was random horizontal flip. Class imbalance was addressed by weighting the probability to draw a sample by its relative class occurrence in the training set. Convergence typically occurred within ten hours.

Region Detection: After training, we evaluated the generalisation of our networks on a test set consisting of three previously unseen subjects' examinations, with a total number of 24,500 frames. The detailed classification scores of each network on the test set are summarised in Table 1. The best performing network was ResNet18-SP. To further illustrate the results of this network, we show precision/recall curves for each anatomical region and the region confusion matrix in Fig. 3. The confusion matrix is a valuable indication on how the network is behaving in a real case scenario.

Region Localisation: We evaluated the correctness of the localisation task. We computed the IoU metric between predicted and ground truth bounding boxes on a randomised sub-selection of the test set, totalling 4,300 frames. The average IoU between all classes for the four architectures is reported in the last column of Table 1. Detection and localisation results using ResNet18-SP and VGG13-SP for each class are shown in Fig. 4. Additionally, we illustrate in the last column some examples of mis-classifications of the networks.

Table 1. Detailed detection scores (Accuracy) for the four SP- modified architectures on the test set for each class and their average. The last column shows the localisation scores (Intersection over Union), averaged over all classes.

Arch	Abdo	Head	Limbs	Plac	Spine	Thorax	Avg.	IoU
resnet18-sp	0.941	0.922	0.852	0.968	0.840	0.947	**0.912**	0.393
resnet34-sp	0.945	0.933	0.686	0.966	0.871	0.946	0.891	0.378
vgg13-sp	0.930	0.921	0.767	0.978	0.833	0.899	0.891	**0.424**
vgg16-sp	0.948	0.908	0.785	0.996	0.839	0.899	0.896	0.415

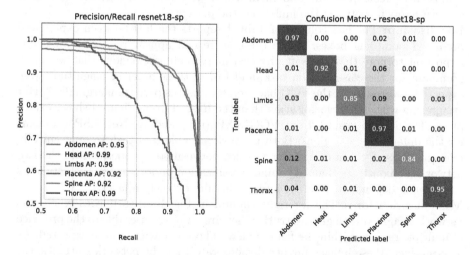

Fig. 3. Classification results for the ResNet18-SP network. Left: Precision/recall curves for each class. Right: Normalised confusion matrix. Figure best viewed in colour.

5 Discussions

Detection: Table 1 shows relatively high detection accuracy over the different regions considered. ResNet18-SP demonstrates marginally higher performance.

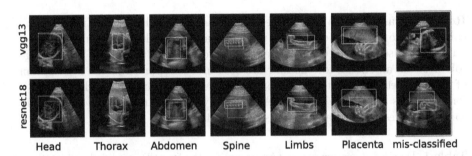

Fig. 4. Localisation results of VGG13-SP (top) and ResNet18-SP (bottom) for different anatomical regions. The far right column shows mis-classified examples. Images are superimposed by the soft proposal map corresponding to the predicted label. Expert bounding box is shown in white, and predicted in color. Figure best viewed in colour.

Interestingly, deeper networks do not seem to increase performance, and can even demonstrate overfitting in the ResNet case. The limbs and spinal regions appear to be less trivial to categorise. This is partly explained by the fact that they often appear in conjunction with other regions in the field of view. The confusion matrix in Fig. 3 illustrates further this difficulty. The network can be confused between spine and abdomen, which are often seen together. A similar pattern happens between the limbs and the placenta.

Localisation: The last column of Table 1 reports the IoU between expert and predicted bounding boxes. While these score can appear relatively low, it is important to note that the soft proposal maps highlight regions that were discriminant for the classification task, and IoU of these order of magnitude were expected. Interestingly, the VGG backbones networks perform marginally better at agreeing with expert localisation than the ResNet ones. Figure 4 shows example of localisation results from VGG13-SP (top) and ResNet18-SP (bottom) for the different fetal regions. Both network are able to attach to anatomically relevant parts of the image. Discrepancies between soft proposal from the two networks demonstrate that, at similar classification performances, the network's attention is dependent from the internal feature extraction layer.

Mis-classifications: The far right column in Fig. 4 shows images where the network disagreed with ground truth. They are for most cases due to the presence of multiple regions within the field of view. Those behaviours were expected. As a bi-product, these images further demonstrate that the network's attention is focusing on relevant anatomical regions.

Known Limitations: Our work does not yet account for images with multiple anatomical regions at training. This situation does however occur frequently. This limitation is partly addressed in our choice of loss function but may be misleading the network in difficult cases. To fully address this issue, we will investigate the introduction of multi-labelled images at training. Another limitation of this work is the relatively small number of subjects used for training. This was however balanced by the large variability of appearances per class even within a subject, as we allow categorisation of an anatomical region from any possible angle, resulting in 9,000 images per class per subject on average.

6 Conclusion

In this paper, we augmented classification network architectures with soft proposal layers, and adapted them for the specific task of fetal region detection and localisation in real-time 2D ultrasound imaging. We showed that the proposed network achieves high accuracy for automatic annotation of arbitrary 2D fetal ultrasound images. Furthermore, the network is capable of localising relevant anatomical structures characteristic of each anatomical region, while there was no localisation provided at training. The ability to semantically categorise arbitrary US images could play a key role to developing navigation systems, or guide non-expert sonography scanning. Furthermore, this work could aid subsequent tasks such as scan plane detection, semantic segmentation or biometry estimation in a multi-task framework.

Acknowledgments. This work was supported by the Wellcome/EPSRC Centre for Medical Eng. [WT203148/Z/16/Z], and the Wellcome IEH Award [102431].

References

1. Baumgartner, C.F., et al.: Sononet: real-time detection and localisation of fetal standard scan planes in freehand ultrasound. IEEE Trans. Med. Imaging **36**(11), 2204–2215 (2017)
2. UK National Screening Committee et al.: Fetal Anomaly Screening: Programme Handbook. Public Health England, London (2015)
3. He, K., Zhang, X., Ren, S., Sun, J.: Deep residual learning for image recognition. In: Proceedings of the IEEE Conference on Computer Vision and Pattern Recognition (CVPR), pp. 770–778 (2016)
4. Ioffe, S., Szegedy, C.: Batch normalization: accelerating deep network training by reducing internal covariate shift. In: ICML, pp. 448–456 (2015)
5. Oquab, M., Bottou, L., Laptev, I., Sivic, J.: Is object localization for free? weakly-supervised learning with convolutional neural networks. In: CVPR, pp. 685–694 (2015)
6. Ren, S., He, K., Girshick, R., Sun, J.: Faster R-CNN: towards real-time object detection with region proposal networks. In: Advances in Neural Information Processing Systems, pp. 91–99 (2015)
7. Sarris, I., et al.: Intra-and interobserver variability in fetal ultrasound measurements. Ultrasound Obstet. Gynecol. **39**(3), 266–273 (2012)
8. Simonyan, K., Zisserman, A.: Very deep convolutional networks for large-scale image recognition. arXiv preprint arXiv:1409.1556 (2014)
9. Yaqub, M., Kelly, B., Papageorghiou, A.T., Noble, J.A.: Guided random forests for identification of key fetal anatomy and image categorization in ultrasound scans. In: Navab, N., Hornegger, J., Wells, W.M., Frangi, A.F. (eds.) MICCAI 2015. LNCS, vol. 9351, pp. 687–694. Springer, Cham (2015). https://doi.org/10.1007/978-3-319-24574-4_82

10. Zhou, B., Khosla, A., Lapedriza, A., Oliva, A., Torralba, A.: Learning deep features for discriminative localization. IEEE Comput. Vis. Pattern Recognit. **2016**, 2921–2929 (2016)
11. Zhu, Y., Zhou, Y., Ye, Q., Qiu, Q., Jiao, J.: Soft proposal networks for weakly supervised object localization. arXiv preprint arXiv:1709.01829 (2017)

PIMMS: Permutation Invariant Multi-modal Segmentation

Thomas Varsavsky[1(✉)], Zach Eaton-Rosen[1,2(✉)], Carole H. Sudre[1,2,3(✉)],
Parashkev Nachev[4(✉)], and M. Jorge Cardoso[1,2(✉)]

[1] CMIC, University College London, London, UK
{ucabtmv,z.eaton-rosen,carole.sudre.12}@ucl.ac.uk
[2] School of Biomedical Engineering and Imaging Sciences,
King's College London, London, UK
m.jorge.cardoso@kcl.ac.uk
[3] Dementia Research Centre, University College London, London, UK
[4] Institute of Neurology, University College London, London, UK
p.nachev@ucl.ac.uk

Abstract. In a research context, image acquisition will often involve a
pre-defined static protocol and the data will be of high quality. If we are
to build applications that work in hospitals without significant operational changes in care delivery, algorithms should be designed to cope
with the available data in the best possible way. In a clinical environment, imaging protocols are highly flexible, with MRI sequences commonly missing appropriate sequence labeling (e.g. T1, T2, FLAIR). To
this end we introduce PIMMS, a Permutation Invariant Multi-Modal
Segmentation technique that is able to perform inference over sets of
MRI scans without using modality labels. We present results which show
that our convolutional neural network can, in some settings, outperform
a baseline model which utilizes modality labels, and achieve comparable
performance otherwise.

1 Introduction

Over the years, public medical imaging datasets have emerged which enable
researchers to benchmark the performance of their algorithms [1]. Data is mostly
acquired from patients who have volunteered to be part of a clinical research
study and are subject to a strict study protocol. If the study involves the acquisition of Magnetic Resonance Imaging (MRI) scans, the study protocol might dic-
tate the scanner choice as well as the acquisition parameters to be used [4]. In the
real unconstrained clinical setting however, MRIs are more likely to be acquired
from different machines under different acquisition protocols and parameters.
There is no guarantee that a particular sequence will be available, no guarantee on the number of available modalities, no guarantee that modalities will be
unique (e.g. same sequence acquired with different orientations and contrasts),
and no guarantee that any of the modalities will be labeled appropriately for

© Springer Nature Switzerland AG 2018
D. Stoyanov et al. (Eds.): DLMIA 2018/ML-CDS 2018, LNCS 11045, pp. 201–209, 2018.
https://doi.org/10.1007/978-3-030-00889-5_23

algorithmic use. If hospitals are to benefit from advances in neuroimaging, algorithms that can cope with this lack of available modalities are necessary. We argue that an algorithm which is to be deployed in this setting should have two key properties: (1) permutation invariance, i.e permuting the order of the input images should not affect the output and (2) robustness to missing modalities. To this end we propose a segmentation model, with neural networks as building blocks, which can learn with limited data and segment scans without MR modality labels. In this work we focus on the task of segmenting white matter hyperintensities (WMH). In studies involving WMH segmentation the most common modalities are T1, T2 and T2-FLAIR which provide complementary information about the imaged tissue. Although T1 and T2 modalities are created from different underlying physical signals (longitudinal and transverse relaxation time respectively) the scans produced will almost always be a combination of both (hence the name attribute - weighted). By varying the acquisition parameters, such as the echo and relaxation times, these underlying physical signals are observed in different proportions [3]. Modality labels are a discrete approximation of a continuous acquisition parameter landscape and we use this as inspiration for the model we present.

In order to address missing modalities, research has focused mostly on generative models where missing MRI scans are synthesized or imputed [2,8]. In the work of [6] the authors handle missing modalities without using generative models of MR modalities. Instead of synthesizing the missing modalities, their model, Hetero-modal Image Segmentation (HeMIS), is trained to handle missing input modalities. More details about HeMIS can be found in Sect. 2. Although HeMIS is successful at dealing with missing modalities, it assumes that the MR modalities in a test case will be labeled. The authors of [10] tackle the issue of generalizing to unseen protocols and scanners. In order to be robust to different scanners and protocols, they propose a tuning of the batch normalization parameters of a CNN. However, their method still requires approximately four scans with their associated segmentations from the unseen protocol to perform well.

We introduce a model that learns to build intermediate representations of the images as a linear combination of the available inputs which are more continuous than their original labels. The proposed model does not assume the modality is known and has the ability to generalize to unseen scanners/protocols, taking in N unordered input scans with no modality labels to produce accurate segmentation masks. We provide results on a variety of datasets featuring WMH with large variability in scanner type and acquisition parameters and show that our model is both permutation invariant and robust to missing modalities. We demonstrate that it can perform comparatively well with an algorithm which utilizes the modality labels having never seen an image from that particular protocol. Furthermore, our model can outperform the baseline method (HeMIS) in the case where it has seen MR modality labels of the same protocol it is being tested on.

2   Methods

HeMIS. In HeMIS each available modality, $x_1, \ldots, x_M$, is embedded with a modality specific function $\phi_m(x_m) \in \mathbb{R}^{D \times K}$ denoted the "back-end" to produce embeddings. An"abstraction" layer then operates on these embeddings by computing the mean and variance across their K dimensions and concatenating the two resulting vectors $\phi_\alpha = [\hat{\mathrm{E}}(\phi(\mathbf{x})), \hat{\mathrm{Var}}(\phi(\mathbf{x}))]$, where $\mathbf{x} \in \mathbb{R}^{D \times M}$ M is the number of modalities and D is the spatial dimensions of the input. Let ϕ_α be a fixed dimensional tensor which represents an input of variable size. This forms the input to the final portion of the network referred to as the "frontend" which will output a semantic segmentation map. The network is trained using a Dice loss, first proposed in [11] as a loss function for training neural networks.

During training, random modalities are set to zero, encouraging robustness to missing modalities. HeMIS, shown in Fig. 1, forms part of our architecture.

Our Approach. We propose a method which at test time takes in an arbitrary number of N scans (denoted X) which do not have corresponding MR modality labels and produces a permutation invariant representation that is also robust to missing modalities. In theory this common representation could be applied to a variety of tasks. In this paper we focus on white matter hyperintensity segmentation.

The inputs are fed into an MR modality classifier f_{mod} which outputs a distribution over modalities for a given scan as its prediction. These modality scores $\mathcal{S} \in \mathbb{R}^{M \times N}$ are combined with the inputs, X, to produce modified inputs denoted as $\hat{X} \in \mathbb{R}^{D \times M}$. In the attention literature a distinction is drawn between "soft" and"hard" attention [14]. Soft attention generally involves a probabilistic weighted sum whilst a hard attention is a categorical argmax over the inputs. With this in mind, we explore two methods for performing $X \to \hat{X}$: f_{soft} and f_{hard}. The function f_{soft} is defined as,

$$f_{soft}(X, \mathcal{S}) = \sum_{n=1}^{N} \mathcal{S}_{mn} x_n = \hat{x}_m \tag{1}$$

Each component $\hat{x}_m$ of the modified input $\hat{X}$ is formed by taking a weighted sum of each input x_n according to the probabilities provided by $\mathcal{S}$. f_{hard} is defined as,

$$f_{hard}(X, \mathcal{S}) = \sum_{n=1}^{N} \mathbb{1}(\arg \max_{m^*} \mathcal{S}_{m^*n} = m) x_n = \hat{x}_m \tag{2}$$

The modified input $\hat{X}$ now consists of a finite number of modalities. The mapping $f : X \to \hat{X}$ is illustrated in the blue block in Fig. 1.

Each MR modality is designed to capture fundamentally different physical properties which justifies having individual feature extractors, ϕ_m, for each $\hat{x}_m$

modality representation. The output of these modality-specific feature extractors is collected into one tensor by taking the mean and the variance across modalities and concatenating the result to give $\phi_\alpha \in \mathbb{R}^{D \times K}$ where K is given by the choice of filter depth in ϕ_m. This feeds into a final network, ϕ_{seg} which produces a segmentation prediction. This use of modality specific models, pooling and a separate segmentation network is the same as HeMIS and is illustrated in the grey block in Fig. 1.

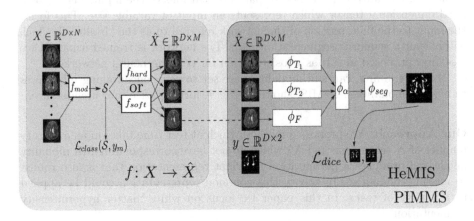

Fig. 1. Diagram showing the network architecture. During training the inputs are $X \in \mathbb{R}^{D \times N}$ and the corresponding ground truth binary segmentation $y \in \mathbb{R}^{D \times 2}$. A function f_{mod} takes each scan as input and outputs a modality score S which produces the representation $\hat{X} \in \mathbb{R}^{D \times M}$. The weights of ϕ_{T_1}, ϕ_{T_2}, ϕ_F and ϕ_{seg} are learned by differentiating with respect to $\mathcal{L}_{seg}$ and the weights of f are learned by differentiating with respect to $\mathcal{L}_{class}$. y_m is a one-hot encoded modality label.

A convolutional neural network was used for f_{mod}. A network with 36 layers using skip connections and ReLU non-linearities inspired by the residual network (ResNet) proposed in [7] is used. The network was trained with the categorical cross-entropy loss which we refer to as $\mathcal{L}_{class}$. where y_{mi} is a one-hot encoded modality label and S_{mi} is the modality score. Each of the branches ϕ_m as well as ϕ_{seg} were two convolutional layers with ReLU non-linearities (more details in Sect. 2). The parameters of ϕ_m and ϕ_{seg} were found by minimizing $\mathcal{L}_{seg}$ which is the binary Dice Loss.

For two of our variants these losses were trained separately (or "offline"). However, we also trained an "online" variant where the parameters of the modality classifier are learned using a multi-objective loss function. This loss is defined as, $\mathcal{L}_{tot} = \mathcal{L}_{seg} + \lambda \mathcal{L}_{class}$, where λ is some choice of weighting or parametrized weighting function. Although the loss consists of multiple objectives this should not be considered "multi-task learning". There is no conditional independence between the tasks and no representation sharing — instead this can be seen as a differentiable attention mechanism. The four variants trained are summarized below,

HeMIS - $X \rightarrow \hat{X}$ using labels, f_{mod} trained separately from $\phi_{seg}, \phi_{T_1}, \phi_{T_2}$ & ϕ_F
Soft - f_{soft} used to create $\hat{X}$, f_{mod} trained separately from $\phi_{seg}, \phi_{T_1}, \phi_{T_2}$ & ϕ_F,
Hard - f_{hard} used to create $\hat{X}$, f_{mod} trained separately from $\phi_{seg}, \phi_{T_1}, \phi_{T_2}$ & ϕ_F,
Online - f_{soft} used to create $\hat{X}$, f_{mod} trained jointly with $\phi_{seg}, \phi_{T_1}, \phi_{T_2}$ & ϕ_F.,

Implementation Details. It is important to note that the network architecture takes in 2D patches from the image as was done in [6]. Specifically we take patches of size 100×100 from 3D scans which have all been resampled to $1 \, mm \times 1 \, mm \times 1 \, mm$. This theoretical framework permits any spatial dimension D and future work will train and run inference in full 3D.

All results were obtained using the NiftyNet framework [5], which is a wrapper around TensorFlow designed for medical imaging. f_{mod} uses a standard ResNet design with nine blocks per resolution, each with three convolutions and ReLU activations. The network is trained using the Adam optimizer with a learning rate of 3×10^{-4}. A batch size of 64 was used on this network and weight decay regularization of 1×10^{-4}.

For each ϕ_m and ϕ_{seg} the implementation details from [6] were recreated. Two convolutional layers with 48 filters, 5×5 kernel sizes, zero-padding and ReLU activation were used followed by a max pooling layer with kernel size $(2, 2)$ and a stride of 1 this preserves the spatial resolution of the image. For ϕ_{seg} two convolutional layers were used, one with 16 filters, 5×5 kernel sizes, zero padding and ReLU activation the last convolutional layer had 2 filters, a kernel size of 21×21, zero padding and a softmax activation which provided the per class predictions. We also utilized the pseudo-curriculum learning approach from HeMIS. Random modalities are set to zero but the chance of setting only one or no modalities to zero is higher. The online model was harder to train than the offline ones. The joint training lead to odd dynamics between the classification loss and the segmentation loss. To help stabilize the training an exponential decay weighting was used on the classification loss in order to encourage training it towards the start and remove its importance later on so that the model could experiment with representations which do not match the provided labels and not be punished by $\mathcal{L}_{class}$. Our best performing "online" model used $\lambda(i) = e^{-\gamma i}$ where i is the current iteration and γ is a decay constant hyperparameter set to 1×10^{-4}.

This same ResNet architecture was used as f_{mod} in the online case in order to make a fair comparison in terms of number of parameters. However, in the online setting, the batch size had to be reduced as a practical consideration as the combination of both modality and backend models proved too large to fit in GPU memory. All experiments were run on a single NVIDIA Titan Xp.

3   Experiments and Results

Data used in this work comes from a variety of sources, chosen to try and capture the acquisition variability observed in a practical setting due to multiple MRI scanners/protocols. A subset of 973 subjects each with T1 and FLAIR scans were obtained from the Alzheimer's Disease Neuroimaging Initiative (ADNI) database [9]. The data in this study was collected from multiple scanners, but used the same protocol for setting the acquisition parameters. We therefore deem this dataset one of relatively low variance between subjects. We also utilise data collected from the longitudinal SABRE study [13]. The data contains one cohort of 586 subjects with T1, T2 and FLAIR obtained using the same scanner (low variance) and another of 1263 with T1, T2 and FLAIR obtained from multiple scanners with multiple settings (high variance). Additionally we use a dataset of 626 patients with T1 and FLAIR obtained from multiple scanners using multiple field strengths. As no manual annotations were available for this large collection of MRI scans, the outputs of BaMoS [12], a fully unsupervised WM lesion segmentation algorithm, were quality controlled by an experienced human rater and subsequently used as silver-standard training labels. Additionally, we evaluate our trained models on a manually annotated dataset from the MICCAI 2017 White Matter Hyperintensity Challenge [1].

The split between training, validation and test sets was chosen in order to measure the ability of our method at generalizing to unseen scanners and protocols. Three separate holdouts were created, defined as follows,

Silver Protocol Holdout - ADNI: 973 subjects with silver standard labels.
Gold Protocol Holdout - MICCAI2017: 60 subjects with human rater labels.
Mixed Holdout - Random 10% subset of the full data minus Silver/Gold.

Overall there was a 80/10/10 split between training, validation and test using the 2474 subjects that are not in the gold or silver protocol holdouts. All four models described in Sect. 2 were trained with this subset.

Table 1. Dice scores of the different models on different combinations of available modalities. Modalities present are denoted by ● and those that are missing are denoted by ○. Bold numbers are results which outperform the baseline model, HeMIS, with statistical significance $p < 0.01$ as provided by a Wilcoxon test. Presentation of table inspired by the one in [6]

Mixed Holdout

Modalities			Dice Score				Avg. Symmetric Distance			
T_1	T_2	F	HeMIS	Soft	Hard	Online	HeMIS	Soft	Hard	Online
●	●	●	0.47	**0.51**	0.48	**0.54**	0.71	0.65	0.71	1.9
●	●	○	0.3	**0.39**	0.3	0.24	2.32	**1.92**	2.36	4.21
○	●	●	0.26	**0.32**	**0.26**	**0.4**	0.77	0.82	0.76	3.32
●	○	●	0.44	**0.45**	**0.45**	**0.52**	0.61	0.63	0.62	2.06
●	○	○	0.1	**0.1**	0.1	**0.19**	3.42	3.76	3.51	4.48
○	●	○	0.08	**0.08**	0.07	**0.09**	4.07	4.13	4.53	7.48
○	○	●	0.16	**0.18**	**0.16**	**0.41**	0.56	0.61	**0.54**	3.31

Modalities			Dice Score				Avg. Symmetric Distance			
T_1	T_2	F	HeMIS	Soft	Hard	Online	HeMIS	Soft	Hard	Online
			Silver Protocol Holdout							
●	○	●	0.48	0.46	0.46	0.44	0.68	0.72	1.12	3.52
●	○	○	0.11	0.11	0.08	**0.21**	0.79	0.79	1.63	5.17
○	○	●	0.25	0.16	0.24	**0.5**	0.69	**0.68**	0.8	2.77
			Gold Protocol Holdout							
●	○	●	0.59	0.64	0.62	0.61	0.76	**0.57**	0.72	1.18
●	○	○	0.41	0.35	0.42	**0.47**	0.8	**0.44**	**0.77**	2.18
○	○	●	0.38	0.38	0.26	**0.45**	1.01	1.75	20.75	3.63

For the mixed holdout it was found that the classification accuracy was 99% between all three modalities. For unseen protocols the accuracy was lower, 88% for ADNI and 87% for MICCAI17 which showed that the inter-scanner variance was harder to model than the inter-subject variance. For each of the holdout sets, results are presented on all possible subsets of the available modalities. The quantitative and qualitative results are shown in Table 1 and Fig. 2, respectively. The brains shown are selected from the 95%, 50% and 20% percentile of Dice score on the dataset holdout for a model shown all available modalities. We note that the samples of very high Dice score are often the ones with large lesions which the algorithm has managed to capture well and there is poor performance when the contrast settings are significantly different.

We utilise the Wilcoxon signed-rank test to test whether the Dice scores from each of our models outperforms the baseline (HeMIS). Bold values in Tables 1 denotes that the model is better than HeMIS with a statistical significance of $p < 0.01$. We compare ground truths and predictions using the Dice score as well as the average symmetric distance in order to provide a geometric evaluation.

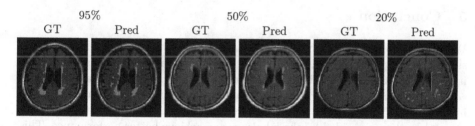

Fig. 2. Qualitative results showing white matter lesion segmentations on the mixed holdout set. Images show the ground truth on the left and the network predictions on the right. Red shows the predicted segmentation. The results were chosen to highlight the 95th, 50th, and 20th percentile in terms of Dice score for a model which is trained on all available scans but does not use modality labels.

4 Discussion

The "hard" setting converges to HeMIS as the accuracy of the modality classifier tends to 1. This is observed in practice. Note that the results of HeMIS are similar to "hard" in the mixed holdout set where the modality classifier has had access to the test set distribution and consistently worse in the Silver Protocol holdout. It does comparatively better on the Gold Protocol as the modality classifier has better performance on these scans than on Silver. The "soft" version matches or improves on the performance of HeMIS and "hard" on the mixed holdout, but does not outperform HeMIS on other holdouts. The fact that "soft" outperforms "hard" is evidence towards our hypothesis that mixing the input images can lead to better representations which improve performance on a visual task.

This can be interpreted as a coarse attention mechanism as the transformation from X to $\hat{X}$ is linear with few degrees of freedom.

The "online" model outperforms the baseline in the mixed holdout set with statistical significance in 6/7 cases when using the Dice score. Although the median average symmetric distance (ASD) is higher, the average is lower in 4/7 cases with a much lower 95 percentile. There is some improvement over the baseline model even in the protocol holdout but the gains seen in Dice score are not reflected in the ASD. Qualitatively this is explained by the "online" method overpredicting the positive class leading to a higher Dice score and yet missing lesions altogether leading to a larger ASD. This gives us insights as to how we can improve the model.

Future work will extend the "online" model to an unsupervised setting in terms of scan labels. This is appealing not only due to the lack of modality labels currently available in certain hospital databases but also in order to go *beyond* the information contained in the modality label and towards a representation which is more true to the underlying physical structure.

5   Conclusion

We have presented PIMMS, a segmentation algorithm for MRI scans which simultaneously addresses the problem of missing modalities and missing modality labels in a clinical setting. We present three variants which all include a convolutional neural network and are trained to perform modality classification in a supervised setting. We argue that by mixing the input modalities in ratios other than those provided by the labels we can achieve better performance. This could be due to more accurately capturing the underlying distribution of physical quantities, but future work is needed to make this claim. Evidence is presented with statistical significance which suggests that a model which mixes inputs can perform better than one which does not with all other factors kept identical.

The results show that the modality classifier almost replicates modality labels when trained and tested on the same protocol while the categorical accuracy reaches 88% when protocols differ at training and testing times. Our model serves as a proof of concept for a system that could utilize all the MR scans associated with a patient in a hospital and provide accurate segmentation predictions.

Acknowledgements. We gratefully acknowledge the support of NVIDIA Corporation with the donation of the Titan Xp GPU used for this research. Zach Eaton-Rosen is supported by the EPSRC Doctoral Prize. Carole H. Sudre is supported by the Biomedical Junior Fellowship from Alzheimer's Society. Parashkev Nachev is funded by the Wellcome Trust and the UCLH NIHR Biomedical Research Centre. Jorge Cardoso is funded by Wellcome Trust.

References

1. White Matter Segmentation Grand Challenge at MICCAI 2017
2. Chartsias, A.: Multimodal MR synthesis via modality-invariant latent representation. IEEE Trans. Med. Imaging **37**(3), 803–814 (2017)
3. Fischl, B., et al.: Sequence-independent segmentation of magnetic resonance images. Neuroimage **23**, S69–S84 (2004)
4. Ghafoorian, M., et al.: Location sensitive deep convolutional neural networks for segmentation of white matter hyperintensities. CoRR abs/1610.04834 (2016)
5. Gibson, E., et al.: Niftynet: a deep-learning platform for medical imaging. arXiv preprint arXiv:1709.03485 (2017)
6. Havaei, M., Guizard, N., Chapados, N., Bengio, Y.: HeMIS: hetero-modal image segmentation. In: Ourselin, S., Joskowicz, L., Sabuncu, M.R., Unal, G., Wells, W. (eds.) MICCAI 2016. LNCS, vol. 9901, pp. 469–477. Springer, Cham (2016). https://doi.org/10.1007/978-3-319-46723-8_54
7. He, K., Zhang, X., Ren, S., Sun, J.: Identity mappings in deep residual networks. In: Leibe, B., Matas, J., Sebe, N., Welling, M. (eds.) ECCV 2016. LNCS, vol. 9908, pp. 630–645. Springer, Cham (2016). https://doi.org/10.1007/978-3-319-46493-0_38
8. Iglesias, J.E., Konukoglu, E., Zikic, D., Glocker, B., Van Leemput, K., Fischl, B.: Is synthesizing MRI contrast useful for inter-modality analysis? In: Mori, K., Sakuma, I., Sato, Y., Barillot, C., Navab, N. (eds.) MICCAI 2013. LNCS, vol. 8149, pp. 631–638. Springer, Heidelberg (2013). https://doi.org/10.1007/978-3-642-40811-3_79
9. Jack, C.R.: The Alzheimer's disease neuroimaging initiative (ADNI): MRI methods. J. Magn. Reson. Imaging **27**(4), 685–691 (2008)
10. Karani, N., et al.: A lifelong learning approach to brain MR segmentation across scanners and protocols. arXiv:1805.10170 (2018)
11. Milletari, F., et al.: V-Net: fully convolutional neural networks for volumetric medical image segmentation. In: 3DV, pp. 565–571. IEEE (2016)
12. Sudre, C.H.: Bayesian model selection for pathological neuroimaging data applied to white matter lesion segmentation. IEEE TMI **34**(10), 2079–2102 (2015)
13. Tillin, T.: Southall and brent revisited: cohort profile of Sabre, a UK population-based comparison of cardiovascular disease and diabetes in people of European, Indian Asian and African Caribbean origins. IJEpid **41**(1), 33–42 (2010)
14. Xu, K., et al.: Show, attend and tell: neural image caption generation with visual attention. In: International Conference on Machine Learning, pp. 2048–2057 (2015)

Unsupervised Feature Learning for Outlier Detection with Stacked Convolutional Autoencoders, Siamese Networks and Wasserstein Autoencoders: Application to Epilepsy Detection

Zara Alaverdyan[✉], Jiazheng Chai, and Carole Lartizien

Univ Lyon, INSA-Lyon, Université Claude Bernard Lyon 1, UJM-Saint Etienne, CNRS, Inserm, CREATIS UMR 5220, U1206, 69621 Lyon, France
zaruhi.alaverdyan@creatis.insa-lyon.fr

Abstract. In this study we tackle the problem of detecting subtle epilepsy lesions in multiparametric (T1w, FLAIR) MR images considered as normal during a visual examination by a neurologist (MRI *negative*). We cast this problem as an outlier detection problem and adapt the framework proposed in [1]. It consists in learning a oc-SVM model for each voxel in the brain volume. We generalize this approach by proposing unsupervised deep architectures as feature extracting mechanisms in order to learn representations characterizing healthy subjects. We hypothesize that such architectures may capture features that allow to distinguish pathological voxels from the normal cases used in the training. As such, we exploit and compare three architectures, a novel configuration of siamese networks, stacked convolutional autoencoders and Wasserstein autoencoders. The models are trained on 75 healthy subjects and validated on 21 patients (with 18 MRI *negatives*) with confirmed epilepsy lesions achieving the best sensitivity of 62%.

Keywords: Wasserstein autoencoders · Siamese networks · Unsupervised learning · Epilepsy detection · Anomaly detection

1 Introduction

Computer aided diagnosis (CAD) systems assist clinicians in various tasks such as organ or lesion segmentation, detection of abnormal regions in a medical image, etc. The vast majority of the existing CAD systems are built upon methods developed in supervised settings, using either manually designed features or currently ubiquitous deep learning architectures. However, when the number of labeled pathological cases in the training set is not sufficient to account for the complexity of the task, supervised learning becomes infeasible. To bypass the problem of insufficient labeled data, some authors formulate lesion detection

© Springer Nature Switzerland AG 2018
D. Stoyanov et al. (Eds.): DLMIA 2018/ML-CDS 2018, LNCS 11045, pp. 210–217, 2018.
https://doi.org/10.1007/978-3-030-00889-5_24

tasks in semi-supervised settings, by accounting for both labeled and unlabeled data in a deep architecture for MS lesion segmentation [2] or by exploiting weak labels (the number of lesions in a scan) to detect enlarged perivascular spaces in the basal ganglia [3].

Another recent tendency goes even further and casts lesion detection problem as an anomaly detection task. Anomaly detection, also referred to as outlier detection, consists in learning the boundary of the normal class in order to later identify the observations that lay outside of it. Over the recent years the challenging topic of outlier detection has been studied extensively and many algorithms have been proposed for outlier detection depending on the nature of the data and the type of anomalies [4]. In computer vision, recent works investigated approaches based on deep architectures such as autoencoders or Generative Adverserial Networks (GANs) coupled with various outlier detection algorithms [5]. In the medical imaging domain, [6,7] proposed a model defining a score function that measures how anomalous a given sample is based on the reconstruction and discrimination losses estimated by a GAN architecture trained on normal samples only. In [8,9], a latent representation of normal samples is first learned with deep unsupervised networks and then fed to a one-class support vector machine (oc-SVM) model to estimate the boundaries of the normal examples.

In this work we build on the framework proposed in [9] for the challenging application of epilepsy lesion detection in patients with *MRI negative* exams, meaning that the lesions were not visually identified by clinicians on the MR scans [10]. We propose to exploit three unsupervised deep learning architectures as feature extracting mechanisms in the outlier detection context. We consider stacked convolutional autoencoders, a novel configuration of siamese networks [9] and Wasserstein autoencoders [11] that have been shown to combine the advantages of both standard generative adversarial networks (GAN) and variational autoencoders (VAE) in generating synthetic natural images without compromising the stability of the training. We couple these architectures with voxel-level oc-SVM models and compare their performances on the epilepsy lesion detection task.

2   Method

2.1   Unsupervised Feature Extraction with Autoencoders

The first step of the proposed system is to learn patch-level representations of healthy subjects by exploiting the three types of architectures below.

Stacked Convolutional Autoencoders (sCAE) are a variation of autoencoders that first map the input $\mathbf{x} \in \mathcal{X}$ to a latent representation space $\mathcal{Z}$ through a series of convolutional and max-pooling operations (encoder E) and later map it back to the original input space with a series of de-convolutions and up-poolings by producing a reconstruction $\tilde{\mathbf{x}}$ of the input (decoder G). The

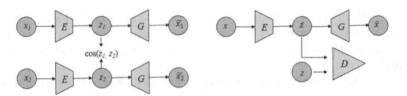

Fig. 1. Left: Siamese neural network composed of stacked convolutional autoencoders as sub-networks (sCAE). The input consists of a pair of patches $(\mathbf{x_1}, \mathbf{x_2})$ of 2 different subjects centered at the same voxel in the brain. The encoder E maps $\mathbf{x}$ to the latent representation $\mathbf{z}$ while the decoder G maps it back to the input space producing a reconstruction $\tilde{\mathbf{x}}$. Right: Wasserstein autoencoder (WAE) composed of an encoder E, a decoder G and an adversary discriminator D.

parameters are iteratively updated to minimize the deviation between the output $\tilde{\mathbf{x}}$ and the input $\mathbf{x}$. A sCAE is illustrated on Fig. 1 as the top sub-network of the architecture on the left.

Regularized Siamese Autoencoders (rSN), as proposed in [9], consist of two identical (same architecture, shared parameters) stacked convolutional autoencoders with K hidden layers and a cost module (shown on Fig. 1). The siamese network receives a pair of patches $(\mathbf{x_1}, \mathbf{x_2})$ at input, then each patch is propagated through the corresponding subnetwork yielding representations $(\mathbf{z_1}, \mathbf{z_2})$ respectively in the middle layer which are then passed to the loss function 1 below. The network is trained to maximize the cosine similarity of the representations of patches centered at the same voxel and belonging to different healthy subjects, at the same time imposing the subnetworks to produce reconstructions close to the original input. The loss function for a single pair hence is:

$$L_{rSN}(\mathbf{x_1}, \mathbf{x_2}; \Theta_{rSN}) = \sum_{t=1}^{2} ||\mathbf{x_t} - \tilde{\mathbf{x}}_\mathbf{t}||_2^2 - \alpha \cdot cos(\mathbf{z_1}, \mathbf{z_2}) \qquad (1)$$

where $\tilde{\mathbf{x}}_\mathbf{t}$ is the reconstructed output of the patch $\mathbf{x_t}$ produced by sub-network t while $\mathbf{z_t}$ is its (vectorized) representation in the middle layer and α is a coefficient that controls the tradeoff between the two terms. Θ_{rSN} denotes the parameter set.

Wasserstein Autoencoders (WAE) have been recently introduced as generative models combining the best properties of Wasserstein GANs and Variational Autoencoders [12]. As shown on Fig. 1, a Wasserstein auto-encoder consists of three components: an encoder E mapping an input patch from the data space $\mathcal{X}$ to the latent space $\mathcal{Z}$, a decoder G mapping a latent code from the latent space $\mathcal{Z}$ to the data space $\mathcal{X}$, and an adversary network D that tries to distinguish the prior distribution of the latent code P_Z from the latent distribution Q_Z produced by the encoder. The resulting loss function can be expressed as

$$L_{WAE}(X;\Theta_{WAE}) = \frac{1}{N}\sum_{i=1}^{N} c(\mathbf{x_i}, \tilde{\mathbf{x}}_i) + \lambda \cdot D_Z(P_z, Q_z) \tag{2}$$

where D_Z measures the discrepancy between a given distribution P_z and Q_z for the dataset $X = \{\mathbf{x_i}\}_{1,..,N}$ and c measures the reconstruction error. λ is a coefficient that controls the tradeoff between the two terms and Θ_{WAE} denotes the parameter set. The generic form of the WAE loss allows different reconstruction error functions and regularizers. We used the standard reconstruction error $c(\mathbf{x_i}, \tilde{\mathbf{x}}_i) = ||\mathbf{x} - \tilde{\mathbf{x}}_i||_2^2$ and the Jenssen-Shanon divergence as D_Z.

2.2 Voxel-Level Outlier Detection with Oc-SVM Classifiers

A oc-SVM classifier [13] is an outlier detection method that seeks to find the optimal hyperplane that separates the given points from the origin in a dot product space defined by some kernel function ϕ. The latent representations $\mathbf{z}$ learnt by each of the networks proposed above was used to train oc-SVM classifiers at voxel level. For a given voxel v_i, the associated oc-SVM model C_i is trained on the matrix $M_i = [\mathbf{z_{i1}}, ..., \mathbf{z_{in}}]$ where $\mathbf{z_{ij}}$ is the feature vector corresponding to the patch centered at v_i of subject j and n is the number of subjects. For a new patient, each voxel v_i is matched against the corresponding model C_i and is assigned the signed score output by C_i. This yields a *distance map* D_p for the given patient. This map is later normalized by the estimated voxel-level standard deviation (computed on the healthy subjects with 1-fold evaluation). We keep the most negative scores up to the score corresponding to a pre-chosen *p-value* in the patient's distance score distribution and apply a 26-connectivity rule to identify connected components which we refer to as *clusters* (and the map - *cluster map*). The *clusters* are what we refer to as *detections* by the proposed method. The clusters are then ranked according to the size and the average score of their voxels. Such ranking favors large clusters with the most negative average score. Finally, we keep the top n detections and discard the rest. When a cluster overlaps significantly with the ground truth of a patient we consider it a *true positive* and *false positive* otherwise.

3 Experiments and Results

3.1 Dataset Description and Pre-processing

The study was approved by our institutional review board with approval numbers 2012-A00516-37 and 2014-019 B and a written consent was obtained for all participants.

Our database consists MR images (T1-weighted and FLAIR) of 75 healthy subjects and 21 patients acquired on a 1.5T Sonata scanner (Siemens Healthcare, Erlangen, Germany). All the volumes were normalized to the standard brain template of the Montreal Neurological Institute (MNI) [14] using a voxel size of $1 \times 1 \times 1$ mm with the unified segmentation algorithm [15] implemented in

SPM12 also correcting for magnetic field inhomogeneities. This spatial normalization assures a voxel-level correspondence between the subjects. We removed top 1% intensities and scaled the images between 0 and 1 at image level before feeding the patches to the networks.

The method has been validated on 21 patients admitted to our clinical center with confirmed medically intractable epileptogenic lesions: 2 of them were visually detected on the FLAIR images and only 1 lesion was identified on both T1w and FLAIR scans. The remaining 18 patients are confirmed *MRI negative* patients. The *MRI negative* patients had surgeries and have been seizure-free since. The ground truth annotations used in the performance evaluation were obtained by outlining the visible zones of the *MRI positive* patients and by combining the information of post-surgical MR images and the resected zones for *MRI negative* patients.

3.2   Feature Extraction with sCAE, rSN and WAE

As shown on Fig. 1, the three architectures consist of the same encoder E and decoder G (the stacked convolutional autoencoder is identical to the upper sub-network of the siamese network). The architecture details are shown on Fig. 2a. The encoder E takes as input an $18 \times 18 \times 2$ patch (the third dimension corresponds to the two modalities-T1 and FLAIR) and outputs a latent representation z of dimension 64. LeakyReLU was used as activation in the WAE discriminator with scale 0.02 for negative input values. ReLU was used in the generator and the encoder (except for the last layer of G where sigmoid is applied). We varied the λ parameter values in loss 2 among 1, 5, 10, 20 and 100.

All the three networks were trained on the same data set of patches extracted from healthy subjects' images with a stride 8. In the case of the siamese network, each patch of a subject was randomly matched with a 'similar pair' among the remaining subjects. The α parameter in the loss 1 is set to 0 during the first 10 epochs, then grows linearly for 15 epochs until it reaches 0.5 and then plateaus for 5 more epochs. The Adam optimizer was used with the learning rate set to 0.001 with a training batch size of 128.

3.3   oc-SVM Classifier Design

We used oc-SVM classifiers with RBF kernel by setting the kernel width γ for each voxel v_i individually to the estimated median of the standardized euclidean pairwise distances of the corresponding matrix M_i (see Sect. 2.2) as in [16]. The allowed fraction of outliers for all models was set to 0.03 (this parameter does not impact the results).

3.4   Results and Discussion

Below we evaluate the performance of the system on 21 patients with confirmed epilepsy lesions. Figure 2b shows the performance obtained with each of the architectures: the y-axis shows the detection rate among the top n clusters, ranked according to their average score and size. The rSN features seem to outperform the features learnt with WAE and sCAE, WAE performing better than sCAE for certain values of λ ($\lambda = 1$ and $\lambda = 100$ did not yield a good performance). The latter confirms our hypothesis that the reconstruction error, when enhanced with a regularization, fits better to the anomaly detection context. The WAE performance is still inferior to that of rSN which might be due to a limitation of the model itself or the experimental choice of the hyper-parameters (we can see how the performance is affected by the choice of λ; the value 20 is less successful, probably since it prioritizes too much the adversarial term; the value 100 entirely degraded the results and, hence, is not shown). Figure 3 shows the output of the system with the considered architectures. The patient has a visible lesion outlined in green. The detection quality varies, especially WAE with $\lambda = 20$ almost misses the lesion.

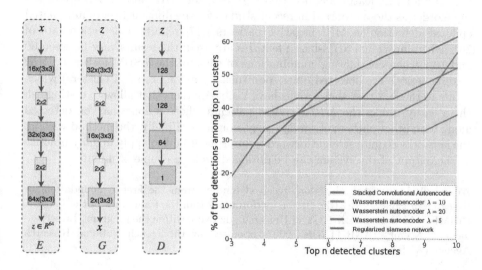

Fig. 2. (a) The encoder, decoder and discriminator architectures respectively. Red/green/violet boxes denote convolutional/deconvolutional/fully connected layers respectively. Orange/yellow boxes stand for maxpooling/uppooling. (b) The performance of the CAD system with sCAE, WAE and rSN features. x-axis: Top n clusters, y-axis: Detection rate among the top n clusters. Ranking based on average score and size. (Color figure online)

Unlike most recent studies that focus on a single epilepsy type (FCD) and use handcrafted features characterizing it [1,17–20], our method seeks to find more complex features in an unsupervised manner in order to identify lesions with rather unknown signatures. Naturally, such an approach, when applied to a specific pathology, is likely to produce more false positive detections. Although a fair comparison with the published results is difficult because of the differences in the patient groups, the obtained results (62% sensitivity for 9 false positives

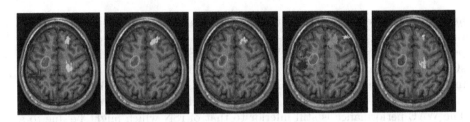

Fig. 3. CAD output for a MRI positive patient with sCAE, WAE $\lambda = 5$, WAE $\lambda = 10$, WAE $\lambda = 20$ and rSN features respectively. The images show the maximum intensity projections of the cluster maps onto an MRI transverse slice (ground truth is outlined in green circles). The maps show the top 6, 2, 2, 6 and 3 clusters, respectively. (Color figure online)

per scan for rSN features and between 52–58% for WAE and sCAE) are of the same order as those reported in recent studies for the difficult task of automated epilepsy detection in MRI negative patients ([17] reports a detection rate of 70% when individual SBM-based features are used; the results vary between 60 and 70% when considering combinations of some of these SBM features). *MRI positive* lesions are detected quite soon (usually among top 2–4 clusters) which is due to the fact that such lesions have visible markers that allow to distinguish them easily unlike the *MRI negative* patients whose lesions may be detected along with other outliers of similar 'suspiciousness'. Finally, the method with all the networks is quite straightforward to implement and to apply in daily practice as the output of the system can be obtained under a couple of minutes.

Acknowledgements. This work received funding from the French Foundation for Research in Epilepsy (FFRE). It was performed within the framework of the LABEX PRIMES (ANR-11-LABX-0063) of Université de Lyon, within the program "Investissements d'Avenir" (ANR-11-IDEX-0007) operated by the French National Research Agency (ANR).

References

1. El Azami, M., Hammers, A., Jung, J., Costes, N., Bouet, R., Lartizien, C.: Detection of lesions underlying intractable epilepsy on t1-weighted MRI as an outlier detection problem. PloS ONE **11**(9), e0161498 (2016)
2. Baur, C., Albarqouni, S., Navab, N.: Semi-supervised deep learning for fully convolutional networks. In: Descoteaux, M., Maier-Hein, L., Franz, A., Jannin, P., Collins, D.L., Duchesne, S. (eds.) MICCAI 2017. LNCS, vol. 10435, pp. 311–319. Springer, Cham (2017). https://doi.org/10.1007/978-3-319-66179-7_36
3. Dubost, F., et al.: GP-Unet: lesion detection from weak labels with a 3D regression network. In: Descoteaux, M., Maier-Hein, L., Franz, A., Jannin, P., Collins, D.L., Duchesne, S. (eds.) MICCAI 2017. LNCS, vol. 10435, pp. 214–221. Springer, Cham (2017). https://doi.org/10.1007/978-3-319-66179-7_25
4. Chandola, V., Banerjee, A., Kumar, V.: Anomaly detection: a survey. ACM Comput. Surv. **41**(3), 15:1–15:58 (2009)

5. Kiran, B.R., Thomas, D.M., Parakkal, R.: An overview of deep learning based methods for unsupervised and semi-supervised anomaly detection in videos. J. Imaging **4**(2), 36 (2018)
6. Schlegl, T., Seeböck, P., Waldstein, S.M., Schmidt-Erfurth, U., Langs, G.: Unsupervised Anomaly detection with generative adversarial networks to guide marker discovery. In: Niethammer, M., et al. (eds.) IPMI 2017. LNCS, vol. 10265, pp. 146–157. Springer, Cham (2017). https://doi.org/10.1007/978-3-319-59050-9_12
7. Zenati, H., Foo, C.S., Lecouat, B., Manek, G., Chandrasekhar, V.R.: Efficient GAN-based anomaly detection
8. Erfani, S.M., Rajasegarar, S., Karunasekera, S., Leckie, C.: High-dimensional and large-scale anomaly detection using a linear one-class svm with deep learning. Pattern Recogn. **58**, 121–134 (2016)
9. Alaverdyan, Z., Jung, J., Bouet, R., Lartizien, C.: Regularized Siamese neural network for unsupervised outlier detection on brain multiparametric magnetic resonance imaging: application to epilepsy lesion screening. In: First Conference on Medical Imaging with Deep Learning (MIDL 2018)
10. Kini, L.G., Gee, J.C., Litt, B.: Computational analysis in epilepsy neuroimaging: a survey of features and methods. Neuroimage **11**, 515–529 (2016)
11. Tolstikhin, I., Bousquet, O., Gelly, S., Schoelkopf, B.: Wasserstein auto-encoders. arXiv preprint arXiv:1711.01558 (2017)
12. Tolstikhin, I., Bousquet, O., Gelly, S., Schoelkopf, B.: Wasserstein auto-encoders. ArXiv e-prints, November 2017
13. Schölkopf, B., Platt, J.C., Shawe-Taylor, J., Smola, A.J., Williamson, R.C.: Estimating the support of a high-dimensional distribution. Neural Comput. **13**(7), 1443–1471 (2001)
14. Mazziotta, J., et al.: A probabilistic atlas and reference system for the human brain: International Consortium for Brain Mapping (ICBM). Philos. Trans. Roy. Soc. Lond. B Biol. Sci. **356**(1412), 1293–1322 (2001)
15. Ashburner, J., Friston, K.: Unified segmentation. Neuroimage **26**, 839–851 (2005)
16. Caputo, B., Sim, K., Furesjo, F., Smola, A.: Appearance-based object recognition using SVMs: which kernel should I use? In: Proceedings of NIPS Workshop on Statistical Methods for Computational Experiments in Visual Processing and Computer Vision, vol. 2002. Whistler (2002)
17. Ahmed, B., Thesen, T., Blackmon, K.E., Kuzniekcy, R., Devinsky, O., Brodley, C.E.: Decrypting "cryptogenic" epilepsy: semi-supervised hierarchical conditional random fields for detecting cortical lesions in MRI-negative patients. J. Mach. Learn. Res. **17**(112), 1–30 (2016)
18. Thesen, T.: Detection of epileptogenic cortical malformations with surface-based MRI morphometry. PloS ONE **6**(2), 16430 (2011)
19. Hong, S.-J., Kim, H., Schrader, D., Bernasconi, N., Bernhardt, B.C., Bernasconi, A.: Automated detection of cortical dysplasia type II in MRI-negative epilepsy. Neurology **83**(1), 48–55 (2014)
20. Gill, R.S., et al.: Automated detection of epileptogenic cortical malformations using multimodal MRI. In: Cardoso, M.J., et al. (eds.) DLMIA/ML-CDS -2017. LNCS, vol. 10553, pp. 349–356. Springer, Cham (2017). https://doi.org/10.1007/978-3-319-67558-9_40

Semi-automated Extraction of Crohns Disease MR Imaging Markers Using a 3D Residual CNN with Distance Prior

Yechiel Lamash[✉], Sila Kurugol, and Simon K. Warfield

Boston Children's Hospital and Harvard Medical School, Boston, USA
shilikster@gmail.com

Abstract. We propose a 3D residual convolutional neural network (CNN) algorithm with an integrated distance prior for segmenting the small bowel lumen and wall to enable extraction of pediatric Crohns disease (pCD) imaging markers from T1-weighted contrast-enhanced MR images. Our proposed segmentation framework enables, for the first time, to quantitatively assess luminal narrowing and dilation in CD aimed at optimizing surgical decisions as well as analyzing bowel wall thickness and tissue enhancement for assessment of response to therapy. Given seed points along the bowel lumen, the proposed algorithm automatically extracts 3D image patches centered on these points and a distance map from the interpolated centerline. These 3D patches and corresponding distance map are jointly used by the proposed residual CNN architecture to segment the lumen and the wall, and to extract imaging markers. Due to lack of available training data, we also propose a novel and efficient semi-automated segmentation algorithm based on graph-cuts technique as well as a software tool for quickly editing labeled data that was used to train our proposed CNN model. The method which is based on curved planar reformation of the small bowel is also useful for visualizing, manually refining, and measuring pCD imaging markers. In preliminary experiments, our CNN network obtained Dice coefficients of $75 \pm 18\%$, $81 \pm 8\%$ and $97 \pm 2\%$ for the lumen, wall and background, respectively.

1 Introduction

Magnetic resonance enterography (MRE) has emerged as a most effective method for imaging the small bowel in patients with Crohns disease (CD) [1]. Extracting CD biomarkers is essential for staging disease, selecting treatment, and assessing therapeutic response. Moreover, our ability to segment diseased bowel will facilitate automated computation of quantitative imaging markers such as length of involvement, wall thickness, lumen narrowing, stricture length, upstream dilation and tissue contrast enhancement. Several methods [2–5] have been proposed for segmenting the small bowel wall. However, all these methods segment the wall and lumen together from their background instead of each compartment alone. In addition, they do not provide the small bowel's tube structure that is

© Springer Nature Switzerland AG 2018
D. Stoyanov et al. (Eds.): DLMIA 2018/ML-CDS 2018, LNCS 11045, pp. 218–226, 2018.
https://doi.org/10.1007/978-3-030-00889-5_25

necessary for computing disease markers such as wall thickness or lumen narrowing. Instead they mark disjoint tissue segments with Crohns disease. Deep learning algorithms, in particular, convolutional neural networks, have rapidly become a methodology of choice for analyzing medical images [6]. Thanks to its unique capability of learning hierarchical feature representations solely from data, deep learning has achieved record-breaking performance in a variety of artificial intelligence applications and grand challenges [7]. Such networks generally have large number of parameters and training them requires a correspondingly large dataset. However, there is not enough publicly available datasets and it is labor intensive to manually label images for segmentation. Moreover, in our problem specifically, there is no training data available at all.

Our first contribution in this work is the development of an efficient software platform for semi-automated segmentation and labeling of pCD accomplished with curved planar reformation (CPR) of small bowel segments. Our proposed software platform generates segmentation of the bowel wall and lumen using a graph-cuts algorithm given a series of seed points located on the lumens centerline. The tool also allows for efficient and quick manual editing of the segmentation results on straightened CPR views as well as visualizing the entire diseased bowel region in a stretched CPR view. We used this semi-automated tool to generate training data for our proposed segmentation algorithm. Our second contribution is a 3D residual CNN network with a distance prior for improved segmentation of the bowel lumen and wall, and extraction of quantitative imaging markers.

2 Method

2.1 Efficient Semi-automated Software for Generating Labeled Training Data for Pediatric Crohn's Disease

To generate a labeled dataset efficiently, we perform the following steps shown in Fig. 1: First, we generate a CPR platform that flattens the small bowel segment. Next, we use a graph cut segmentation [8,9] to obtain an initial segmentation of the bowel wall boundaries. We then manually refine the segmentation contours on straightened CPR images using the proposed tool. Last, we generate a tetrahedral mesh to transfer the segmentations represented by the contours in the straightened CPR views into a volumetric representation. The sections below describe each of these steps.

Generation of CPR Views for the Small Bowel. The first step entails placing seed points along the lumens centerline. We developed a practical and robust platform to perform this task such that seeds can be placed in coronal, sagittal and axial views that are automatically synchronized to the users cursor location. This enables the operator to select seed points in the most visible cross-section along the curved lumen. In the event the lumen is completely obstructed, we select seed points in the middle of the obstruction. We then interpolate between the seed points to obtain a curve $r(t) = [x(t), y(t), z(t)]$. Next, we perform arclength parameterization [10] to obtain an equally sampled curve. For generating a stretched CPR view, we perform the following steps: (1) select a plane that transverses through the two extreme points of the centerline as well as an additional, interactively selected point; (2) project the curve onto that plane; (3) perform arclength parameterization [10] of the projected curve; and (4) interpolate the stretched CPR image by traversing along the projected curve at equal speed where each step is a ray perpendicular to the projected curve.

For straightened CPR view, we set the Frenet-Serret frame [11] along the curve and interpolate images on the curves normal planes. Before calculating the Frenet-Serret frame vectors, we applied Savitzky-Golay filtering [12] to smooth the centerline curve as well as the orthogonal vectors along it.

Graph Cut Segmentation. A graph cut algorithm is used to segment the bowel lumen and wall in the CPR volume. Due to the axis-symmetric representation of the bowel in the reconstructed straightened CPR volume, we define the connectivity of the graph to be between pixels represented in cylindrical coordinates $[r, z, \theta]$. We therefore sample straightened CPR images every 5 degrees to generate a volume where each image represents a slice that passes through the center at a specific angle θ. Using this representation, we segment the volume into five classes: upper background, upper wall, lumen, lower wall, and lower background. After obtaining the segmentation results, we extract the contours of the wall and the lumen and then manually refine the results using the visual interface. The editing is performed on six discrete angles and with interpolation in between.

Projection of the Labeling onto Coronal Images. We use a method similar to [13]. Given the segmentation boundaries in the CPR view, we construct a tetrahedral mesh. We then assign the voxels of each tetrahedron in the mesh with either lumen or wall label. To do so, we perform the following: Given a tetrahedron T, any point $p \in T$ divides it into four sub tetrahedrons such that the vector e of the point p with respect to vertex v can be expressed by $e = \alpha e_i + \beta e_j + \gamma e_k$, where the barycentric coordinates $(\alpha, \beta, \gamma) \in (0, 1)$ are the volume ratios between each sub-tetrahedron and tetrahedron T.

$$\alpha = \frac{\det(e, e_j, e_k)}{\det(e_i, e_j, e_k)}; \beta = \frac{\det(e_i, e, e_k)}{\det(e_i, e_j, e_k)}; \gamma = \frac{\det(e_i, e_j, e)}{\det(e_i, e_j, e_k)} \tag{1}$$

e_i, e_j, e_k are the tetrahedron edge vectors with respect to vertex v.

To find the inner voxels surrounded by each tetrahedron, we take the grid pixels of the minimal box that bounds the tetrahedron and looked up the pixels whose barycentric coordinates apply: $\alpha, \beta, \gamma \geq 0$ and $\alpha + \beta + \gamma \leq 1$.

2.2 Segmentation of the Bowel Lumen and Wall Using a 3D Residual CNN with Distance Prior

Our motivation for using a 3D CNN segmentation algorithm is based on the observation that the highly variable bowel appearance and shape requires a

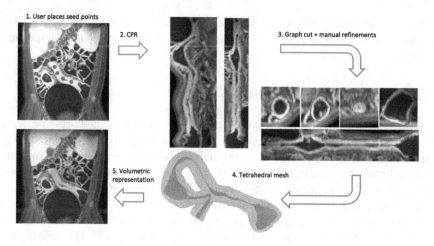

Fig. 1. Generation of labeled dataset of Crohns disease segments.

supervised algorithm that can learn feature representations and a classifier from a large set of augmented training patches for solving this difficult problem. We perform the segmentation in the original coronal image volumes instead of using CPR views to eliminate the dependency of the performance on the initial centerline delineation. The segmentation of the small bowel is challenging because one diseased section of the wall can be adjacent to either part of the same diseased segment, or part of a distal healthy segment. In addition, the lumen and the mesentery might have similar intensities such that from a patch perspective, it may be unclear whether a region is inside the lumen or between two walls. To overcome this ambiguity, we added a distance map prior to the input data. Accordingly, the distance prior is computed as the shortest distance of each voxel from the interpolated centerline seed points-positioned in the lumen.

Our CNN network, shown in Fig. 2, has a 3D fully connected U-Net architecture [14] with residual units [15]. The network has three contracting layers; three expanding layers; and a final convolution layer (with kernel size one) followed by softmax. Each residual layer has two sets of batch normalization (BN), leaky ReLU activation, and convolution as suggested by [15]. Down-sampling and up-sampling of features is done using strided convolutions and transpose convolutions, respectively. The input to the network consists of two channel patches $64 \times 64 \times 32$ in size. The first channel patches were taken from the contrast-enhanced T1-weighted MR images after resampling to isotropic resolution. Before cropping the patches, the images are normalized to have zero mean and a standard deviation equal to 1. In the training, the patches were centered on randomly selected lumen or wall pixels. We scale the distances to the range of $[-1, 1]$ after truncating the max value to 32. We trained the network with a stochastic gradient descent with momentum of 0.9 and L_2 regularization with $\lambda = 10^{-3}$. To augment the training data, we added Gaussian noise, random rotations over the x-axis, random scaling of $\pm 10\%$, and random flips in each of the three dimensions. The augmentation generated >2 million patches - each contains a short tube segment of the small bowel in an arbitrary shape and orientation.

3   Experiments and Results

We used contrast-enhanced T1-weighted MR images of 23 pediatric patients with Crohns disease. The images were scanned in coronal planes with voxel size of about 0.75 × 0.75 × 2 mm. We interpolated the image to isotropic sampling of 0.75 m before the analysis. We generated a labeled dataset of the small bowel lumen and wall as described above. We divided the dataset into a training set of 15 patients and a test set of 8 patients from which we extract 3D patches for training and testing the proposed segmentation network, respectively. To evaluate the accuracy of the segmentation, we computed the Dice Similarity Coefficient (DSC) of the lumen wall and background classes. In addition, we computed the distances between the CNN boundary contours and the label boundary contours.

Figure 3 demonstrates the results of the proposed lumen and wall segmentation algorithm on 4 patients compared to the ground truth labels in the original coronal plane and after reformation of the segmentation results into the straightened CPR views. Table 1 summarizes the performance of our model in segmenting the small bowel lumen and wall. When integrating the proposed distance prior into the proposed 3D Residual U-Nets architecture, the Dice coefficients increased from 55% to 75% for the lumen and from 60% to 81% for the wall segment. The median distance between the automated and manually labeled contours reduced from 1.70 mm to 0.85 mm and from 1.6 mm to 1.0 mm for the lumen-wall and wall-background boundaries, respectively.

Figure 4 shows surface rendering of diseased bowel loops and their corresponding imaging markers from 4 patients. The upper row shows the lumen radius and the lower row shows the thickness of the bowel wall. Figure 4 cases (a) and (d) shows diseased areas with strictures that have a very narrow lumen

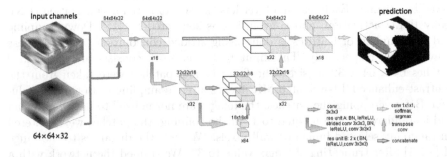

Fig. 2. The networks input patches and its architecture. (To better demonstrate, the two input channels are depicted one above the other, and the residual U-Nets concatenating channels are depicted alongside one another.)

and thickened bowel wall. These markers are useful for surgical planning (a, d) and for quantitatively evaluating disease severity (b, c).

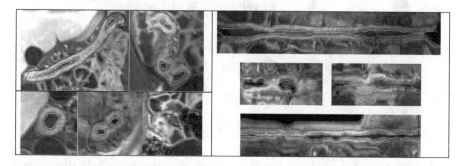

Fig. 3. The results of the proposed segmentation algorithm of the lumen and wall of 4 patients compared to the labels in coronal planes (left) and in straightened CPR views (Right). Color coding: lumen-wall contours CNN (yellow) vs. label (red). Wall-background contours CNN (blue) vs. label (green). (Color figure online)

Table 1. Performance of the network in segmenting the small bowel lumen and wall. DSC-Dice Similarity Coefficient, BD- Boundaries Distance (between the CNN result and the label).

	DSC [%] lumen	DSC [%] wall	DSC [%] back-ground	Cross entropy	Median BD [mm] lumen	Median BD [mm] wall	Average BD [mm] lumen	Average BD [mm] wall
Single input channel	55 ± 25	60 ± 17	93 ± 4	0.33	0.83 ± 2.8	1.7 ± 4.0	1.6 ± 2.8	3.4 ± 4.0
Distance prior concatenated at the final layer	70 ± 19	75 ± 10	95 ± 4	0.22	0.83 ± 1.8	1.8 ± 3.1	1.2 ± 1.8	3.1 ± 3.1
Distance channel prior (proposed)	75 ± 18	81 ± 8	97 ± 2	0.13	0.83 ± 1.5	0.85 ± 2.3	1.0 ± 1.5	1.8 ± 2.3

Table 2. Comparison to Crohns disease small bowel segmentation prior work.

Method	Provide the entire disease segment?	Provide disease mark-ers?	DSC [%] lumen	DSC [%] wall	DSC [%] back-ground	DSC [%] lumen+wall vs. background
SL [2]	No	No	N/A	N/A	N/A	86.5 ± 2.3
SS-AL [4]	No	No	N/A	N/A	N/A	92.1
AS [3]	No	No	N/A	N/A	N/A	90 ± 4
AL [5]	No	No	N/A	N/A	N/A	92.7
CNN (ours)	Yes	Yes	75 ± 18	81 ± 8	97 ± 2	N/A

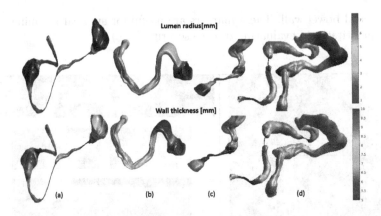

Fig. 4. Surface rendering of the lumen boundary with colormaps indicating lumen radius [mm] (upper row) and wall thickness [mm] (lower row) obtained using the proposed method. Cases (a) and (d) has diseased areas with strictures that have a very narrow lumen and a very thickened bowel wall that may indicate surgical therapy.

4   Discussion and Conclusions

We propose a novel algorithm for segmenting both the bowel lumen and wall in T1-weighted, contrast-enhanced MR images and extracting imaging markers of pediatric Crohns disease including bowel wall thickness and lumen radius. Our algorithm is based on a 3D residual CNN with a distance prior that improved the performance compared to a 3D residual CNN without the distance prior. The performance when adding the distance map as an additional channel was superior to that seen when integrating the distance prior at the final layer -an observation that implies that integrating spatial information to the learned filters will improve overall performance. Such spatial informative channels may improve the performance in other image segmentation applications as well. We observed that, there were several locations where the algorithm delineated the boundaries more accurately than the labeled data. For cases that require manual refinement, our proposed editing software enables efficient and quick manual editing of the segmentations on CPR views before computing the disease markers. All prior works with reported segmentation performance segment the wall and lumen together from their background instead of each compartment alone. These works provide small tissue segments with Crohns disease instead of tube structure and therefore cannot extract the wall thickness or lumen narrowing (Table 2). The limitation of our method, however, is the difficulty in placement of seed points along the centerline in images with high motion artifacts, insufficient bowel preparation or severe disease condition where the lumen path is barely visible. We anticipate the proposed method and the automatically extracted imaging markers will facilitate comprehensive assessment of diseased bowel lumen and wall in pediatric Crohns disease.[1]

References

1. Bruining, D.H., Zimmermann, E.M., Loftus, E.V., Sandborn, W.J., Sauer, C.G., Strong, S.A.: Consensus recommendations for evaluation, interpretation, and utilization of computed tomography and magnetic resonance enterography in patients with small bowel Crohns disease. Gastroenterology **154**(4), 1172–1194 (2018)
2. Mahapatra, D., Schueffler, P., Tielbeek, J.A.W., Buhmann, J.M., Vos, F.M.: A supervised learning based approach to detect Crohn's disease in abdominal MR volumes. In: Yoshida, H., Hawkes, D., Vannier, M.W. (eds.) ABD-MICCAI 2012. LNCS, vol. 7601, pp. 97–106. Springer, Heidelberg (2012). https://doi.org/10.1007/978-3-642-33612-6_11
3. Mahapatra, D.: Automatic detection and segmentation of Crohn's disease tissues from abdominal MRI. IEEE Trans. Med. Imaging **32**(12), 2332–2347 (2013)
4. Mahapatra, D., Schüffler, P.J., Tielbeek, J.A.W., Vos, F.M., Buhmann, J.M.: Semi-supervised and active learning for automatic segmentation of Crohn's disease. In: Mori, K., Sakuma, I., Sato, Y., Barillot, C., Navab, N. (eds.) MICCAI 2013. LNCS, vol. 8150, pp. 214–221. Springer, Heidelberg (2013). https://doi.org/10.1007/978-3-642-40763-5_27
5. Mahapatra, D., et al.: Active learning based segmentation of Crohn's disease using principles of visual saliency. In: 2014 IEEE 11th International Symposium on Biomedical Imaging (ISBI), pp. 226–229. IEEE (2014)
6. Litjens, G.: A survey on deep learning in medical image analysis. Med. Image Anal. **42**, 60–88 (2017)
7. Shen, D., Guorong, W., Suk, H.-I.: Deep learning in medical image analysis. Annu. Rev. Biomed. Eng. **19**, 221–248 (2017)
8. Boykov, Y., Funka-Lea, G.: Graph cuts and efficient ND image segmentation. Int. J. Comput. Vis. **70**(2), 109–131 (2006)
9. Bagon, S.: Matlab wrapper for graph cut, December 2006. http://www.wisdom.weizmann.ac.il/~bagon
10. Willmore, T.J.: An Introduction to Differential Geometry. Courier Corporation (2013)
11. Weatherburn, C.E.: Differential Geometry of Three Dimensions, vol. 1. Cambridge University Press, Cambridge (2016)
12. Orfanidis, S.J.: Introduction to signal processing. **7458**, 168–383 (1996). Prentice-Hall, Inc. Upper Saddle River
13. Lamash, Y., Fischer, A., Carasso, S., Lessick, J.: Strain analysis from 4-D cardiac CT image data. IEEE Trans. Biomed. Eng. **62**(2), 511–521 (2015)

---

[1] This work is supported by Crohns and Colitis Foundation of Americas Career Development Award, AGA-Boston Scientific Technology & Innovation Pilot Research Award, and the National Institute of Diabetes and Digestive and Kidney Diseases (NIDDK) of the NIH under award R01DK100404.

14. Ronneberger, O., Fischer, P., Brox, T.: U-Net: convolutional networks for biomedical image segmentation. In: Navab, N., Hornegger, J., Wells, W.M., Frangi, A.F. (eds.) MICCAI 2015. LNCS, vol. 9351, pp. 234–241. Springer, Cham (2015). https://doi.org/10.1007/978-3-319-24574-4_28

15. He, K., Zhang, X., Ren, S., Sun, J.: Deep residual learning for image recognition. In: Proceedings of the IEEE Conference on Computer Vision and Pattern Recognition, pp. 770–778 (2016)

Learning Optimal Deep Projection of ^{18}F-FDG PET Imaging for Early Differential Diagnosis of Parkinsonian Syndromes

Shubham Kumar[1,2], Abhijit Guha Roy[1,3], Ping Wu[4], Sailesh Conjeti[1,5],
R. S. Anand[2], Jian Wang[6], Igor Yakushev[7], Stefan Förster[7],
Markus Schwaiger[7], Sung-Cheng Huang[8], Axel Rominger[9], Chuantao Zuo[4(✉)],
and Kuangyu Shi[1,9]

[1] Computer Aided Medical Procedures, Technical University of Munich,
Munich, Germany
[2] Indian Institute of Technology, Roorkee, India
[3] Artificial Intelligence in Medical Imaging (AI-Med), KJP, LMU Munich, Munich,
Germany
[4] PET Center, Huashan Hospital, Fudan University, Shanghai, China
zuochuantao@fudan.edu.cn
[5] German Center for Neurodegenerative Diseases (DZNE), Bonn, Germany
[6] Department of Neurology, Huashan Hospital, Fudan University, Shanghai, China
[7] Department of Nuclear Medicine, Technical University of Munich,
Munich, Germany
[8] Department of Molecular and Medical Pharmacology, University of California,
LA, USA
[9] Department of Nuclear Medicine, University of Bern, Bern, Switzerland

Abstract. Several diseases of parkinsonian syndromes present similar symptoms at early stage and no objective widely used diagnostic methods have been approved until now. Positron emission tomography (PET) with ^{18}F-FDG was shown to be able to assess early neuronal dysfunction of synucleinopathies and tauopathies. Tensor factorization (TF) based approaches have been applied to identify characteristic metabolic patterns for differential diagnosis. However, these conventional dimension-reduction strategies assume linear or multi-linear relationships inside data, and are therefore insufficient to distinguish nonlinear metabolic differences between various parkinsonian syndromes. In this paper, we propose a Deep Projection Neural Network (DPNN) to identify characteristic metabolic pattern for early differential diagnosis of parkinsonian syndromes. We draw our inspiration from the existing TF methods. The network consists of a (i) compression part: which uses a deep network to learn optimal 2D projections of 3D scans, and a (ii) classification part: which maps the 2D projections to labels. The compression part can be pre-trained using surplus unlabelled datasets. Also, as the classification part operates on these 2D projections, it can be trained end-to-end effectively with limited labelled data, in contrast to 3D approaches. We show that DPNN is more effective in comparison to existing state-of-the-art and plausible baselines.

© Springer Nature Switzerland AG 2018
D. Stoyanov et al. (Eds.): DLMIA 2018/ML-CDS 2018, LNCS 11045, pp. 227–235, 2018.
https://doi.org/10.1007/978-3-030-00889-5_26

1   Introduction

Approximately 7 to 10 million people worldwide are suffering from Parkinson's disease (PD). On the other hand, very similar clinical signs can appear in patients with atypical parkinsonian syndromes, such as multiple system atrophy (MSA) and progressive supranuclear palsy (PSP) and these conditions account for approximately 25–30% of all cases of parkinsonian syndromes [1]. Diagnosis of parkinsonian patients based on longitudinal clinical follow up remains problematic with a large number of misdiagnoses in early stage [2]. Thus, early differential diagnosis is essential for determining adequate treatment strategies and for achieving the best possible outcome for these patients [3].

Positron emission tomography (PET) captures neuronal dysfunction of PD using specific *in-vivo* biomarkers [4–8] and has been shown to be more advantageous in early diagnosis, far before structural damages to the brain tissue occurs [7,9–11]. Automated approaches such as Principal component analysis (PCA) has been successfully applied on ^{18}F-FDG PET to extract PD-related pattern (PDRP), MSA-related pattern (MSARP), and PSP-related pattern (PSPRP) [12,13]. These patterns have been found as effective surrogates to discriminate between classical PD, atypical parkinsonian syndromes and healthy control subjects [13]. To account for heterogeneous physiology and enable individual pattern visualization, a tensor-factorization based method was developed by projecting the 3D data into 2D planes containing the discriminative information [3]. However, these conventional dimension-reduction based methods assume linear or multi-linear relationship inside data. In contrast, different subtypes of parkinsonian syndromes, caused by different protein aggregation (α-synuclein or Tau), show a non-linear relationship to the anatomical changes. Thus difference of metabolic patterns between PD, MSA and PSP can be nonlinear due to these diverse pathological manifestations and heterogeneous propagation among complex brain connectomes. Therefore, either PCA or tensor factorization is insufficient to identify nonlinear metabolic differences of various parkinsonian syndromes, and is susceptible to providing sub-optimal solutions.

Deep learning based approaches have recently been shown to be very effective in discovering non-linear characteristic patterns within data in an end-to-end fashion [14,15]. It has been shown to surpass human performance in different complicated tasks, like image classification. It has also gained a lot of popularity in the bio-medical community [16] for computerized diagnosis on medical imaging, such as differential diagnosis [15,17,18]. Inspired by these recent successes, we use a deep learning based architecture for early diagnosis of parkinsonism.

One of the major challenge associated with this task is that our input data is 3D in nature, with limited amount of labelled training samples. Standard approaches of going for 3D based CNN models (very high number of learnable parameters) are prone to overfitting when trained on limited samples. To circumvent this issue, we draw inspiration from the existing approaches which uses Tensor Factorization (TF) to project the 3D scans to 2D, and use them for diagnosis. Towards this end, we propose a deep projection neural network (DPNN), which has two parts, (i) Compression Part and (ii) Classification Part. The Compression Part basically mimics TF projection from 3D to 2D. This part can be pre-trained on a large amount of unlabelled dataset, which is easily available. This pre-trained model is added to the 2D-CNN based Classification part (lower model complexity), which is trained end-to-end with limited annotated data. Although in this paper, we present its application for PET scans, the concept is fairly generic and can be easily extended to any 3D data.

2 Materials and Methods

2.1 Data Preparation and Preprocessing

A cohort of 257 patients (Dataset-1) with clinically suspected parkinsonian features were included in this study. The patients were referred for ^{18}F-FDG PET imaging and then assessed by blinded movement disorders specialists for more than 2 years. Finally 136 of them were diagnosed with PD, 91 with MSA and 30 with PSP. All the 3D PET volumes were preprocessed using intensity-normalized by global mean and spatially normalized to Montreal Neurological Institute (MNI) space using SPM8[1] according to a standard PET processing procedure [3]. For optimizing deep networks, the limited availability of PET images of patients at early stage of parkinsonism could be a bottleneck. Therefore, a database of 1077 subjects (Dataset-2) with 41 various non-parkinsonian neurological diseases with brain FDG PET images is further included to enhance the data pool.

2.2 DPNN Architecture

We draw our inspiration from prior work which estimated tensor factorized projection of 3D PET scans and processed them for classification task. In this regard, we formulated to solve the problem in two parts: (i) Learn a separate network to mimic the tensor factorization from 3D data, *i.e.* learning to compress the data (Compression Part), and (ii) Learn a 2D CNN model to map the compressed input to one of the classes (Classification Part). A detailed description of both the parts are provided below with the architectural design in Fig. 1.

Compression Part: Given a 3D PET scan $I_P \in \mathbb{R}^{H \times W \times D}$, here we estimate a function $f_p(\cdot)$ which compresses the data to a 2D projection map P_t, so that $f_p : I_P \to P_t$, where $P_t \in \mathbb{R}^{H \times W}$. This non-linear function $f_p(\cdot)$ is approximated by a series of blocks consisting of a 3×3 convolutional layer, batch normalization and a ReLU activation function. A set of 5 such blocks are stacked together, which compresses I_P sequentially to P_t. The final block uses a sigmoidal nonlinearity instead of ReLU to rescale the activations between $[0, 1]$.

Classification Part: This part takes P_t, the compressed projection map as input. It learns a mapping $f_c(\cdot)$, which maps P_t to the one of the class labels y. The first 5 blocks consist of a 3×3 convolutional layer, batch norm, ReLU

---

[1] Statistical Parametric Mapping, http://www.fil.ion.ucl.ac.uk/spm/software/spm8/, 2009.

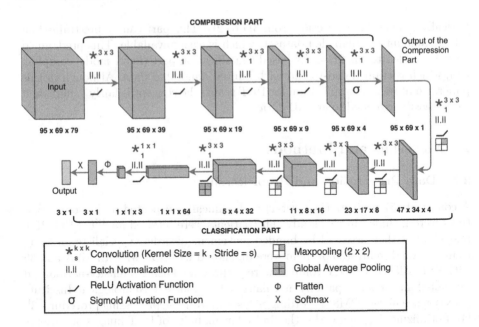

Fig. 1. Illustration of the overall model architecture of deep projection neural network (DPNN). All the architectural details regarding the network are shown here.

activation and a max pooling layer, reducing the spatial dimensions by a factor of 2 at every step. The final block consists of a global average pooling instead of max pooling, squeezing the feature map along spatial dimensions. This is followed by a 1×1 convolutional layer, softmax layer to project the learnt features to the label probalility space $\mathbb{R}^3$, from where y is estimated as the class with highest probability. More details regarding the size of intermediate feature maps and stride are indicated in Fig. 1.

2.3   Training Procedure

To tackle the issue of learning such a highly complex model with limited training data, we propose to address the training procedure in two stages: (i) We leverage unlabelled PET data corpus to pre-train the Compression Part, (ii) limited labelled data is used to learn the weights of the Classification Part, with the Compression Part initialized to the pre-trained weights.

Pretraining: In this part, we use the unlabelled Dataset-2 $\{I_i\}$ for pre-training. We compute the tensor factorized 2D maps of all the volumes as $\{\mathcal{G}_i\}$. In this stage, we train the compression part $f_p(\cdot)$, using this dataset, with the goal of mimicking $\{\mathcal{G}_i\}$ as the output of the network. We hypothesize that this provides a strong initialization to the network for the classification stage. The network is learnt by jointly optimizing a combination of Mean Square Error (MSE) and Structural Similarity Index (SSIM) between the target and prediction, defined as,

$$\mathcal{L} = \underbrace{\frac{1}{2N_p} \sum_{\mathbf{r}} (\mathcal{P}(\mathbf{r}) - \mathcal{G}(\mathbf{r}))^2}_{\text{MSE}} - \underbrace{\frac{1}{N_w} \sum_{\mathbf{w}} \text{SSIM}(\mathbf{w}_p, \mathbf{w}_g)}_{\text{SSIM Index}}, \tag{1}$$

$$\text{SSIM}(\mathbf{w}_p, \mathbf{w}_g) = \frac{(2\mu_p\mu_g + C_1)(2\sigma_{pg} + C_2)}{(\mu_p^2 + \mu_g^2 + C_1)(\sigma_p^2 + \sigma_g^2 + C_2)}, \tag{2}$$

where, $\mathcal{P}$, $\mathcal{G}$, $\mathbf{r}$ and N_r are the predicted map, target projection map, pixel-position, and the total number of pixels respectively. $\mathbf{w}_p$ and $\mathbf{w}_g$ represent a local 6×6 window in $\mathcal{P}$ and $\mathcal{G}$, and N_w is the total number of such windows. SSIM is calculated on all the N_w windows and their average value is used in the cost function. μ_p, σ_p^2, and σ_{pg} are the mean of $\mathbf{w}_p$, the variance of $\mathbf{w}_p$, and the covariance of $\mathbf{w}_p$ and $\mathbf{w}_g$, respectively. C_1 and C_2 are set to $\sim 10^{-4}$ and $\sim 9 \times 10^{-4}$, respectively. We use SSIM based loss function to preserve the quality of the predicted map similar to actual Tensor Factorized map. The weights of the convolutional kernels are initialized using Xavier initialization and Adam optimizer with a learning rate of 10^{-4} is used for the weight updates. The β_1, β_2 and ϵ parameters of the optimizer are set to 0.9, 0.999, and 10^{-8}, respectively. The training is continued until the validation-cost saturates.

Fine-Tuning: In this stage, the pre-trained compression network is combined with the classification part, and the weights of the classification part are initialized using Xavier initialization. The whole network is trained in an end-to-end fashion, minimizing 3-class Cross-Entropy loss function using Adam optimizer with β_1, β_2 and ϵ set to 0.9, 0.999, and 10^{-8}, respectively. The learning rate used for the classification part is 10^{-4}, while for the compression part it is kept 10^{-5}. The learning rate of the compression part is kept one order low to prevent high perturbation in those layer. The weights are regularized with a decay constant of 10^{-5}, preventing over-fitting. A mini-batch of 10 PET scans are used. The training is continued until the convergence of the validation loss.

3   Experiments and Results

Experiments: We evaluate our proposed DPNN model by a 5-fold cross-validation experiment on Dataset-1. An equal distribution of each of samples from the three classes were ensured in each of the folds. For evaluation, we used the standard metrics, (i) True Positive Rate (TPR), (ii) True Negative Rate (TNR), (iii) Positive Predictive Value (PPV), and (iv) Negative Predictive Value (NPV), consistent with [3].

Baselines: We compare our proposed method against state-of-the-art method which uses Tensor Factorization (TF), followed by SVM for classification [3]. Apart from this, we define two other baselines to substantiate our claims:

1. **BL-1:** DPNN, with pre-training using only MSE, to observe the effect of including SSIM in the cost function.

2. **BL-2:** DPNN, without pre-training, trained end-to-end, to observe the effect of pre-training.

For all the experiments we used five-folded cross-validation for evaluation. All the networks were trained on NVIDIA Titan-Xp GPU with 12 GB RAM.

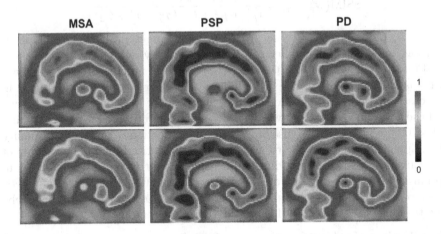

Fig. 2. Projection of 3D PET Volumes generated by the Compression Part of the fine-tuned DPNN. We can visually observe the distinct patterns exhibited by the three sub-types MSA, PSP and PD, which not only aids clinicians for inference, but also aids the Classification part in automated decision making.

Results: Table 1 reports the results of our proposed model (DPNN), with defined baselines and state-of-the-art method, in terms of the mentioned evaluation metrics. Comparing with state-of-the-art [3], DPNN outperforms it in most of the evaluation scores (8 out of 12). Comparing with **BL-1**, DPNN outperforms it. This substantiates our previous hypothesis that MSE+SSIM based pre-training is more effective in providing stronger initialization than MSE alone, which fails to capture the quality based features in the compression stage. It can be attributed to the fact that SSIM applies stricter constraint on similarity which forces the network to learn better representations. Also, comparing to **BL-2**, we prove our previous claim that pre-training is necessary when training such a complicated model with limited annotated data. It has improved the specificities of MSA by 0.79%, PSP by 17.97% and PD by 14.37%, which can play a critical role for differential diagnosis. It is worth noting that DPNN shows consistent good performance across all the metrics for the PD class which has the highest number of samples (*viz.* 136). While all the models show greatest inconsistency in the scores for PSP class, which has just 30 representative samples in the dataset. This is indicative of the fact that given enough data the performance of DPNN can be increased to an ideal level.

Next, we take a closer look at the learnt Projection Maps in Fig. 2, which shows example pattern images of MSA, PSP and PD. Patterns similar to tensor-factorization have been observed in the DPNN Projection results, for example, visible cerebellum and striatum activities in PD, vanishing cerebellum and striatum activities in MSA and decreasing striatum activity and visible cerebellum activity in PSP [3]. This confirms that DPNN is capable of extracting physiologically meaningful patterns, and use it for final decision making.

Table 1. Classification results of our proposed DPNN, in comparison to comparative methods and Baselines.

Model	Metrics											
	MSA				PSP				PD			
	TPR	TNR	PPV	NPV	TPR	TNR	PPV	NPV	TPR	TNR	PPV	NPV
DPNN	84.56	**94.58**	89.63	**91.83**	90.00	**96.93**	79.29	**98.67**	**94.87**	**93.33**	**94.28**	**94.24**
BL-1	76.78	93.98	89.83	88.52	86.67	96.04	76.9	98.24	92.65	86.67	89.44	91.57
BL-2	75.67	93.40	87.90	87.97	80.00	96.48	79.25	97.40	91.96	83.33	86.87	90.46
TF+SVM [3]	86.35	93.79	92.85	88.86	97.87	78.96	97.30	85.07	92.44	78.96	89.14	85.73

4 Conclusion

We developed a deep learning method to extract characteristic metabolic pattern for differential diagnosis of parkinsonian syndrome. In contrast to linear or multi-linear data-reduction methods of the state-of-the-art, the proposed DPNN, processes 3D-data using 2D-convolutions, can explore the non-linear metabolic differences between the subtypes. Furthermore, we introduced a training procedure based on the optimization of SSIM along with MSE which leverages tensor-factorized maps of inputs, from a domain similar to the task-input domain, to overcome the difficulties posed by a small dataset. With limited amount of data, the novel method has already achieved superior accuracy compared to the state-of-the-art. The advanced pre-training strategies play a critical role in the success of this novel method, which prevent the abort of cutting-edge developments before approaching to a large data-bank. The positive performance of deep learning in this study encourages a multi-center study, which is actively in preparation. Although the DPNN patterns extracted in this proof-of-concept study look similar to the previous tensor factorization, an extensive inspection by clinicians may discover the characteristic difference matching to improve accuracy. With the increase of data access, the ability of the deep learning methods to discover new discriminative features will be enhanced, which may provide the potential for a diagnosis at even earlier stage before motor impairment appears, i.e. at prodromal parkinsonian stage such as rapid eye movement (REM) sleep behavior disorder (RBD).

References

1. Hughes, A.J., Ben-Shlomo, Y., Daniel, S.E., Lees, A.J.: What features improve the accuracy of clinical diagnosis in Parkinson's disease: a clinicopathologic study. Neurology **57**(10 Suppl 3), S34–8 (2001)
2. Fahn, S., et al.: Levodopa and the progression of Parkinson's disease. N. Engl. J. Med. **351**(24), 2498–508 (2004)
3. Li, R., et al.: Pattern visualization and recognition using tensor factorization for early differential diagnosis of Parkinsonism. In: Descoteaux, M., Maier-Hein, L., Franz, A., Jannin, P., Collins, D.L., Duchesne, S. (eds.) MICCAI 2017. LNCS, vol. 10435, pp. 125–133. Springer, Cham (2017). https://doi.org/10.1007/978-3-319-66179-7_15
4. Gao, F., Liu, H., Shi, P.: Patient-adaptive lesion metabolism analysis by dynamic PET images. In: Ayache, N., Delingette, H., Golland, P., Mori, K. (eds.) MICCAI 2012. LNCS, vol. 7512, pp. 558–565. Springer, Heidelberg (2012). https://doi.org/10.1007/978-3-642-33454-2_69
5. Xu, Z., Bagci, U., Seidel, J., Thomasson, D., Solomon, J., Mollura, D.J.: Segmentation based denoising of PET images: an iterative approach via regional means and affinity propagation. In: Golland, P., Hata, N., Barillot, C., Hornegger, J., Howe, R. (eds.) MICCAI 2014. LNCS, vol. 8673, pp. 698–705. Springer, Cham (2014). https://doi.org/10.1007/978-3-319-10404-1_87
6. Bagci, U., et al.: Joint segmentation of anatomical and functional images: applications in quantification of lesions from PET, PET-CT, MRI-PET, and MRI-PET-CT images. Med. Image Anal. **17**(8), 929–945 (2013)
7. Jiao, J., Searle, G.E., Tziortzi, A.C., Salinas, C.A., Gunn, R.N., Schnabel, J.A.: Spatio-temporal pharmacokinetic model based registration of 4d PET neuroimaging data. NeuroImage **84**, 225–235 (2014)
8. Bi, L., Kim, J., Feng, D., Fulham, M.: Multi-stage thresholded region classification for whole-body PET-CT lymphoma studies. In: Golland, P., Hata, N., Barillot, C., Hornegger, J., Howe, R. (eds.) MICCAI 2014. LNCS, vol. 8673, pp. 569–576. Springer, Cham (2014). https://doi.org/10.1007/978-3-319-10404-1_71
9. Zhang, D., Shen, D.: Multi-modal multi-task learning for joint prediction of multiple regression and classification variables in Alzheimer's disease. Neuroimage **59**(2), 895–907 (2012)
10. Zhou, L., et al.: MR-less surface-based amyloid estimation by subject-specific atlas selection and Bayesian fusion. In: Ayache, N., Delingette, H., Golland, P., Mori, K. (eds.) MICCAI 2012. LNCS, vol. 7511, pp. 220–227. Springer, Heidelberg (2012). https://doi.org/10.1007/978-3-642-33418-4_28
11. Lu, S., Xia, Y., Cai, W., Fulham, M.J., Feng, D.D.: Early identification of mild cognitive impairment using incomplete random forest-robust support vector machine and FDG-PET imaging. Comp. Med. Imag. Graph. **60**, 35–41 (2017)
12. Eidelberg, D.: Metabolic brain networks in neurodegenerative disorders: a functional imaging approach. Trends Neurosci. **32**(10), 548–57 (2009)
13. Tang, C.C., et al.: Differential diagnosis of pParkinsonism: a metabolic imaging study using pattern analysis. Lancet Neurol. **9**(2), 149–58 (2010)
14. LeCun, Y., Bengio, Y., Hinton, G.: Deep learning. Nature **521**(7553), 436–44 (2015)
15. Ithapu, V.K., Singh, V., Okonkwo, O.C., Chappell, R.J., Dowling, N.M., Johnson, S.C.: Imaging-based enrichment criteria using deep learning algorithms for efficient clinical trials in mild cognitive impairment. Alzheimers Dement **11**(12), 1489–99 (2015)

16. Litjens, G.: A survey on deep learning in medical image analysis. Med. Image Anal. **42**, 60–88 (2017)

17. Zhou, L., Wang, Y., Li, Y., Yap, P.T., Shen, D.: Hierarchical anatomical brain networks for MCI prediction by partial least square analysis. In: CVPR, pp. 1073–1080 (2011)

18. Suk, H.I., Lee, S.W., Shen, D.: Latent feature representation with stacked auto-encoder for AD/MCI diagnosis. Brain Struct. Funct. **220**(2), 841–59 (2015)

Learning to Segment Medical Images with Scribble-Supervision Alone

Yigit B. Can[1], Krishna Chaitanya[1], Basil Mustafa[1,3], Lisa M. Koch[2], Ender Konukoglu[1], and Christian F. Baumgartner[1(✉)]

[1] Computer Vision Lab, ETH Zürich, Zürich, Switzerland
baumgartner@vision.ee.ethz.ch
[2] Computer Vision and Geometry Group, ETH Zürich, Zürich, Switzerland
[3] University of Cambridge, Cambridge, UK

Abstract. Semantic segmentation of medical images is a crucial step for the quantification of healthy anatomy and diseases alike. The majority of the current state-of-the-art segmentation algorithms are based on deep neural networks and rely on large datasets with full pixel-wise annotations. Producing such annotations can often only be done by medical professionals and requires large amounts of valuable time. Training a medical image segmentation network with weak annotations remains a relatively unexplored topic. In this work we investigate training strategies to learn the parameters of a pixel-wise segmentation network from scribble annotations alone. We evaluate the techniques on public cardiac (ACDC) and prostate (NCI-ISBI) segmentation datasets. We find that the networks trained on scribbles suffer from a remarkably small degradation in Dice of only 2.9% (cardiac) and 4.5% (prostate) with respect to a network trained on full annotations.

1 Introduction

Convolutional neural networks (CNN) have been used for semantic segmentation on medical images with great success [2]. For the most part, these methods rely on fully annotated images to train the network. Although CNN-based segmentation algorithms keep evolving and improving, the amount of available training data still has a substantial effect on the performance [9]. However, it is difficult to obtain large scale fully annotated data for medical images since it requires an expert to spend considerable time and effort.

To address this limitation, a number of works have proposed interactive image segmentation methods relying on weak annotations such as bounding boxes [12], or scribbles [4,6]. However, in these works, the annotations need to be provided for each new test image. Recently, a number of works have demonstrated that it is feasible to train fully-automatic, learning-based algorithms using exclusively weak labels [5,9–11]. Despite being trained on weak labels, these methods can produce full segmentation masks on test images. Of the above works only [11] was

Basil Mustafa contributed to this work during a research internship at ETH.

© Springer Nature Switzerland AG 2018
D. Stoyanov et al. (Eds.): DLMIA 2018/ML-CDS 2018, LNCS 11045, pp. 236–244, 2018.
https://doi.org/10.1007/978-3-030-00889-5_27

demonstrated on medical images. The authors proposed to train a segmentation network for fetal structures from bounding box annotations only.

In this paper we present a scribble-based weakly-supervised learning framework for medical images. Scribbles have been recognized as particularly user-friendly form of supervision [9] and may be better suited for nested structures, when compared to bounding boxes. Furthermore, they require only a fraction of the annotation time compared to full pixel-wise annotations. Following previous works, the proposed framework is an iterative two-step procedure in which a segmentation network is trained on the scribble annotations, then this network is used in conjunction with a conditional random field (CRF) to relabel the training set. This in turn is used for an additional training *recursion*[1]. We show that this procedure, under some assumptions, can be interpreted as expectation maximization (EM). We investigate multiple strategies for relabeling the training dataset, estimating the CRF parameters, and quantifying uncertainty in the relabeling step. An overview of the method is shown in Fig. 1.

We evaluate the framework and its individual components on the public cardiac ACDC dataset [2] and the NCI-ISBI 2013 prostate segmentation challenge data [3]. We show that despite the inherently very sparse nature of the annotations the proposed methods achieve a segmentation accuracy within 95% of a baseline network trained with full supervision. To our knowledge, this is the first demonstration of training a pixel-wise segmentation network with scribble supervision on medical image data.

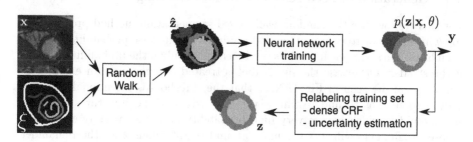

Fig. 1. Overview of the proposed training framework.

2   Methods

The aim of our proposed method is to learn the parameters θ of a CNN-based segmentation network $\mathbf{y} = f(\mathbf{x}; \theta)$ such that it predicts a generally unknown segmentation mask $\mathbf{y} \in \{0, \dots, L\}^N$ for an input image $\mathbf{x} \in \mathbb{R}^N$, where N is the number of pixels. During training, rather than full pixel-wise annotations, we are only provided with a ground truth annotation ξ for a small number of pixels (i.e. the scribbles). Note that this also includes a background scribble

---

[1] We refer to this as recursion rather than iteration to avoid confusion with single mini-batch gradient descent steps, which are also often referred to as iteration.

(see examples in Fig. 2). The proposed framework consists of a repeated estimation of the network parameters and subsequent relabeling of the training dataset by combining the network prediction with a CRF. We investigate two different CRF inference strategies: the dense CRF approach proposed in [8], and a recent extension thereof in which the CRF is formulated as a recurrent neural network (RNN) and the CRF parameters can be learned end-to-end [13]. Moreover, we investigate a novel strategy for incorporating prediction uncertainty in the relabeling step based on [7]. For all investigated strategies we perform an initial region growing step described in the following.

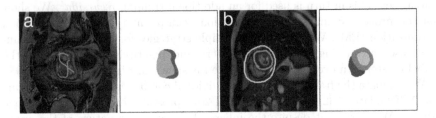

Fig. 2. Example images and scribbles on the left and ground truth segmentations on the right for the (a) prostate and (b) cardiac datasets, respectively.

2.1   Generation of Seed Areas by Region Growing

For this step we use the random walk-based segmentation method proposed by [6], which (similar to neural networks) produces a pixel-wise probability map for each label. We assign each pixel its predicted value only if the probability exceeds a threshold τ. Otherwise the pixel-label is treated as *unknown*. An example of this step can be seen in Fig. 1. Note that the threshold is intentionally chosen very high such as to underestimate the true extent of the structures and only include pixels which have a very high probability of being correctly estimated. Those assignments will serve as new "ground truth" labels $\hat{z}$ for the remainder of the steps and will be referred to as seed areas. The uncertain pixels z are treated as unlabeled, i.e. they are the latent variables of our model.

2.2   Separate CRF and Network Training

We propose a hard expectation maximization (EM) approximation to learn the network parameters θ in an iterative fashion. The algorithm consists of alternatingly estimating the best parameters of the neural network given a labeling obtained using the current parameters θ^{old} (M step), and estimating the optimal labeling of the latent variables given an updated θ (E step). We assume the following graphical model

$$p(\mathbf{z}, \hat{\mathbf{z}} | \mathbf{x}, \theta) = p(\mathbf{z} | \mathbf{x}, \theta) p(\hat{\mathbf{z}} | \mathbf{z}, \mathbf{x}), \tag{1}$$

where $p(\mathbf{z}|\mathbf{x}, \theta)$ is modeled using a neural network $f(\mathbf{x}; \theta)$. Following the standard EM approach, we write the expectation of the complete-data log likelihood as

$$Q(\theta, \theta^{old}) = \sum_{\mathbf{z}} p(\mathbf{z}|\hat{\mathbf{z}}, \mathbf{x}, \theta^{old}) \ln p(\mathbf{z}, \hat{\mathbf{z}}|\mathbf{x}, \theta). \tag{2}$$

In the E step of the algorithm we estimate the mode of $p(\mathbf{z}|\hat{\mathbf{z}}, \mathbf{x}, \theta^{old})$ as

$$\mathbf{z}^* = \arg \max_{\mathbf{z}} p(\mathbf{z}|\hat{\mathbf{z}}, \mathbf{x}, \theta^{old}) = \arg \max_{\mathbf{z}} \frac{p(\mathbf{z}, \hat{\mathbf{z}}|\mathbf{x}, \theta^{old})}{p(\hat{\mathbf{z}}|\mathbf{x})} = \arg \max_{\mathbf{z}} p(\mathbf{z}, \hat{\mathbf{z}}|\mathbf{x}, \theta^{old}), \tag{3}$$

using the fact that $p(\hat{\mathbf{z}}|\mathbf{x})$ does not depend on $\mathbf{z}$.

By assuming a complete dependency graph between all $\mathbf{z}, \hat{\mathbf{z}}$, the conditional joint distribution can be factorized and the E step can be written as the following CRF optimization problem:

$$\mathbf{z}^* = \arg \min_{\mathbf{z}} \sum_{i \in \mathcal{C}_u(\mathbf{z})} \psi_u(z_i|\mathbf{x}, \theta^{old}) + \sum_{i \in \mathcal{C}_u(\hat{\mathbf{z}})} \hat{\psi}_u(\hat{z}_i)$$

$$+ \sum_{i,j \in \mathcal{C}_p(\mathbf{z})} \psi_p(z_i, z_j|x_i, x_j) + \sum_{i,j \in \mathcal{C}_p(\hat{\mathbf{z}})} \psi_p(\hat{z}_i, \hat{z}_j|x_i, x_j) + \sum_{i,j \in \mathcal{C}_p(\mathbf{z}, \hat{\mathbf{z}})} \psi_p(z_i, \hat{z}_j|x_i, x_j), \tag{4}$$

where $\mathcal{C}_u(\cdot)$ denotes the set of all unary cliques of a set of variables and $\mathcal{C}_p(\cdot)$ denotes the set of all pairwise cliques. The unary potential function ψ_u acting on the latent variables is defined using the current network output as

$$\psi_u(z|\mathbf{x}, \theta^{old}) = -\ln p(z_i|\mathbf{x}, \theta^{old}) = -\ln f(x; \theta^{old}). \tag{5}$$

The unary potential function $\hat{\psi}_u$ acting on the seed regions $\hat{\mathbf{z}}$ is defined as 0 for labellings matching the ground truth and infinity otherwise, effectively preventing the initially grown regions from changing. Furthermore, we use the pairwise potential function ψ_p proposed in [8]:

$$\psi_p(z_i, z_j|x_i, x_j) = \mu(z_i, z_j) \left(w_1 \exp \left(-\frac{dist(x_i, x_j)^2}{2\sigma_\alpha^2} - \frac{|x_i - x_j|^2}{2\sigma_\beta^2} \right) \right.$$

$$\left. + w_2 \exp \left(-\frac{dist(x_i, x_j)^2}{2\sigma_\gamma^2} \right) \right), \tag{6}$$

where the label compatibility function is given by the Potts model $\mu(z_i, z_j) = [z_i \neq z_j]$, and $dist(\cdot, \cdot)$ denotes the Euclidean distance between the pixel locations. We estimate the hyperparameters $w_1, w_2, \sigma_\alpha, \sigma_\beta, \sigma_\gamma$ in a grid search on the validation set. In order to optimize Eq. 4 we use the approach in [8]. We also consider a simple modification of this procedure as a baseline in which we set the pairwise terms to zero and only use the unary terms $\psi_u, \hat{\psi}_u$.

In the M step, after we have found the optimal labeling of the latent variables $\mathbf{z}^*$ using the network parameters θ^{old} we can rewrite Eq. 2 as

$$Q(\theta, \theta^{old}) \approx \sum_{\mathbf{z}} \delta(\mathbf{z} = \mathbf{z}^*|\hat{\mathbf{z}}, \mathbf{x}, \theta^{old}) \ln p(\mathbf{z}, \hat{\mathbf{z}}|\mathbf{x}, \theta)$$

$$= \ln p(\mathbf{z}^*|\mathbf{x}, \theta) + \ln p(\hat{\mathbf{z}}|\mathbf{z}^*, \mathbf{x}), \tag{7}$$

where δ is the Dirac delta function, the approximate equality is due to the hard EM approximation and we substituted Eq. 1 to obtain the equality. Since $\ln p(\hat{\mathbf{z}}|\mathbf{z}, \mathbf{x})$ does not depend on θ the optimization can be written as

$$\theta^* = \arg\max_{\theta} \ln p(\mathbf{z}^*|\mathbf{x}, \theta). \tag{8}$$

We find the parameters θ that maximize the likelihood of predicting the labels $\mathbf{z}^*$ by minimizing the pixel-wise cross entropy function between the labels $\mathbf{z}^*$ and the network output using the ADAM optimizer with an initial learning rate of 0.001 which is multiplied by 0.9 every 3000 iterations. We use the modified U-Net segmentation network used in [1] in all experiments. The network parameters θ for each recursion are initialized with θ^{old}. The E and the M steps get repeated until convergence, which typically occurs within 3 recursions or less.

In the first recursion, we set the cross-entropy loss to zero in all locations where the random walk is "uncertain" (probabilities below τ), allowing the network to predict any label in those regions. We also explore a strategy to identify uncertain regions in subsequent iterations, which will be discussed in Sect. 2.4

2.3   Integrated Network Training and (CRF-RNN)

Here, we investigate estimation of the CRF parameters as part of the network training. To that end we use the CRF-RNN layer proposed in [13] which learns individual kernel weights for each class and a more flexible compatibility matrix.

To obtain a new labeling $\mathbf{z}^*$ we simply run a forward pass through the network. Next, in order to prevent the original seed regions $\hat{\mathbf{z}}$ from changing, we simply reset those values to their original label. In future work, we aim to include this constraint directly into the CRF-RNN formulation.

In the subsequent network optimization step, we directly learn to predict those $\mathbf{z}^*$. Here we use the following training scheme: the network parameters are trained as above for 10 mini-batch iterations while keeping the RNN parameters constant. Every 10 iterations, the RNN parameters are updated with a learning rate of 10^{-7}, while freezing the remainder of the network parameters. As before, the label estimation and training steps are repeated until convergence.

2.4   Quantifying Segmentation Uncertainty

In order to prevent segmentation errors from early recursions from propagating we investigate the following strategy to reset labels predicted with insufficient certainty after each E step. We add dropout with probability 0.5 to the 5 innermost blocks of our U-Net architecture during training. In order to estimate the new optimal labeling $\mathbf{z}^*$ we perform 50 forward passes with dropout similar to [7]. Rather than a single output this yields a distribution of logits and softmax outputs for each pixel and label. We then compare the logits distributions of the label with the highest and second highest softmax mean for each pixel using a Welch's t-test. If the logits come from a distribution with the same mean with $p \geq 0.05$ we conclude that the label was not predicted with sufficient certainty and reset its labeling to "uncertain". Thus, in the subsequent M-step the network will be free to predict any label in that location. Otherwise, we set the pixel to the label with the highest probability.

3   Experiments and Results

We trained and evaluated the methods on two publicly available datasets: the ACDC cardiac segmentation challenge data [2] for which the Myocardium (Myo), the left and right ventricles (LV and RV) have been annotated, and the NCI-ISBI 2013 prostate segmentation challenge data [3] for which reference annotations of the central gland (CG) and the peripheral zone (PZ) were available. For the cardiac data we split the data into 160 training volumes and 40 validation volumes, and evaluated the algorithms on 100 images using the challenge server. For the prostate data we split 29 available training volumes into 12 training, 7 validation and 10 testing volumes. Training was performed on 2D slices.

We used $\tau = 0.99$ for the cardiac and $\tau = 0.90$ for the prostate experiments. For the separate CRF we used $w_1 = 5, w_2 = 10, \sigma_\alpha = 2, \sigma_\beta = 0.1, \sigma_\gamma = 5$ for the cardiac experiments and $w_1 = 6, w_2 = 10, \sigma_\alpha = 3, \sigma_\beta = 0.01, \sigma_\gamma = 2, \tau = 0.9$ for the prostate, and for the CRF-RNN we used $\sigma_\alpha = 160$, for the cardiac data, $\sigma_\alpha = 250$ for the prostate, and $\sigma_\beta = 3, \sigma_\gamma = 10$ for both datasets.

In the following experiments, the simple recursive training strategy which does not make use of pairwise terms in Eq. 4, nor uncertainty estimation, is called *base*. We evaluated the performance with and without the components discussed above. Additionally, we also investigated the same segmentation architecture on the fully labeled data to obtain an upper bound on the performance, and a version of *base* in which we did not perform any recursions, but used the network parameters learned directly on the seed regions $\hat{z}$.

The Dice scores with respect to the reference annotations for all the examined methods and structures are shown in Table 1. Note that ACDC challenge server did not allow for higher precision Dice reporting in the post-challenge phase. Example segmentations for the two best performing methods are shown in Fig. 3 for the cardiac and prostate data, respectively.

We observe that (a) the recursive training regime led to substantial improvements over non-recursive training, (b) the dropout based uncertainty was responsible for the largest improvements, (c) additional CRF led to further, albeit smaller improvements, (d) using CRF-RNN without uncertainty led to similar results as the separate CRF with uncertainty, (e) applying dropout uncertainty in conjunction with the CRF-RNN did not lead to additional improvements and performed slightly worse on the prostate. We believe this is due to the CRF-RNN module leading to unusual logit distributions at its input. On average, the training frameworks with (1) CRF-RNN, and with (2) separate CRF and uncertainty performed the best and similar to each other. Future work on integrating uncertainty with the CRF-RNN may lead to further improvements.

Table 1. Dice scores on Cardiac and Prostate datasets.

	Cardiac dataset				Prostate dataset		
	LV	RV	Myo	Avg	PZ	CG	Avg
Base (no recursion)	0.895	0.875	0.825	0.865	0.631	0.827	0.729
Base	0.905	0.880	0.835	0.873	0.670	0.829	0.750
Base + separate CRF	0.890	0.880	**0.840**	0.870	0.698	0.837	0.767
Base + CRF-RNN	**0.915**	0.885	**0.840**	**0.880**	0.698	**0.863**	**0.781**
Base + uncertainty	0.910	**0.890**	**0.840**	**0.880**	0.720	0.837	0.778
Base + sep. CRF & unc.	0.910	**0.890**	**0.840**	**0.880**	**0.722**	0.839	0.780
Base + CRF-RNN & unc.	**0.915**	0.885	**0.840**	**0.880**	0.710	0.834	0.772
Fully supervised	0.935	0.905	0.895	0.912	0.746	0.889	0.818

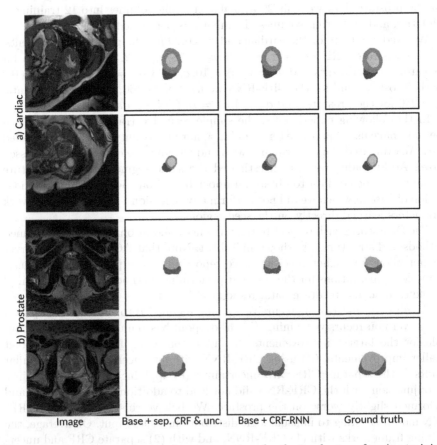

Fig. 3. Randomly sampled example segmentations for the two best performing training strategies for the (a) cardiac and (b) prostate data.

Most importantly, the results show that our proposed training strategy allows to learn a pixel-level segmentation network using scribble supervision alone with a remarkably small degradation compared to the fully supervised upper bound. For instance, the performance of the CRF-RNN method is only 4.5% worse on the prostate, and 2.9% worse on the cardiac data compared to fully supervised training. These results are also confirmed by the qualitative analysis. We believe this is likely an acceptable error margin for certain quantification studies where precise border delineation is of secondary importance such as automatic estimation cardiac ejection fractions [2].

4   Conclusion

In this paper, we investigated training strategies to train a fully automatic segmentation network with scribble supervision alone. We demonstrated the feasibility of the techniques on two publicly available medical image datasets and showed that only a remarkably small performance degradation is incurred with respect to fully supervised upper bound networks.

Acknowledgements. This work was partially supported by the Swiss Data Science Center. One of the Titan X Pascal used for this research was donated by the NVIDIA Corporation.

References

1. Baumgartner, C.F., Koch, L.M., Pollefeys, M., Konukoglu, E.: An exploration of 2D and 3D deep learning techniques for cardiac MR image segmentation. In: Pop, M., et al. (eds.) STACOM 2017. LNCS, vol. 10663, pp. 111–119. Springer, Cham (2018). https://doi.org/10.1007/978-3-319-75541-0_12
2. Bernard, O., et al.: Deep learning techniques for automatic MRI cardiac multi-structures segmentation and diagnosis: is the problem solved? IEEE Trans. Med. Imaging (2018)
3. Bloch, N., Madabhushi, A., Huisman, H., et al.: NCI-ISBI 2013 challenge: automated segmentation of prostate structures (2015)
4. Criminisi, A., Sharp, T., Blake, A.: GeoS: geodesic image segmentation. In: Forsyth, D., Torr, P., Zisserman, A. (eds.) ECCV 2008. LNCS, vol. 5302, pp. 99–112. Springer, Heidelberg (2008). https://doi.org/10.1007/978-3-540-88682-2_9
5. Dai, J., He, K., Sun, J.: BoxSup: exploiting bounding boxes to supervise convolutional networks for semantic segmentation. In: Proceedings of the ICCV, pp. 1635–1643 (2015)
6. Grady, L.: Random walks for image segmentation. IEEE Trans. Pattern Anal. **28**(11), 1768–1783 (2006)
7. Kendall, A., Badrinarayanan, V., Cipolla, R.: Bayesian SegNet: model uncertainty in deep convolutional encoder-decoder architectures for scene understanding. arXiv preprint arXiv:1511.02680 (2015)
8. Krähenbühl, P., Koltun, V.: Efficient inference in fully connected CRFs with Gaussian edge potentials. In: Advances in Neural Information Processing Systems, pp. 109–117 (2011)

9. Lin, D., Dai, J., Jia, J., He, K., Sun, J.: ScribbleSup: scribble-supervised convolutional networks for semantic segmentation. In: Proceedings of the CVPR, pp. 3159–3167 (2016)

10. Papandreou, G., Chen, L., Murphy, K., Yuille, A.L.: Weakly- and semi-supervised learning of a DCNN for semantic image segmentation. In: Proceedings of the ICCV 2015 (2015)

11. Rajchl, M.: DeepCut: object segmentation from bounding box annotations using convolutional neural networks. IEEE Trans. Med. Imaging **36**(2), 674–683 (2017)

12. Rother, C., Kolmogorov, V., Blake, A.: "GrabCut": interactive foreground extraction using iterated graph cuts. ACM Trans. Graph. **23**(3), 309–314 (2004)

13. Zheng, S., et al.: Conditional random fields as recurrent neural networks. In: Proceedings of the ICCV, pp. 1529–1537 (2015)

Learning to Decode 7T-Like MR Image Reconstruction from 3T MR Images

Aditya Sharma$^{(\boxtimes)}$, Prabhjot Kaur, Aditya Nigam, and Arnav Bhavsar

School of Computing and Electrical Engineering, Indian Institute of Technology,
Kamand, Mandi, India
adityasharma101993@gmail.com, prabhjot_kaur@students.iitmandi.ac.in,
{aditya,arnav}@iitmandi.ac.in

Abstract. Increasing demand for high field magnetic resonance (MR) scanner indicates the need for high-quality MR images for accurate medical diagnosis. However, cost constraints, instead, motivate a need for algorithms to enhance images from low field scanners. We propose an approach to process the given low field (3T) MR image slices to reconstruct the corresponding high field (7T-like) slices. Our framework involves a novel architecture of a merged convolutional autoencoder with a single encoder and multiple decoders. Specifically, we employ three decoders with random initializations, and the proposed training approach involves selection of a particular decoder in each weight-update iteration for back propagation. We demonstrate that the proposed algorithm outperforms some related contemporary methods in terms of performance and reconstruction time.

Keywords: Autoencoder · Multiple decoders · Low-field MRI
Reconstruction · High-field MRI

1 Introduction

Improvement of trade-off between spatial resolution and signal to noise ratio (SNR) in MR imaging motivates the research from the perspective of both hardware and signal processing. As SNR increases monotonically with the strength of magnetic field, high-field MR scanners (7T, 11.5T) have been designed and are successful in providing higher SNR for the same resolution of images. However, the cost increases exponentially with the magnetic field strength. This leads to the lesser availability of high-field MR scanners across different hospitals and clinical labs and thus doesn't solve the problem in practice. The number of clinical 7T scanners in the world are just ∼40, as compared to ∼20000 3T scanners [5]. Thus, developing algorithms to enhance images from low-field (and low-cost) MR scanners, serve as an important alternative. Indeed, it has been shown that the signal processing techniques can improve the spatial resolution along with significant increment in the SNR [1].

A. Sharma and P. Kaur—The authors have contributed equally in this work.

© Springer Nature Switzerland AG 2018
D. Stoyanov et al. (Eds.): DLMIA 2018/ML-CDS 2018, LNCS 11045, pp. 245–253, 2018.
https://doi.org/10.1007/978-3-030-00889-5_28

The problem to reconstruct the high-field like images from the low-field images is manifold and consists many sub-problems which include (i) increase in resolution leading to enhancement of image details, (ii) contrast improvement, and (iii) increase in signal to noise ratio. Also, those approaches to address such problems are more feasible in clinical practices, which take less time.

One can address the above concerns by learning a highly non-linear mapping from the low field to high field MR images using exemplar low-field (LF) and high-field (HF) MR images. Considering this, Khosro et al. in [2] attempted to construct 7T like MR images from 3T MR images using dictionaries defined in same space, which is estimated by hierarchical application of canonical correlation analysis (CCA), and 7T MR images are reconstructed using the dictionary defined for 7T MR images and the coefficient vector computed by representation of 3T MR images using dictionary of corresponding exemplary 3T MR images. As it tries to capture the non-linearity of the transformation, it performs better than the approaches which solely increase the resolution with SNR [3,4]. However, the non-linearity of transformation is still approximated by linear operations and may have significant fitting errors by degree of the non-linearity.

This is further addressed by the approaches defined in the popular framework of a neural network which can well approximate even the non-linear transformations [5,6]. In [5] the reconstruction of 7T MR images is explored using convolutional neural network (CNN) network with a requirement of anatomical features. Reconstruction, as well as segmentation of the high-field MR images, is performed using a cascaded CNN given the 3T MR images and corresponding segmentation images at the input. Both these approaches divide the image volumes into 3D cubes and execute the algorithm with 3D CNN. Processing 3D cubes can help in reconstruction of local details and consistency in x, y, and z directions, but at the same time it may introduce block artifacts, and importantly, increases the time for reconstruct the test MR volumes.

Considering the ill-posed nature of the problem, and a possibility of multiple good solutions, we propose a merged convolutional autoencoder with three decoders, along with a strategy to update the weights adaptively based on the performance of each decoder at every iteration. The final estimate of the HF image is obtained by averaging the reconstructed images from the three decoders. To make the algorithm better usable in clinical practices, we reduce the reconstruction time of test MR volumes, while achieving better reconstruction and segmentation of the high-field MR images, by processing 2D images, and removing the requirement of any anatomical/segmentation based features.

Thus, our contributions can be summarized as: (a) architecture of convolutional autoencoder with multiple decoders. (b) update criteria for the encoder weights on the basis of decoder performance. (c) merge connections to enhance the reconstruction ability. (d) demonstrating reconstruction and segmentation improvements along with significant reduction in reconstruction time as compared to the state-of-the-art approaches. (e) we demonstrate superior performance across a variety of quantitative metrics such as PSNR, SSIM, sharpness and edge width unlike [5,6].

2   Proposed Approach

In this work, we employ the convolutional autoencoder which tries to learn compact representative features of the image data. The problem to construct HF-like MR images from LF MR images involves the non-linear transformation, which the convolutional autoencoder learns at in latent space at multiple scales of the image obtained by upsampling and downsampling layers. The salient aspects of the proposed approach are detailed below:

2.1   One Encoder with Multiple Decoders

For the image reconstruction task, being an ill-posed problem, many solutions (HF images) may exist for the transformation of LF image to the HF image estimate. The transformation in our case depends on the filter weights which ideally should be representative enough to construct image details of complex structures, and discriminative enough to be able to learn the differences between details of HF and LF image. While, such a transformation can be learnt with a simple convolutional autoencoder (single encoder and decoder), considering that the transformation can be highly non-linear, there could be different weight combinations that can provide good estimates of such a transformation. The proposed multi-decoder model is thoughtfully designed with a notion that decoders initialized randomly, and updated using individual distinct costs, are likely to learn different weights via the different optimization paths. The random initializations can yield diverse solutions that can easily be collated for better PSNR. The distinctness between the learnt weights can be observed in Fig. 2 via activation maps at same layers of different decoders.

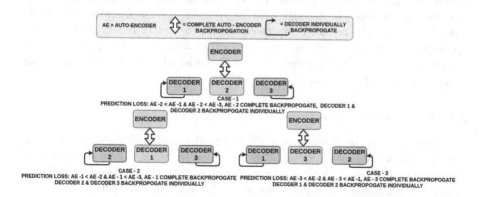

Fig. 1. Selective auto-encoder backpropagation

While there can be different configurations of multiple decoders, as an example, in this work we consider three decoders, integrated with a single encoder in the proposed architecture (Fig. 2). In this architecture, a selective backpropagation approach (as elaborated next) (Fig. 1) is proposed to enable the weight updates across the three paths, by selecting one decoder out of the three based on their losses, in each weight-update iteration (i.e. for each batch, with multiple batches considered within an epoch).

2.2   Updating the Weights

As indicated above, the weights of the architecture are updated in a three-fold manner which involves the selection of one of the three decoders, in each iteration. The selection is based on the minimum loss. Suppose $\mathbf{E}_i$ represents the error of the network at the ith decoder, such that $\mathbf{E}_i = g(\mathbf{W}_E, \mathbf{W}_{D_i})$, with encoder weights $\mathbf{W}_E$ and decoder weights $\mathbf{W}_{D_i}$, $(i = 1, 2, 3.)$. The weight update of the encoder is represented as $\Delta\mathbf{W}_E \propto \min_i(\mathbf{E}_i)$. In this way, in every iteration the encoder weights have three open but guided paths to move on, and the optimal one (with minimum loss) is chosen.

While the encoder weights are updated with the minimum decoder loss, for updating the decoder weights, we update all the decoders using their respective losses, i.e. $\Delta\mathbf{W}_{D_i} \propto \mathbf{E}_i$. We observe that simultaneously updating the decoders helps in minimizing the training loss faster, even as compared to a single encoder and decoder model, and also yields an improved performance.

2.3   Merge Connections

We define the proposed architecture with blocks of subsequent filter layers followed by a max pooling layer in the encoder section as shown in Fig. 2. To reconstruct the original size of image at output, an upsampling layer is introduced in each block of the decoders. While upsampling, there may be some artifacts introduced due to missing details in downsampled input of decoder. Hence, we concatenate the input of decoder with its upscaled version from the encoder in order to provide the nature of upscaled details for better reconstruction while upsampling in decoder. Indeed, we observe that adding the merge connections yield a significant PSNR improvement (of the order of 5db). This setting of our architecture is inspired from [7].

2.4   Proposed Architecture

The proposed approach employs a single encoder and multiple decoder architecture with a single channel input as described in Fig. 2. Three convolutional layers are used in each block of an encoder and all the three decoders, followed by a batch normalization layer to maintain the numerical stability.

The first convolutional block in the encoder has 32 filters and the number of filters doubles after each convolutional block. In all the decoders the first convolutional block has 256 filters and the number of filters are halved after each block. We use a filter size of 3-by-3 in all convolutional blocks.

We use Rectified Linear Unit (ReLU) as an activation function in all the layers except the final layer. Since our data is normalized between 0 and 1, a Sigmoid activation function is used at the final layer.

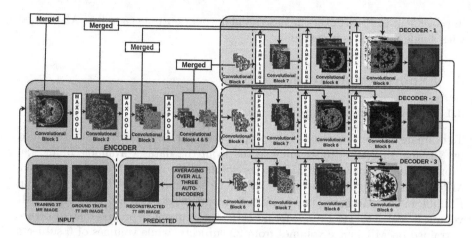

Fig. 2. Proposed Architecture (Better viewed in color)

The pixel values greater than zero (brain area) are passed to the next layer and rest of the pixels (outer part of the brain) are squashed to zero. This phenomenon is clearly visible in the initial layers of the encoder and the last layers of all the three decoders, through the activation maps in Fig. 2.

It is well known that local image details at various scales play a significant role in image reconstruction. The proposed architecture considers images at different scales using hierarchical layers for downsampling (maxpooling) and upsampling (each for a factor of 2) in encoder and decoders, respectively. The encoded representation obtained after three downsampling operations brings the data from a high dimension input to a latent space representation.

As the training proceeds, after every epoch the model is validated on 20% of the unseen validation data. The auto-encoder with minimum mean square error in training data, predicts on the validation data, and using the predicted output we calculate PSNR on the validation data and save the best weights corresponding to the maximum PSNR across epochs. The test reconstructions are then computed on these weights. Further, we have observed experimentally that the minimum strategy for backpropagation gives better results as compared to maximum strategy.

To aid a faster convergence we reduce the learning rate by 10% of its value after every 20 epochs. We also observe that using learning rate decay, the loss value converges to a smaller value than the case without using learning rate decay. The initial value for learning rate is set to be 1e-3. The model is trained for 500 epochs, which is observed to be more than sufficient to ensure convergence.

Finally, in the testing phase, the three reconstruction estimates on the test data are obtained at the three decoder outputs, and we take an average of all the three predictions which improves the results quantitatively. We observe that averaging the predicted outputs also helps in reducing the noise-*like* effects, with preservation of local features in the reconstructed images, and hence the improvement in PSNR over the individual decoder outputs as well as AE trained with single decoder is observed.

3   Experimental Results

3.1   Experimental Setup

To evaluate the performance of the proposed algorithm, real MR images scanned by 3T and 7T MR scanner are selected from the dataset available online [8]. From a pool of volumes 39 MR image volumes are randomly selected and 3T MR images are registered with 7T MR image volumes using FLIRT software in FSL [9], in order to have pixel to pixel correspondence. Further, each of the MR volume is scaled to 0 to 1 range for numerical stability. The proposed architecture is trained on MR image volumes from 22 subjects, while volumes of 6 subjects are used for validation and 11 are used for testing. We cross validate across 3 trails involving random sets of training, validation and test data.

For comparison with existing approaches, we re-implement the 3D CNN approach defined in [5]. As some of the parameters are not mentioned in their work, we have used the same parameters as used in proposed work for e.g. learning rate, learning rate decay strategy, optimizer, batch size. To consider a complementary framework, the sparse-representation approach is also used for comparison [4]. For training all approaches we use 207 images from each subject volume. However, due to insignificant information in first and last 20 slices, we select central 167 slices per volume for reconstruction. All implementations are on a system with Nvidia 1080 Ti GPU Xeon e5 GeForce processor with 32 GB RAM.

3.2   Reconstruction Results

The test 7T MR image volumes are constructed using proposed approach and other existing works and two images are randomly selected to illustrate the quality comparison between different approaches. It can be observed from Figs. 3 and 4, that sparse based approach [4] is able to construct the details but with diffused tissue boundary. 3DCNN performs well in terms of tissue boundary but is unable to restore smaller differences in voxel values. Both these aspects are improved upon by the proposed approach.

The improvement is reflected in the quantitative results in Table 1 with higher PSNR and SSIM values. To compute the performance in terms of blurriness of the edges, two parameters i.e. sharpness and edge width are computed as defined in [10]. We observe that the algorithm may change the dynamic range of the data. Thus to be consistent for comparing quality of images reconstructed, we first match the histogram (HM) of reconstructed image with the corresponding 3T image. However, we also show the results for the proposed method without HM. The values for parameters are computed over non-background pixels of reconstructed images scaled to their original range.

3T Image   Zoomed 3T   ScSR[4]   3D-CNN[5] Single decoder   Proposed   7T Image

Fig. 3. Example reconstructions and comparison visualized at a finer scale.

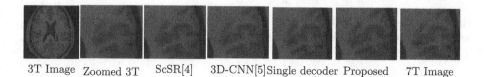

3T Image   Zoomed 3T   ScSR[4]   3D-CNN[5] Single decoder   Proposed   7T Image

Fig. 4. Example reconstructions and comparison visualized at a finer scale.

3.3 Segmentation Results

High quality images helps in improving segmentation of the tissues required for medical analysis. Thus, we compare segmentation labels for images reconstructed by different algorithms, with FAST software of FSL for gray matter(GM), white matter(WM) and CSF. The dice-ratio improvements in segmentation with reconstruction using the proposed approach is clear from Table 2. The work in [5] has outperformed the sparse based reconstruction, thus we do not provide segmentation results for the latter.

Table 1. Quantitative comparison of proposed approach

Approaches	ScSR with HM [4]	3D-CNN with HM [5]	Single decoder with HM	Proposed approach with HM	Proposed approach w/o HM
PSNR (dB)	35.96 ($\pm$0.93)	34.20 ($\pm$0.81)	36.96 ($\pm$0.92)	37.45 ($\pm$1.00)	39.25 ($\pm$1.46)
Average SSIM	0.7092	0.7094	0.7371	0.7432	0.8253
Sharpness [10]	0.3967	0.4043	0.4092	0.4179	0.4001
Edge width [10]	0.0989	0.0945	0.0947	0.0919	0.0959

3.4 Computational Complexity

Here, we stress the computational advantage of the proposed approach in terms of run-time for reconstruction, as compared to the approach of [5]. The 3D CNN approach [5] takes 137 min to construct 11 subject image volume. The proposed algorithm contrarily is computationally simple and takes less than 2 min to do

Table 2. Dice ratio for segmentation of images reconstructed by different algorithms

Approaches	3T MR images	3D-CNN with HM [5]	Proposed approach
CSF	0.8836 (±0.0081)	0.8766 (±0.0053)	0.9149 (±0.0042)
White matter	0.9372 (±0.0086)	0.9279 (±0.0100)	0.9528 (±0.0068)
Gray matter	0.9503 (±0.0083)	0.9216 (±0.0157)	0.9602 (±0.0087)

the same task. To justify, we note that the amount of multiplications in the architecture of [5] is 2145 times than that in the proposed one. This is largely due to unpadded 3D convolution in [5].

4 Conclusion

We reported a novel convolutional single encoder with three decoder framework for reconstructing 7T-like MR images from 3T MR image as inputs. The proposed approach employs single-channel input (i.e. does not require anatomical and segmentation features as an input), and yet achieves a superior reconstruction quality over some contemporary methods. It also has a significant computational advantage. We also show that the reconstructed 7T-like MR images when segmented have better dice ratio compared to the comparative approaches.

References

1. Plenge, E., et al.: Super-resolution methods in MRI: can they improve the trade-off between resolution, signal-to-noise ratio, and acquisition time? Magn. Reson. Med. **68**(6), 1983–1993 (2012). https://doi.org/10.1002/mrm.24187
2. Bahrami, K., Shi, F., Zong, X., Shin, H.W., An, H., Shen, D.: Reconstruction of 7T-like images from 3T MRI. IEEE Trans. Med. Imaging **35**(9), 2085–2097 (2016)
3. Roy, S., Carass, A., Prince, J.L.: Magnetic resonance image example based contrast synthesis. IEEE Trans. Med. Imaging **32**(12), 2348–2363 (2013)
4. Yang, J., Wright, J., Huang, T.S., Ma, Y.: Image super-resolution via sparse representation. IEEE Trans. Image Process. **19**(11), 2861–2873 (2010)
5. Bahrami, K., Shi, F., Rekik, I., Shen, D.: Convolutional neural network for reconstruction of 7T-like images from 3T MRI using appearance and anatomical features. In: Carneiro, G., et al. (eds.) LABELS/DLMIA -2016. LNCS, vol. 10008, pp. 39–47. Springer, Cham (2016). https://doi.org/10.1007/978-3-319-46976-8_5
6. Bahrami, K., Rekik, I., Shi, F., Shen, D.: Joint reconstruction and segmentation of 7T-like MR images from 3T MRI based on cascaded convolutional neural networks. In: Descoteaux, M., Maier-Hein, L., Franz, A., Jannin, P., Collins, D.L., Duchesne, S. (eds.) MICCAI 2017. LNCS, vol. 10433, pp. 764–772. Springer, Cham (2017). https://doi.org/10.1007/978-3-319-66182-7_87
7. Ronneberger, O., Fischer, P., Brox, T.: U-net: convolutional networks for biomedical image segmentation. In: Navab, N., Hornegger, J., Wells, W.M., Frangi, A.F. (eds.) MICCAI 2015. LNCS, vol. 9351, pp. 234–241. Springer, Cham (2015). https://doi.org/10.1007/978-3-319-24574-4_28

8. https://www.humanconnectome.org/study/hcp-young-adult/document/1200-subjects-data-release
9. Shi, F., Wang, L., Dai, Y., Gilmore, J.H., Lin, W., Shen, D.: LABEL: pediatric brain extraction using learning-based meta-algorithm. NeuroImage **62**(3), 1975–1986 (2012)
10. Guan, J., Zhang, W., Gu, J., Ren, H.: No-reference blur assessment based on edge modeling. J. Vis. Commun. Image Represent. **29**, 1–7 (2015)

Nonlinear Adaptively Learned Optimization for Object Localization in 3D Medical Images

Mayalen Etcheverry[✉], Bogdan Georgescu, Benjamin Odry, Thomas J. Re, Shivam Kaushik, Bernhard Geiger, Nadar Mariappan, Sasa Grbic, and Dorin Comaniciu

Digital Technology and Innovation, Siemens Medical Solutions, Princeton, NJ, USA
Mayalen.Irene.Catherine.Etcheverry@siemens-healthineers.com

Abstract. Precise localization of anatomical structures in 3D medical images can support several tasks such as image registration, organ segmentation, lesion quantification and abnormality detection. This work proposes a novel method, based on deep reinforcement learning, to actively learn to localize an object in the volumetric scene. Given the parameterization of the sought object, an intelligent agent learns to optimize the parameters by performing a sequence of simple control actions. We show the applicability of our method by localizing boxes (9 degrees of freedom) on a set of acquired MRI scans of the brain region. We achieve high speed and high accuracy detection results, with robustness to challenging cases. This method can be applied to a broad range of problems and easily generalized to other type of imaging modalities.

Keywords: Deep reinforcement learning
Nonlinear parameter optimization · 3D medical images
Object localization

1 Introduction

Localization of anatomical structures in medical imaging is an important prerequisite for subsequent tasks such as volumetric organ segmentation, lesion quantification and abnormality detection. Ensuring consistency in the local context is one of the key problems faced when training the aforementioned tasks.

In this paper, we investigate a new approach, to simplify upstream localization of the region of interest. In particular, a deep reinforcement-learning agent is trained to learn the search strategy that maximizes a reward for accurately localizing the sought anatomy. The benefit of the proposed method is that it eliminates exhaustive search or the use of generic nonlinear optimization techniques by learning optimal convergence path. The method is demonstrated for localizing a specific box around the brain in head MRI, achieving performances in the range of the inter-observer variability with an average processing time of 0.6 s per image.

© Springer Nature Switzerland AG 2018
D. Stoyanov et al. (Eds.): DLMIA 2018/ML-CDS 2018, LNCS 11045, pp. 254–262, 2018.
https://doi.org/10.1007/978-3-030-00889-5_29

2   Related Work

2.1   Object Localization in 3D Medical Imaging

Several methods have been proposed for automatic localization of anatomical structures in the context of 3D data.

Atlas-based registration methods [1] solve the object localization task by registering input data to a set of images present in an atlas database. By transforming these images to a common standard space the known shapes of the atlas can be aligned to match the input unseen data. These methods require complex non-rigid registration and are hardly scalable to large 3D-volumes.

Regression-based methods [2,3] directly learn the non-linear mapping from voxels to parameters by formulating the localization as a multivariate regression problem. These methods are difficult to train, especially in problems where the dataset has a large variation in the field of view, limiting the applicability in 3D medical imaging.

Classification-based methods are usually done in two steps: discretization of the parametric space in a large set of hypotheses and exhaustive testing through a trained classifier. The hypothesis with the maximum confidence score is kept as detection result. Marginal Space Learning (MSL) [4,5], widely used approach, reduces the search by decoupling the task in three consecutive stages: location, orientation and size. This method manually imposes dependencies in the parametric search space. It can lead to suboptimal solutions and is hard to generalize.

Recent work [10] proposes to apply faster R-CNN [9] techniques to medical imaging analysis. Faster R-CNN jointly performs object classification and object localization in a single forward pass, significantly decreasing the processing time. However, this architecture requires very large annotated datasets to train and can be hardly generalizable to the variety of input clinical cases.

2.2   Deep Reinforcement Learning as a Search Strategy

In contrast to traditional approaches, Ghesu et al. [6] use reinforcement learning to identify the location of an anatomical landmark in a set of image data. They reformulate the detection problem as a sequential decision task, where a goal-directed intelligent agent can navigate inside the 3D volume through simple linear translation actions. However the framework is limited to finding a set of coordinates (x, y, z). We build upon their work and propose to extend the method to a wider range of image analysis applications by expanding the search space to an nonlinear multi-dimensional parametric space.

In this paper, we develop a deep reinforcement learning-based method to automatically estimate the 9 parameters (position, orientation and scale) of an anatomical bounding box.

3   Method

The sought object is modeled with a set of D independent parameters $\{x_i\}_{i=1}^{D}$. Reachable parameter values form a D-dimensional space where an instance is uniquely represented as a point of coordinates $(x_1, \ldots, x_D)$. The goal is to locate an object in an input 3D scan, or equivalently to find an optimal parameter vector $x^* = (x_1^*, \ldots, x_D^*)$ in the parameter space.

This work deploys an artificial intelligent agent that can navigate into the D-dimensional parametric space with the goal of reaching the targeted position x^*. Based on its own experience, the autonomous agent actively learns to cope with the uncertain environment (volumetric image signal) by performing a sequence of simple control actions. To optimize the control strategy of the agent inside this D-dimensional space, an adaptive sequential search across different scale representations of the environment is proposed. As in [6], our work follows the concepts of deep reinforcement learning and multi-scale image analysis but extended for a search in high-dimensional nonlinear parametric spaces. Figure 1 gives an overview of the proposed method.

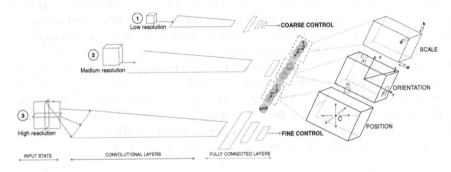

Fig. 1. Schematic illustration of the proposed control strategy. Measurement from the image (input state) drive the output of the deep-Q-network which itself drive the agent decisions. In the proposed MDP, the agent follows a multi-scale progressive control strategy and has D = 9 degrees of freedom to transform the box (3 for position, 3 for orientation and 3 for scale).

3.1   Object Localization as a Markov Decision Process

The D-dimensional parametric space is discretized into regular intervals in every dimension, giving the set of reachable positions by the agent.

We model the problem as a Markov Decision Process (MDP), defined by a tuple of objects (S, A, p, R, γ) where S is the set of possible states, p is the transition probability distribution, A is the set of possible actions, R is a scalar reward function, and γ is the discount factor. The states, actions and reward of the proposed MDP are described below.

State representation s: At each time step t, the 3D-volume environment returns the observed *state* of the world s_t as the current visible region by the agent. The current parameters x^t define a certain region in the physical space. We set the *visibility* of the agent to be the content of this region plus a fixed margin of voxels to provide additional context. We resample it to match a fixed-size grid of voxels that we use as input state s_t of the network. This operation involves rotation and scaling of the 3D volume, and is performed at each agent step.

Control actions a: At each time step, the agent can choose between $2D$ *move* actions to modify the current object geometry x^t or to terminate the search with the *stop* action. The agent movements in the parametric space are represented as unit-length steps along one of the of the of the basis vectors $(-e_1, +e_1, \ldots, -e_D, +e_D)$, where e_d denotes the vector with a 1 in the dth coordinate and 0's elsewhere.

Reward function r: The agent learns a strategy policy with the goal of maximizing the cumulative future reward over one episode $R = \sum_{t=0}^{T} \gamma^t r_t$. We define a distance-based reward:
$$r_t = \begin{cases} dist(x_t, x^*) - dist(x_{t+1}, x^*) & if \ a_t \in \{1, \ldots, 2D\} \\ \left(\frac{dist(x_t, x^*) - d_{min}}{d_{max} - d_{min}} - 0.5\right) * 6 & if \ a_t = 2D + 1 \\ -1 & if \ s_{t+1} \ not \ legal \ state \end{cases}$$
where $dist(x, x')$ defines a metric distance between two objects x and x' in the parametric space. The reward gives the agent an evaluative feedback each time it chooses an action a_t from the current state s_t. Intuitively, the reward is positive when the agent gets closer to the ground truth target and negative otherwise. If one *move* action leads to a *non-legal* state s_{t+1}, the agent receives a negative reward -1. A state is non legal if one of the parameters is outside of a predefined allowed search range. Finally, if the agent decides to stop, the closer it is from the target the greater reward it gets and reversely. The reward is bounded between $[-1; 1]$ for choosing a *move* action and between $[-3; 3]$ for the *stop* action. Possible metric distances include the ℓ_p-norm family, the intersection over union and the average corner-to-corner distance.

Deep Reinforcement Learning to Find the Optimal control Strategy:

We use Q-learning combined with a neural network function approximator due to the lack of prior knowledge about the state-transition and the reward probability distributions (model-free setting) and to the high-dimensionality of the input data (continuous volumetric images). This approach, introduced by Mnih et al. [7], estimates the optimal action-value function using a deep Q-network (DQN): $Q^*(s, a) \approx Q(s, a, \theta)$. The training uses Q-learning to update the network by minimizing a sequence of loss functions $L_i(\theta_i)$ expressing how far $Q(s, a; \theta_i)$ is from its target y_i: $L_i(\theta_i) = \mathbb{E}_{s,a,r,s'} (y_i - Q(s, a; \theta_i))^2$. For effective training of the DQN, the proposed concepts of experience replay, ε-greedy exploration and loss clipping are incorporated. At the difference of traditional random exploration, we constrain it to positive directions (actions leading to positive reward) to accelerate the agent's discovery of positive reward trajectory. We also use double Q-learning [8] with a "frozen" version of the online network as target network $Q_{target} = Q(\theta_{i'}), i' < i$.

3.2 Multi-scale Progressive Control Strategy

Ghesu et al. [6] propose a multi-scale sampling of the global image context for an efficient voxel-wise navigation within the three-dimensional image space. In this work, we take a step further by proposing a progressive spanning-scheme of the nonlinear D-dimensional search space. The goal is for the agent to develop an optimal control strategy with incremental precision across scales.

Discretization of the continuous volumetric image: The "context" in which evolves the agent (continuous 3D volumetric image) is downsampled into a multi-scale image pyramid with increasing image resolution $L_1, L_2, \ldots, L_N$.

Discretization of the parametric search space: At each scale level L_i of the image pyramid, the D-dimensional parametric space is discretized into a regular grid of constant scale cells $\Delta^{(i)} = (\Delta x_1^{(i)}, \ldots, \Delta x_D^{(i)})$ where $\Delta^{(i)}$ determines the precision of the agent control over the parameters. The agent starts the search with both coarse field-of-view and coarse control. Following the sampling scheme of the global image context, the agent gains finer control over the parameter each time it transitions to a finer scale level L_{i+1}. This scheme goes on until the finest scale level, where the final agent position is taken as estimated localization result.

The transition between subsequent scale levels is proposed as an additional control action (*stop* action), which also acts as a stopping criterion at the finest scale level L_N. Autonomously learned by the intelligent agent, a timely and robust stopping criterion is ensured. At inference, if the maximum number of steps is exceeded or if two complementaries actions are taken consecutively (placing the agent in an infinite loop), the stop action is forcefully triggered.

4　Experiment and Results

MRI scans of the head region can be acquired along some specific brain anatomical regions to standardize orientations of acquisitions, facilitate reading and assessment of clinical follow-up studies. We therefore propose to localize a standard box from Scout/Localizer images that covers the brain, and aligned along specific orientations. This is a challenging task requiring robustness against variations in the localizer scan orientation, the view of the object and the brain anatomy. In some cases, some of the brain or bone structures may be missing or displaced either by natural developmental variant or by pathology. We reformulate the task as a nonlinear parameter optimization problem and show the applicability of the proposed method.

4.1　Dataset

The dataset consists of 530 annotated MRI scans of the head region. 500 were used for training and 30 for testing. The 30 test cases were annotated twice by different experts to compute the inter-rater variability. 15 additional challenging test cases with pathologies (tumors or fluid swelling in brain tissue), in plane rotation of the head, thick cushion of the head rest, or cropped top of the skull were selected to evaluate the robustness of the method.

The scale space is discretized into 4 levels: 16 mm (L_1), 8 mm (L_2), 4 mm (L_3) and 2 mm (L_4). The images, of input resolution (1.6 × 1.5625 × 1.5625), were isotropically down-sampled to 16, 8, 4 and 2 mm. The voxels intensities were clipped between the 3rd and 97th percentile and normalized to the [0; 1] range.

Ground-truth boxes have been annotated based on anatomical structures present in the brain region. The orientation of the box is determined by positioning the brain midsagittal plane (MSP), separating the two brain hemispheres and going through the Crista Galli, Sylvian Aqueduct and Medulla Oblongata. The rotational alignment within the MSP is based on two anatomical points: the inflection distinguishing the Corpus Callosum (CC) Genu from the CC Rostrum and the most inferior point on the CC Splenium. Given this orientation, the lower margin of the box is defined to intersect the center of C1-vertebrae arches points. The other box extremities define an enclosing bounding box of the brain.

Following the annotation protocol, we define an orthonormal basis (i, j, k) where i is the normal of the MSP and j defines the rotation within the MSP. The orientation of the box is controlled by three angles: α_1 and α_2 which control respectively the yaw and pitch of the MSP, and β_1 which controls the inplane roll around i. The center position is parameterized by its cartesian coordinates $C = (C_x, C_y, C_z)$. The scale is parametrized by the width w, depth d and height h of the box. Control of the box parameters is shown in Fig. 1.

4.2 Results

In our experiments, the very first box is set to cover the whole image at the coarsest scale and is sequentially refined following the agent's decisions. The network architecture and hyper-parameters can be found in appendix. Table 1 shows comparison between the proposed method, human performances (inter-rater variability) and a previous landmark-based method.

The landmark-based method uses the proposed algorithm of [6] to detect 14 landmarks carefully chosen after the box definition. The midsagital plane is consequently initialized with RANSAC robust fitting. Finally a box is fitted with a gradient descent algorithm to minimize angular and positional errors with respect to the detected landmarks. 8 out of the 14 landmarks are associated with the angles α_1 and α_2, therefore achieving good results for these measures. On the other hand, due to the fewer landmarks associated to β_1 (2), this angle is not robust to outliers.

The proposed method however, achieves performances in the range of the inter-observer variability for every measure. Performing a direct optimization on the box parameters, this work does not rely on the previous detection of specific points. For recall the finer scale level is set to 2 mm, meaning that our method achieves an average accuracy of 1–2 voxels precision.

Table 1. Absolute mean and maximal errors of the 30 test cases with respect to ground truth boxes. α_1 and α_2 are the angles between the i vectors projected into the XZ and XY plane. β_1 is the angle between the j vectors projected into the ground truth MSP. δ_R (right), δ_L (left), δ_A (anterior), δ_P (posterior), δ_I (inferior) and δ_S (superior) are the orthogonal distances from the center of the detected face to the ground truth face. The best obtained results are shown in bold.

		Inter-rater	Landmark-based	Our approach (4mm)	Our approach (2mm)
	$\alpha_1(°)$	0.99($\leq$3.50)	0.92($\leq$3.45)	1.28($\leq$3.78)	**0.92($\leq$3.23)**
	$\alpha_2(°)$	1.04($\leq$4.71)	0.99($\leq$4.93)	1.20($\leq$4.46)	**0.97($\leq$2.11)**
	$\beta_1(°)$	1.47($\leq$5.19)	2.00($\leq$6.86)	1.62($\leq$6.35)	**1.39($\leq$5.86)**
	δ_R(mm)	1.32($\leq$3.54)	2.06($\leq$5.78)	2.65($\leq$7.54)	**1.45($\leq$3.30)**
	δ_L(mm)	1.45($\leq$4.75)	1.89($\leq$5.03)	2.20($\leq$8.68)	**1.83($\leq$4.95)**
	δ_A(mm)	2.00($\leq$3.36)	**1.65($\leq$4.93)**	2.46($\leq$6.07)	1.94($\leq$6.08)
	δ_P(mm)	1.48($\leq$3.89)	1.86($\leq$9.62)	3.31($\leq$9.68)	**1.65($\leq$5.68)**
	δ_I(mm)	3.33($\leq$3.61)	**2.22($\leq$6.00)**	3.12($\leq$11.5)	2.74($\leq$8.21)
	δ_S(mm)	1.3($\leq$3.28)	**2.13($\leq$5.74)**	3.04($\leq$7.46)	2.16($\leq$6.31)

We did not observe any major failure over the 15 "difficult" test cases, showing robustness of the method to diverse image acquisitions, patient orientations, brain anatomy and extreme clinical cases (see Fig. 2).

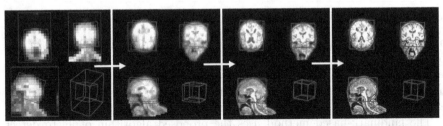

(a) Case with rotation in the localizer scan orientation and tilted patient head.

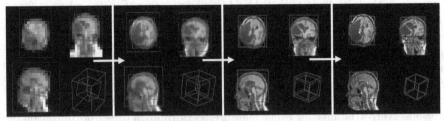

(b) Extreme clinical case with tumor.

Fig. 2. Four samples of the box evolution during inference on challenging cases. The current agent box is depicted in blue and the ground truth reference in green. (Color figure online)

At inference, our algorithm runs in 0.6 s on average on GPU (GEFORCE GT X). We would like to stress that this processing time includes the 4 scale levels navigation. If near real-time performance is desired, the search can be stopped at 4 mm resolution with a minor loss in accuracy, reducing the average runtime to less than 0.15 s.

5   Conclusion

This paper proposes a novel approach, based on deep reinforcement learning, to sequentially search for a target object inside 3D medical images. The method can robustly localize the target object and achieves high speed and high accuracy results. The methodology can learn optimization strategies eliminating the need for exhaustive search or for complex generic nonlinear optimization techniques. The proposed object localization method can be applied to any given parametrization and imaging modality type.

Disclaimer: This feature is based on research, and is not commercially available. Due to regulatory reasons, its future availability cannot be guaranteed.

References

1. Ranjan, S.R.: Organ localization through anatomy-aware non-rigid registration with atlas. In: 2011 IEEE Applied Imagery Pattern Recognition Workshop (AIPR), pp. 1–5. IEEE (2011)
2. Criminisi, A., et al.: Regression forests for efficient anatomy detection and localization in computed tomography scans. Med. Image Anal. **17**(8), 1293–1303 (2013)
3. Cuingnet, R., Prevost, R., Lesage, D., Cohen, L.D., Mory, B., Ardon, R.: Automatic detection and segmentation of kidneys in 3D CT images using random forests. In: Ayache, N., Delingette, H., Golland, P., Mori, K. (eds.) MICCAI 2012. LNCS, vol. 7512, pp. 66–74. Springer, Heidelberg (2012). https://doi.org/10.1007/978-3-642-33454-2_9
4. Zheng, Y., Georgescu, B., Comaniciu, D.: Marginal space learning for efficient detection of 2D/3D anatomical structures in medical images. In: Prince, J.L., Pham, D.L., Myers, K.J. (eds.) IPMI 2009. LNCS, vol. 5636, pp. 411–422. Springer, Heidelberg (2009). https://doi.org/10.1007/978-3-642-02498-6_34
5. Ghesu, F.C., et al.: Marginal space deep learning: efficient architecture for volumetric image parsing. IEEE Trans. Med. Imaging **35**(5), 1217–1228 (2016)
6. Ghesu, F.C., et al.: Multi-scale deep reinforcement learning for real-time 3D-landmark detection in CT scans. IEEE Trans. Pattern Anal. Mach. Intell. (2017)
7. Mnih, V., et al.: Playing atari with deep reinforcement learning. arXiv preprint arXiv:1312.5602 (2013)

8. Van Hasselt, H., Guez, A., Silver, D.: Deep reinforcement learning with double Q-learning. In: AAAI, vol. 16, pp. 2094–2100 (2016)
9. Ren, S., He, K., Girshick, R., Sun, J.: Faster R-CNN: towards real-time object detection with region proposal networks. In: Advances in Neural Information Processing Systems (2015)
10. Akselrod-Ballin, A., Karlinsky, L., Alpert, S., Hasoul, S., Ben-Ari, R., Barkan, E.: A region based convolutional network for tumor detection and classification in breast mammography. In: Carneiro, G., et al. (eds.) LABELS/DLMIA -2016. LNCS, vol. 10008, pp. 197–205. Springer, Cham (2016). https://doi.org/10.1007/978-3-319-46976-8_21

SCAN: Structure Correcting Adversarial Network for Organ Segmentation in Chest X-Rays

Wei Dai[✉], Nanqing Dong, Zeya Wang, Xiaodan Liang, Hao Zhang, and Eric P. Xing

Petuum Inc., Pittsburgh, USA
{wei.dai,nanqing.dong,zeya.wang,xiaodan.liang,
hao.zhang,eric.xing}@petuum.com

Abstract. Chest X-ray (CXR) is one of the most commonly prescribed medical imaging procedures, often with over 2–10x more scans than other imaging modalities. These voluminous CXR scans place significant workloads on radiologists and medical practitioners. Organ segmentation is a key step towards effective computer-aided detection on CXR. In this work, we propose Structure Correcting Adversarial Network (SCAN) to segment lung fields and the heart in CXR images. SCAN incorporates a critic network to impose on the convolutional segmentation network the structural regularities inherent in human physiology. Specifically, the critic network learns the higher order structures in the masks in order to discriminate between the ground truth organ annotations from the masks synthesized by the segmentation network. Through an adversarial process, the critic network guides the segmentation network to achieve more realistic segmentation that mimics the ground truth. Extensive evaluation shows that our method produces highly accurate and realistic segmentation. Using only very limited training data available, our model reaches human-level performance without relying on any pretrained model. Our method surpasses the current state-of-the-art and generalizes well to CXR images from different patient populations and disease profiles.

Keywords: Chest X-ray · Medical image segmentation
Adversarial learning · Deep neural networks

1 Introduction

Chest X-ray (CXR) is one of the most common medical imaging procedures. Due to CXR's low cost and low dose of radiation, hundreds to thousands of

Electronic supplementary material The online version of this chapter (https://doi.org/10.1007/978-3-030-00889-5_30) contains supplementary material, which is available to authorized users.

© Springer Nature Switzerland AG 2018
D. Stoyanov et al. (Eds.): DLMIA 2018/ML-CDS 2018, LNCS 11045, pp. 263–273, 2018.
https://doi.org/10.1007/978-3-030-00889-5_30

CXRs are generated in a typical hospital daily, which create significant diagnostic workloads. In 2015/16 year over 22.5 million X-ray images were requested in UK's public medical sector, constituting over 55% of the total number of medical images and dominating all other imaging modalities such as computed tomography (CT) scan (4.5M) and MRI (3.1M) [4]. Among X-ray images, 8 million are Chest X-rays, which translate to thousands of CXR readings per radiologist per year. The shortage of radiologists is well documented across the world [11,14]. It is therefore of paramount importance to develop computer-aided detection methods for CXRs to support clinical practitioners.

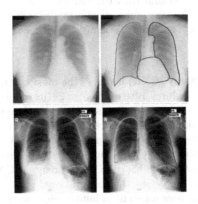

Fig. 1. Two example chest X-ray (CXR) images from two dataset: JSRT (top) and Montgomery (bottom). The left and right columns show the original CXR images and the lung field annotations by radiologists. JSRT (top) additionally has the heart annotation. Note that contrast can vary significantly between the dataset, and pathological lung profiles such as the bottom patient pose a significant challenge to the segmentation problem.

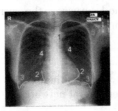

Fig. 2. Important contour landmarks around lung fields: aortic arch (1) is excluded from lung fields; costophrenic angles (3) and cardiodiaphragmatic angles (2) should be visible in healthy patients. Hila and other vascular structures (4) are part of the lung fields. The rib cage contour (5) should be clear in healthy lungs.

An important step in computer-aided detection on CXR images is organ segmentation. The segmentation of the lung fields and the heart provides rich structural information about shape irregularities and size measurements [3] that can be used to directly assess certain serious clinical conditions, such as cardiomegaly (enlargement of the heart), pneumothorax (lung collapse), pleural effusion, and emphysema. Furthermore, explicit lung region masks can also mask out non-lung regions to minimize the effect of imaging artifacts in computer-aided detection, which is important for the clinical use [13].

One major challenge in CXR segmentation is to incorporate the implicit medical knowledge involved in contour determination. For example, the heart and the lung contours should always be adjacent to each other due to definition of the lung boundaries (Sect. 2). Moreover, when medical experts annotate the lung fields, they look for certain consistent structures surrounding the lung fields (Fig. 2). Such prior knowledge helps resolve ambiguous boundaries caused by pathological conditions or poor imaging quality, as can be seen in Fig. 1. Therefore, a successful segmentation model must effectively leverage global structural information to resolve the local details.

Unfortunately, unlike natural images, there are very limited CXR data because of sensitive privacy issues. Even fewer training data have pixel-level annotations, due to the expensive label acquisition involving medical professionals. Furthermore, CXRs exhibit substantial variations across different patient populations, pathological conditions, as well as imaging technology and operation. Finally, CXR images are gray-scale and are drastically different from natural images, which may limit the transferability of existing models. Existing approaches to CXR organ segmentation generally rely on hand-crafted features that can be brittle when applied to different patient populations, disease profiles, or image quality. Furthermore, these methods do not explicitly balance local information with global structure in a principled way, which is critical to achieving realistic segmentation outcomes suitable for diagnostic tasks.

In this work, we propose to use the Structure Correcting Adversarial Network (SCAN) framework that incorporates a critic network to guide the convolutional segmentation network to achieve accurate and realistic organ segmentation in chest X-rays. By employing a convolutional network approach to organ segmentation, we side-step the problems faced by existing approaches based on ad hoc feature extraction. Our convolutional segmentation model alone can achieve performance competitive with existing methods. However, the segmentation model alone cannot capture sufficient global structures to produce natural contours due to the limited training data. To impose regularization based on the physiological structures, we introduce a critic network which learns the higher order structures in the masks in order to discriminate between the ground truth organ annotations from the masks synthesized by the segmentation network. Through an adversarial training process, the critic network effectively transfers this learned global information back to the segmentation network to achieve realistic segmentation outcomes that mimic the ground truth.

Without using any pre-trained models, SCAN produces highly realistic and accurate segmentation even when trained on a very small dataset. With the global structural information, our segmentation model is able to resolve difficult boundaries that require a strong prior knowledge. SCAN improves the state-of-the-art lung segmentation methods [1,12,15] and outperforms strong baselines including U-net [9] and DeepLabV2 [2], achieving performance competitive with human experts. Furthermore, SCAN is more robust than existing methods when applied to different patient populations. To our knowledge, this is the first successful application of convolutional neural networks (CNN) to CXR image segmentation, and our CNN-based method can be readily integrated for clinical tasks such as automated cardiothoracic ratio computation [3]. We note that SCAN is similar to [8] in applying adversarial methods to segmentation. Further related work may be found in supplemental materials.

2 Structure Correcting Adversarial Network

We propose to use adversarial training for segmenting CXR images. Figure 3 shows the overall SCAN framework in incorporating the adversarial process into the semantic segmentation. The framework consists of a segmentation network and a critic network that are jointly trained. The segmentation network makes pixel-level predictions of the target classes, playing the role of the generator in Generative Adversarial Network (GAN) [5] but conditioned on an input image. On the other hand, the critic network takes the segmentation masks as input and outputs the probability that the input mask is the ground truth annotation instead of the prediction by the segmentation network.

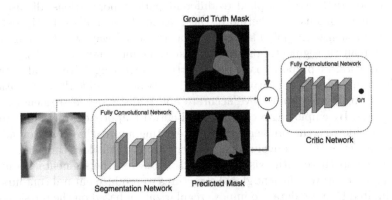

Fig. 3. Overview of the proposed SCAN framework that jointly trains a segmentation network and a critic network through an adversarial process. The segmentation network produces a mask prediction. The critic takes either the ground truth mask or the predicted mask and outputs the probability estimate of whether the input is the ground truth (with training target 1) or predicted mask (with training target 0).

The higher order consistency enforced by the critic is particularly desirable for CXR segmentation. Human anatomy, though exhibiting substantial variations across individuals, generally maintains a stable relationship between physiological structures (Fig. 2). CXRs also pose consistent views of these structures thanks to the standardized imaging procedures. We can, therefore, expect the critic to learn these higher order structures and guide the segmentation network to generate masks more consistent with the learned global structures.

Training Objectives. The networks can be trained jointly through a minimax scheme that alternates between optimizing the segmentation network and the critic network. Let S, D be the segmentation network and the critic network, respectively. The data consist of the input images $\boldsymbol{x}_i$ and the associated mask labels $\boldsymbol{y}_i$, where $\boldsymbol{x}_i$ is of shape $[H, W, 1]$ for a single-channel gray-scale image with height H and width W, and $\boldsymbol{y}_i$ is of shape $[H, W, C]$ where C is the number of classes including the background. Note that for each pixel location (j, k), $y_i^{jkc} = 1$ for the labeled class channel c while the rest of the channels are zero $(y_i^{jkc'} = 0$ for $c' \neq c)$. We use $S(\boldsymbol{x}) \in [0, 1]^{[H, W, C]}$ to denote the class probabilities predicted by S at each pixel location such that the class probabilities sum to 1 at each pixel. Let $D(\boldsymbol{x}_i, \boldsymbol{y})$ be the scalar probability estimate of $\boldsymbol{y}$ coming from the training data (ground truth) $\boldsymbol{y}_i$ instead of the predicted mask $S(\boldsymbol{x}_i)$. We define the optimization problem as

$$\min_S \max_D \left\{ J(S, D) := \sum_{i=1}^N J_s(S(\boldsymbol{x}_i), \boldsymbol{y}_i) - \lambda \Big[J_d(D(\boldsymbol{x}_i, \boldsymbol{y}_i), 1) + J_d(D(\boldsymbol{x}_i, S(\boldsymbol{x}_i)), 0) \Big] \right\},$$

(1)

where $J_s(\hat{\boldsymbol{y}}, \boldsymbol{y}) := \frac{1}{HW} \sum_{j,k} \sum_{c=1}^C -y^{jkc} \ln \hat{y}^{jkc}$ is the multi-class cross-entropy loss for predicted mask $\hat{\boldsymbol{y}}$ averaged over all pixels. $J_d(\hat{t}, t) := -\{t \ln \hat{t} + (1 - t) \ln(1 - \hat{t})\}$ is the binary logistic loss for the critic's prediction. λ is a tuning parameter balancing pixel-wise loss and the adversarial loss. We can solve Eq. (1) by alternating between optimizing S and optimizing D with corresponding loss function. See supplemental materials for details.

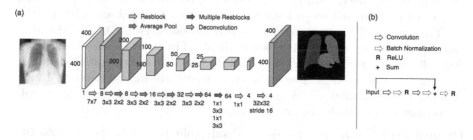

Fig. 4. The segmentation network architecture. (a) Fully convolutional network for dense prediction. (b) The residual block architecture is based on [6]. Further details are in supplementary materials.

Network Architectures. The segmentation network is a fully convolutional network (FCN) [2,7]. Figure 4 details our FCN architecture. The segmentation network contains 271k parameters, 500x smaller than VGG-based FCN [7]. Our FCN is highly parsimonious to adpat to the stringent dataset size of the medical domain: our training dataset of 247 CXR images is orders of magnitude smaller than the dataset in the natural image domains. Furthermore, CXR is gray-scale with consistent viewpoint, which can be captured by fewer feature maps and thus fewer parameters. The parsimonious network construction allows us to optimize it efficiently without relying on any existing trained model, which is not readily available for the medical domain. Figure 5 shows the critic architecture, which has 258k parameters.

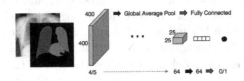

Fig. 5. The critic network architecture. Our critic FCN mirrors the segmentation network (Fig. 4). The training target is 0 for synthetic masks; 1 otherwise. Further details are in supplementary materials.

3   Experiments

We perform extensive evaluation of the proposed SCAN framework and demonstrate that our approach produces highly accurate and realistic segmentation of CXR images.

Dataset and Protocols. We use the following two publicly available datasets to evaluate our proposed SCAN framework. The datasets come from two different countries with different lung diseases, representing diverse CXR samples. **JSRT.** The dataset contains 247 CXRs, among which 154 have lung nodules and 93 have no lung nodule [10,12] (Fig. 1). **Montgomery.** The Montgomery dataset, collected in Montgomery County, Maryland, USA, consists of 138 CXRs, including 80 normal patients and 58 patients with manifested tuberculosis (TB) [1]. The CXR images are 12-bit gray-scale images of dimension 4020×4892 or 4892×4020. Only the lung masks annotations are available (Fig. 1). We scale all images to 400×400 pixels, which retains visual details for vascular structures in the lung fields and the boundaries. The evaluation metrics are Intersection-over-Union (IoU) and Dice Coefficient. We present the details of data processing and evaluation metrics in Supplementary Materials.

Quantitative Comparisons. We randomly split the JSRT dataset into the development set (209 images) and the evaluation set (38 images). We tune our architecture and hyperparameter λ (Eq. (1)) using a validation set within the development set and fix $\lambda = 0.01$. We use FCN to denote the segmentation network only architecture, and SCAN to denote the full framework with the critic.

We investigate how SCAN improves upon FCN. Table 1 shows the IoU and Dice scores using JSRT dataset. We observe that the adversarial training significantly improves the performance. In particular, IoU for the two lungs improves from 92.9% to 94.7%.

Table 1. IoU and Dice scores on JSRT evaluation set for left lung (on the right side of the PA view CXR), right lung (on the left side of the image), both lungs, and the heart. The model is trained on the JSRT development set. ± represents one standard deviation estimated from bootstrap.

		FCN	SCAN
IoU	Left Lung	91.3% ± 0.9%	**93.8% ± 0.8%**
	Right Lung	94.2% ± 0.2%	**95.5% ± 0.2%**
	Both Lungs	92.9% ± 0.5%	**94.7% ± 0.4%**
	Heart	86.5% ± 0.9%	86.6% ± 1.2%
Dice	Left Lung	95.4% ± 0.5%	**96.8% ± 0.5%**
	Right Lungs	97.0% ± 0.1%	**97.7% ± 0.1%**
	Both Lungs	96.3% ± 0.3%	**97.3% ± 0.2%**
	Heart	92.7% ± 0.6%	92.7% ± 0.2%

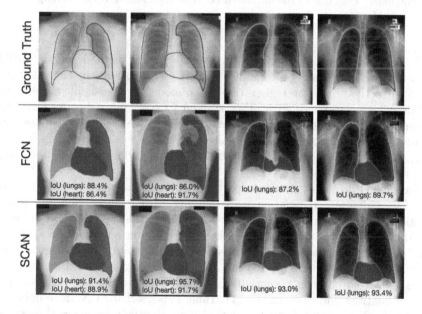

Fig. 6. Visualization of segmentation results on 4 patients, one per column. The left two columns are patients from the JSRT evaluation set with models trained on JSRT development set. The right two columns are from the Montgomery dataset using a model trained on the full JSRT dataset but not Montgomery, which is a much more challenging scenario. Note that only the two patients from JSRT dataset (left two columns) have heart annotations for evaluation of heart area IoU. The contours of the predicted masks are added for visual clarity.

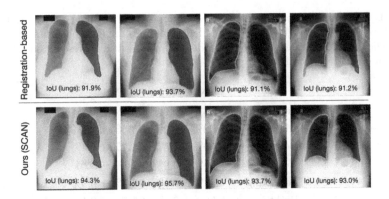

Fig. 7. Comparison with the current state-of-the-art [1]. SCAN produces sharp contours at the costophrenic angles for the left two columns (from the JSRT evaluation set). Furthermore, our model generalizes well to different patient populations and imaging setup, as shown in the Montgomery CXR in the right two columns. [1] struggles on Montgomery data due to the mismatch between train and test patient lung profiles (JSRT and Montgomery dataset, respective).

Table 2 compares our approach to several existing methods on the JSRT dataset, as well as human performance. Our model surpasses the current state-of-the-art method based on registration-based model [1] by a significant margin. Additionally, we compare with other standard CNN approaches for semantic segmentation: DeepLabV2 with ResNet101 [2] and U-Net [9] and demonstrate the advantage of our parsimonious architecture and adversarial training. Importantly, our method is competitive with the human performance for both lung fields and the heart.

For clinical deployment, it is important for the segmentation model to generalize to a different population with different patient population and image qualities, such as when deployed in another country or a specialty hospital with very different disease distributions. We therefore train our model on the full JSRT dataset, which is collected in Japan from a population with lung nodules, and test the trained model on the full Montgomery dataset, which is collected in the U.S. from patients potentially with TB. The two datasets present very different contrast and diseases (Fig. 1). Table 3 shows that FCN alone does not generalize well to a new dataset, but SCAN substantially improves the performance, surpassing [1].

We further investigate the scenario when training on the two development sets from JSRT and Montgomery *combined* to increase variation in the training data. Without any further hyperparameter tuning, SCAN improves the IoU on two lungs to 95.1% ± 0.43% on the JSRT evaluation set, and 93.0% ± 1.4% on the Montgomery evaluation set, a significant improvement compared with when training on JSRT development set alone.

Table 2. Comparison with existing single-model approaches to lung field segmentation on JSRT dataset. Note that [12,15] use different data splits than our evaluation.

	IoU (Lungs)	IoU (Heart)
Human Observer [12]	**94.6%** ± 1.8%	**87.8%** ± 5.4%
Ours (SCAN)	**94.7%** ± 0.4%	86.6% ± 1.2%
Registration-based [1]	92.5% ± 0.4%	–
DeepLabV2 101 [2]	85.7% ± 0.9%	–
U-net [9]	84.4% ± 1.3%	–
ShRAC [15]	90.7% ± 3.3%	–
ASM [12]	90.3% ± 5.7%	79.3% ± 11.9%
AAM [12]	84.7% ± 9.5%	77.5% ± 13.5%
Mean Shape [12]	71.3% ± 7.5%	64.3% ± 14.7%

Qualitative Comparison. Figure 6 shows the qualitative results from these two experiments. The failure cases in the middle row by our FCN reveal the difficulties arising from CXR images' varying contrast across samples. For example, the apex of the ribcage of the rightmost patient's is mistaken as an internal rib bone, resulting in the mask "bleeding out" to the black background, which has a similar intensity as the lung field. Vascular structures near mediastinum and anterior rib bones (which appears very faintly in the PA view CXR) within the lung field can also have similar intensity and texture as the exterior boundary, causing prediction errors in the middle two columns for FCN. SCAN significantly improves all of the failure cases and produces much more realistic outlines of the organs. SCAN also sharpens the segmentation of costophrenic angle (the sharp angle at the junction of ribcage and diaphragm), which are important in diagnosing pleural effusion and lung hyperexpansion, among others.

Figure 7 compares SCAN with the current state-of-the-art [1] qualitatively. We restrict the comparison to lung fields, as [1] only supports lung field segmentation. SCAN generates more accurate lung masks especially around costophrenic angles when tested on the same patient population (left two columns of Fig. 7). SCAN also generalizes better to a different population in the Montgomery dataset (right two columns of Fig. 7) whereas [1] struggles with domain shift.

Our SCAN framework is efficient at test time, as it only needs to perform a forward pass through the segmentation network but not the critic network. Table 4 shows the run time of our method compared with [1] on a laptop with Intel Core i5. [1] takes much longer due to the need to search through lung models in the training data to find similar profiles, incurring linear cost in the size of training data. In clinical setting such as TB screening [14] a fast test time result is highly desirable.

Table 3. Performance on the full Montgomery dataset using models trained on the full JSRT dataset. Compared with the JSRT dataset, the Montgomery dataset exhibits a much higher degree of lung abnormalities and varying imaging quality, testing the transferrability of the models.

	IoU (Both Lungs)
Ours (SCAN)	**91.4%** $\pm$ 0.6%
Ours (FCN)	87.1% $\pm$ 0.8%
Registration [1]	90.3% $\pm$ 0.5%

Table 4. Prediction time for each CXR image (resolution 400×400) from the Montgomery dataset on a laptop with Intel Core i5, along with the estimated human time.

	Test time
Ours (SCAN)	0.84 s
Registration [1]	26 s
Human	$\sim$2 min

References

1. Candemir, S., et al.: Lung segmentation in chest radiographs using anatomical atlases with nonrigid registration. IEEE Trans. Med. Imaging **33**(2), 577–590 (2014)
2. Chen, L.C., et al.: Deeplab: semantic image segmentation with deep convolutional nets, atrous convolution, and fully connected crfs. IEEE TPAMI **40**, 834–848 (2018)
3. Dallal, A.H., et al.: Automatic estimation of heart boundaries and cardiothoracic ratio from chest x-ray images. In: In: SPIE Medical Imaging (2017)
4. NHS England: Diagnostic imaging dataset annual statistical release 2015/16 (2016)
5. Goodfellow, I., et al.: Generative adversarial nets. In: Advances in Neural Information Processing Systems, pp. 2672–2680 (2014)
6. He, K., Zhang, X., Ren, S., Sun, J.: Identity mappings in deep residual networks. In: Leibe, B., Matas, J., Sebe, N., Welling, M. (eds.) ECCV 2016. LNCS, vol. 9908, pp. 630–645. Springer, Cham (2016). https://doi.org/10.1007/978-3-319-46493-0_38
7. Long, J., et al.: Fully convolutional networks for semantic segmentation. In: Proceedings of the IEEE Conference on Computer Vision and Pattern Recognition, pp. 3431–3440 (2015)
8. Luc, P., Couprie, C., Chintala, S., Verbeek, J.: Semantic segmentation using adversarial networks. In: NIPS Workshop on Adversarial Training (2016)
9. Ronneberger, O., Fischer, P., Brox, T.: U-net: convolutional networks for biomedical image segmentation. In: Navab, N., Hornegger, J., Wells, W.M., Frangi, A.F. (eds.) MICCAI 2015. LNCS, vol. 9351, pp. 234–241. Springer, Cham (2015). https://doi.org/10.1007/978-3-319-24574-4_28
10. Shiraishi, J., et al.: Development of a digital image database for chest radiographs with and without a lung nodule: receiver operating characteristic analysis of radiologists' detection of pulmonary nodules. Am. J. Roentgenol. **174**(1), 71–74 (2000)

11. The Royal College of Radiologists: Clinical radiology UK workforce census 2015 report, September 2016
12. Van Ginneken, B., et al.: Segmentation of anatomical structures in chest radiographs using supervised methods: a comparative study on a public database. Med. Image Anal. **10**, 19–40 (2006)
13. Wang, X., et al.: Chestx-ray8: hospital-scale chest x-ray database and benchmarks on weakly-supervised classification and localization of common thorax diseases. arXiv:1705.02315 (2017)
14. World Health Organization: Computer-aided Detection for Tuberculosis (2012)
15. Yu, T., Luo, J., Ahuja, N.: Shape regularized active contour using iterative global search and local optimization. In: CVPR. IEEE (2005)

Monte-Carlo Sampling Applied to Multiple Instance Learning for Histological Image Classification

Marc Combalia[✉][iD] and Verónica Vilaplana[iD]

Universitat Politècnica de Catalunya, Barcelona, Spain
marc.combalia@alu-etsetb.upc.edu, veronica.vilaplana@upc.edu

Abstract. We propose a patch sampling strategy based on a sequential Monte-Carlo method for high resolution image classification in the context of Multiple Instance Learning. When compared with grid sampling and uniform sampling techniques, it achieves higher generalization performance. We validate the strategy on two artificial datasets and two histological datasets for breast cancer and sun exposure classification.

Keywords: Histological image classification · Deep learning
Multiple instance learning · Patch sampling · Monte-Carlo methods

1 Introduction

Deep learning is widely used for image classification with great success [4,9]. However, neural networks can not be directly applied to very high resolution images, such as Whole Slide Tissue images, due to the high computational cost involved. A common solution consists in dividing the image into patches and using patch-level annotations to train a supervised classifier. However, patch-level annotations are not usually available, especially when working with medical datasets. On the contrary, image-level annotations are much easier to obtain so practitioners have used Multiple Instance Learning (MIL) to train patch-level classifiers in a weakly supervised manner, aggregating patch-level predictions into image-level scores [5–7,10].

When the input images are small enough, the MIL formulation can be implemented using a global Max Pooling layer at the output of a Fully Convolutional Network [8]. However, in the case of high resolution images, this implementation is not possible due to memory constraints. This is why patches are usually sampled using a regular grid (with or without overlap) [2,5] before being fed to the neural network. Grid sampling may skip some zones in the image which might be relevant for classification, and concentrate too much effort in zones which are not. In this work we propose a novel patch sampling strategy which extracts knowledge from the network to focus attention on the most discriminative regions in an image for a given instant in the training process, permitting

© Springer Nature Switzerland AG 2018
D. Stoyanov et al. (Eds.): DLMIA 2018/ML-CDS 2018, LNCS 11045, pp. 274–281, 2018.
https://doi.org/10.1007/978-3-030-00889-5_31

better convergence and higher generalization performance. We compare this approach to uniform sampling and conventional grid sampling on two artificial and two histological datasets.

2 Materials and Methods

2.1 Multiple Instance Learning

The Multiple Instance Learning formulation permits training a patch-based classifier with only image-level annotations, aggregating patch level predictions into image-level scores.

Multiple Instance Learning is a type of weakly supervised learning algorithm where training data is arranged in bags, where each bag contains a set of instances $X = \{x_1, x_2, ..., x_M\}$, and there is one single label Y per bag, $Y \in \{0, 1\}$ in the case of a binary classification problem. It is assumed that individual labels $y_1, y_2, ..., y_M$ exist for the instances within a bag, but they are unknown during training. In the standard Multiple Instance assumption (SMI), a bag is considered negative if all its instances are negative. On the other hand, a bag is positive, if at least one instance in the bag is positive [11].

The MIL formulation has been often used to solve the problem of high resolution image classification. An image (bag) is divided into M patches (instances), and the patches pertaining to the same image are treated jointly in the classifier. If an image is positive ($Y = 1$), it will contain at least one positive patch ($y_m = 1$ at least for one m). On the contrary, if the image is negative ($Y = 0$), all its patches will be negative ($y_m = 0$ for all m). Then, the max operator can be used to aggregate patch predictions to obtain an image-wise score: $\hat{Y} = max_m(\hat{y}_m)$, where $\hat{y}_m$ is the prediction for patch m. When using this aggregating function, the weights of the network will be updated with the information of only one patch per image. Other less strict aggregating functions have been proposed in the literature [6,10,11], which use not only the highest scoring patch but an aggregation of more than one patch prediction per image.

2.2 Patch Sampling

Since the neural network will use a small subset of patches to update its weights at every iteration, it is important to select an adequate sampling strategy. The traditional grid-sampling strategy, a sampling strategy based on a uniform random variable, and a novel sampling strategy based on sequential Monte Carlo methods are reviewed in this section.

Grid Sampling: The extraction of patches is performed in a grid-like manner; the image is divided into a regular grid of patches, with or without overlap. Given that the sampling is performed only once in the whole training process, grid sampling is the fastest sampling strategy. However, the subset of patches to train will be the same throughout the epochs. Also, this strategy will sample patches from not discriminative regions in the image even after the network has learned that they are not relevant for classification.

Uniform Sampling: A uniform distribution is applied to select the patches used to train the neural network at every epoch. This means that the neural network will see a different subset of patches every time the image goes through the training loop. As the number of training epochs increases, the network will tend to see all possible patches from every image. Nevertheless, this approach will sample patches from irrelevant regions in the image even after they have been learned to be non-discriminative.

Monte-Carlo Sampling: The objective of this sampling strategy is to concentrate the effort on the most relevant regions of a high resolution image. When a new image is fed into the network, its output probability map is estimated using a variation of a sequential Monte-Carlo method. New patches are obtained from regions around high activations in the output probability map.

1. Initialization: n image points are sampled following a uniform distribution.
2. Evaluation: a patch centered on each point is sampled and forwarded through the network. The output produced by the patch is used to represent the point.
3. Normalization: the point scores are re-scaled between 0 to 1. The points whose value is closer to 1 will be the ones corresponding to patches which have obtained the highest output from the neural network.
4. Re-sampling: the lowest scoring points are removed, and (the same number of) new points are re-sampled on top of the ones which have a higher score. This re-sampling step can be done deterministically (re-sampling the l lowest scoring points) or stochastically (using a random uniform distribution).
5. Displacement: the new points are slightly displaced according to a random 2D Gaussian distribution.
6. Go to step 2 for k iterations.

The proposed method relocates patches which have not been relevant for classification into more discriminative regions in the image, that is, around the patches with higher activations. This process is performed at every batch, since the discriminative regions in the image will vary as the network learns during the training process.

3 Experiments

3.1 Datasets

Artificial Datasets: Two binary artificial datasets named MNIST-Sparse and MNIST-Clustered have been created to test the performance of the various sampling algorithms. Each image of 1024×1024 pixels consists of an aggregation of 28×28 images from the MNIST dataset. A positive image contains at least one MNIST digit corresponding to the class '9', while a negative image contains only digits corresponding to the other classes ('0' to '8'). Digit '9' has been chosen because it can be mistaken for '4' or '5' [6].

The purpose of these datasets is to imitate two different distributions found in histological images. The MNIST-Sparse dataset has the relevant regions (where the target number is localized) spread through the image. On the contrary, the MNIST-Clustered dataset has the target patches concentrated in space. The training and test subsets contain 1000 and 400 images, respectively. Figure 2 shows examples extracted from the two datasets, where the target digits '9' have been highlighted using red squares.

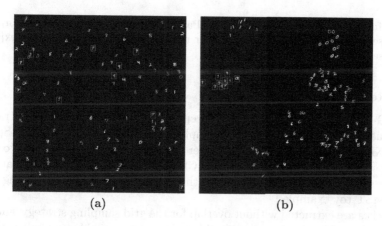

(a)   (b)

Fig. 1. Images extracted from MNIST-Sparse dataset (a) and MNIST-Clustered dataset (b). Target numbers (9) are marked with red squares in both images (Color figure online)

Histological Datasets: The sampling strategies are also evaluated on two histological datasets: the ICIAR Grand Challenge 2018 dataset Part A [1], and the Skin subset of the GTEx dataset [3].

The ICIAR dataset is formed by 400 breast microscopy tissue images divided in 4 different classes: normal, benign, invasive and in-situ carcinoma. For each class, there are 100 different Hematoxylin & Eosin stained images with a dimension of 2048 × 1536 pixels. The images are in RGB color space. We use benign and invasive classes to create a binary problem on which to test the algorithms, which results in 160 images for training and 40 for test. The images have already been pre-cropped from labeled Whole Slide Tissue images, and hence, from a MIL perspective, a large number of patches (instances) that we extract from an image (a bag) are expected to be consistent with the image label.

The Skin subset of the GTEx dataset is composed of approximately 10000 pieces of skin, which correspond to sun-exposed and not sun-exposed tissues. The smallest slide available (8 microns per pixel) is used to train the neural networks. The training and test splits contain 8000 and 2000 images, respectively.

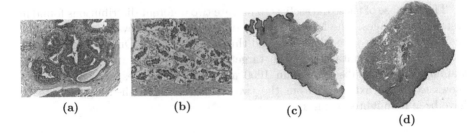

Fig. 2. Images extracted from the ICIAR Part A Dataset for benign (a) and invasive (b) classes; and the GTEx Skin dataset for the sun-exposed (c) and not-sun-exposed (d) classes.

3.2   Results

A VGG-like architecture [9] with a receptive field of 40×40 pixels is trained to evaluate the performance of the sampling algorithms on the MNIST-Sparse and MNIST-Clustered datasets. A higher capacity neural network based on the ResNet [4] architecture is used in the ICIAR Part A and GTEx Skin datasets with a receptive field of 224×224, since these datasets are more challenging than the MNIST toy example.

Patches are extracted without overlap for the grid sampling strategy, and the same number of patches/points is used for the uniform and Monte-Carlo training strategies. This results in a total of 625 patches per image for the MNIST dataset and 54 patches per image for the ICIAR dataset. The number of patches in the case of the GTEx dataset is variable since images have different sizes. One iteration is used on the Monte-Carlo algorithm every time the images go through the training loop, as it was found to be enough to perform a correct estimation of the output probability map of an image.

Patch scores are aggregated using the max operator into an image-level score for the MNIST and the GTEx Skin datasets, since relevant information is expected to be very localized in space. On the other hand, the Top-K (with $K = 10$) aggregating function is used in the ICIAR Part A dataset, since patches are expected to be consistent with the label of the image. The Top-K function will use the top K scoring instances in a bag to obtain the bag-level prediction.

The neural networks are trained with Adam optimization. Grid sampling with 50% overlap is used to sample patches from the images at test time, and the max function is used to aggregate patch scores into image-wise predictions. The accuracy results on the test set for each sampling strategy are shown in Table 1 and the train and validation accuracy curves for the MNIST-Sparse and MNIST-Clustered datasets are presented in Figs. 3 and 4, respectively.

4   Discussion

Figures 3 and 4 illustrate how the sampling strategy used for training can have a very large impact on the final performance of the neural network. This is espe-

Table 1. Test accuracies for the various sampling strategies on the MNIST-Sparse, MNIST-Clustered, ICIAR Part A and GTEx Skin datasets

Test accuracy	MNIST Sparse	MNIST Clust	ICIAR PartA	GTEx Skin
Grid sampling	0.520 ± 0.01	0.523 ± 0.01	0.776	0.826
Uniform sampling	0.759 ± 0.03	0.83 ± 0.01	0.790	0.920
Monte-Carlo sampling	$\mathbf{0.825 \pm 0.02}$	$\mathbf{0.852 \pm 0.03}$	**0.847**	**0.942**

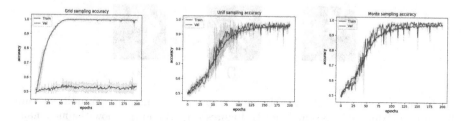

Fig. 3. Train and validation accuracy on the MNIST-Sparse dataset for the proposed sampling strategies: grid (left), uniform (center), Monte-Carlo (right).

cially true in cases where the receptive field of the network is small compared to the spatial extension of the discriminative features, as it is on the MNIST-Sparse and MNIST-Clustered datasets, where target digits are patches of 28×28 pixels and clusters of 40×40 pixels, respectively. In these cases, the grid sampling technique would need a very large overlap between patches to provide a good subset of patches to the network, which would result in a substantial increase in training time. While the neural network trained with the grid sampling strategy is unable to learn the true distribution of the data, the stochastic nature of the uniform and Monte-Carlo sampling strategies permits seeing a different subset of patches at every epoch. This allows the network to correctly find the discriminative regions on the image. In addition, once the network has learned which regions in the image are the relevant ones, the Monte-Carlo strategy samples only from these regions. This results in a higher validation accuracy, especially in the MNIST-Clustered dataset.

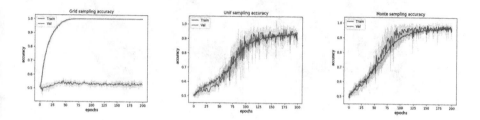

Fig. 4. Train and validation accuracy on the MNIST-Clustered dataset for the proposed sampling strategies: grid (left), uniform (center), Monte-Carlo (right).

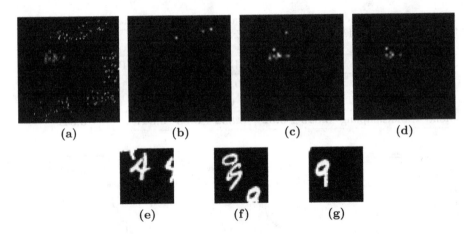

(a)   (b)   (c)   (d)

(e)   (f)   (g)

Fig. 5. Input image (a), output probability map for grid sampling (b), uniform sampling (c) and Monte-Carlo sampling (d). Figures (e), (f) and (g) show the maximally activated patch for grid, uniform and Monte-Carlo sampling, respectively.

Figure 5 shows the output probability maps of one positive image from the MNIST-Clustered database for each sampling strategy. The neural network trained with the grid sampling strategy fails to localize the target digit; the patch with the maximum score contains a '4'. On the other hand, the neural networks trained with the stochastic sampling strategies succeed activating on the regions containing the target digit '9'. The Monte-Carlo sampling strategy produces a more accurate map.

The stochastic sampling approaches outperform the grid sampling also on the histological datasets. This time, however, the neural networks trained with the grid sampling strategy perform correctly. In this case the neural networks have a larger receptive field, and the discriminative image regions are smaller compared to the receptive field. However, the neural networks still benefit from the Monte-Carlo training strategy, which focuses on the relevant regions, improving accuracy. Figure 6 shows how the distribution of samples in the Monte-Carlo

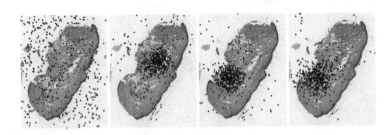

Fig. 6. Black points correspond to points sampled with Monte-Carlo at epochs 2, 6, 8 and 37 during the training process of the neural network for the sun-exposure classification problem.

approach changes as the neural network learns. In the first epochs, the Monte-Carlo strategy behaves very similarly to the uniform sampling strategy. However, as the network keeps learning, the Monte-Carlo sampling strategy further concentrates its effort on the discriminative regions.

5   Conclusions

In this paper we have shown that a simple grid sampling technique can compromise the performance of a network, especially when its receptive field is small compared to the size of the relevant features in the image. We have proposed a sampling strategy based on a sequential Monte-Carlo method for high resolution images which samples from the most relevant regions during the training process, overcoming the problems of grid sampling. We have illustrated its capabilities on two artificial and two histological datasets for breast cancer and sun exposure classification.

Acknowledgments. This work has been partially supported by the project MALE-GRA TEC2016-75976-R financed by the Spanish Ministerio de Economía y Competitividad and the European Regional Development Fund.

References

1. BACH: Iciar 2018 (2018). https://iciar2018-challenge.grand-challenge.org/
2. Campanella, G., Werneck Krauss Silva, V., Fuchs, T.J.: Terabyte-scale deep multiple instance learning for classification and localization in pathology, May 2018
3. Carithers, L.J., et al.: A novel approach to high-quality postmortem tissue procurement: the GTEx project. Biopreservation Biobanking **13**(5), 311–319 (2015)
4. He, K., Zhang, X., Ren, S., Sun, J.: Deep residual learning for image recognition. CoRR abs/1512.03385 (2015). http://arxiv.org/abs/1512.03385
5. Hou, L., Samaras, D., Kurc, T.M., Gao, Y., Davis, J.E., Saltz, J.H.: Patch-based convolutional neural network for whole slide tissue image classification. In: Proceedings of the IEEE Conference on Computer Vision and Pattern Recognition, pp. 2424–2433 (2016)
6. Ilse, M., Tomczak, J.M., Welling, M.: Attention-based deep multiple instance learning. CoRR abs/1802.04712 (2018). http://arxiv.org/abs/1802.04712
7. Mercan, C., Mercan, E., Aksoy, S., Shapiro, L.G., Weaver, D.L., Elmore, J.G.: Multi-instance multi-label learning for whole slide breast histopathology. In: Medical Imaging 2016: Digital Pathology, vol. 9791, p. 979108. International Society for Optics and Photonics (2016)
8. Pathak, D., Shelhamer, E., Long, J., Darrell, T.: Fully convolutional multi-class multiple instance learning. CoRR abs/1412.7144 (2014). http://arxiv.org/abs/1412.7144
9. Simonyan, K., Zisserman, A.: Very deep convolutional networks for large-scale image recognition. CoRR abs/1409.1556 (2014). http://arxiv.org/abs/1409.1556
10. Tomczak, J.M., Ilse, M., Welling, M.: Deep learning with permutation-invariant operator for multi-instance histopathology classification. ArXiv e-prints, December 2017
11. Wang, X., Yan, Y., Tang, P., Bai, X., Liu, W.: Revisiting multiple instance neural networks. Pattern Recogn. **74**, 15–24 (2018)

Automatic Segmentation of Pulmonary Lobes Using a Progressive Dense V-Network

Abdullah-Al-Zubaer Imran[1,2], Ali Hatamizadeh[1,2], Shilpa P. Ananth[2],
Xiaowei Ding[1,2(✉)], Demetri Terzopoulos[1,2], and Nima Tajbakhsh[2]

[1] University of California, Los Angeles, CA 90095, USA
[2] VoxelCloud Inc., Los Angeles, CA 90024, USA
xding@voxelcloud.io

Abstract. Reliable and automatic segmentation of lung lobes is important for diagnosis, assessment, and quantification of pulmonary diseases. The existing techniques are prohibitively slow, undesirably rely on prior (airway/vessel) segmentation, and/or require user interactions for optimal results. This work presents a reliable, fast, and fully automated lung lobe segmentation based on a progressive dense V-network (PDV-Net). The proposed method can segment lung lobes in one forward pass of the network, with an average runtime of 2 s using 1 Nvidia Titan XP GPU, eliminating the need for any prior atlases, lung segmentation or any subsequent user intervention. We evaluated our model using 84 chest CT scans from the LIDC and 154 pathological cases from the LTRC datasets. Our model achieved a Dice score of 0.939 ± 0.02 for the LIDC test set and 0.950 ± 0.01 for the LTRC test set, significantly outperforming a 2D U-net model and a 3D dense V-net. We further evaluated our model against 55 cases from the LOLA11 challenge, obtaining an average Dice score of 0.935—a performance level competitive to the best performing team with an average score of 0.938. Our extensive robustness analyses also demonstrate that our model can reliably segment both healthy and pathological lung lobes in CT scans from different vendors, and that our model is robust against configurations of CT scan reconstruction.

Keywords: Lung lobe segmentation · CT · Progressive dense V-Net
Fissure · 3D CNN

1 Introduction

Human lungs are divided into five lobes. The right lung has three lobes, namely, right upper lobe (RUL), right middle lobe (RML), and right lower lobe (RLL), which are separated by a minor and a major fissure, whereas the left lung has

---

Electronic supplementary material The online version of this chapter (https://doi.org/10.1007/978-3-030-00889-5_32) contains supplementary material, which is available to authorized users.

© Springer Nature Switzerland AG 2018
D. Stoyanov et al. (Eds.): DLMIA 2018/ML-CDS 2018, LNCS 11045, pp. 282–290, 2018.
https://doi.org/10.1007/978-3-030-00889-5_32

two lobes, namely, left upper lobe (LUL) and left lower lobe (LLL), separated by a major fissure. Figure 1 shows the five lobes separated by major and minor fissures in a coronal CT slice. Each of the five lobes is functionally independent as they have separate bronchial and vascular systems.

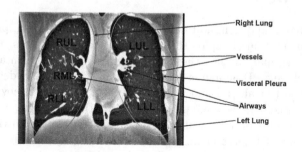

Fig. 1. A coronal lung CT slice with visible fissures. Major fissures are denoted by red arrows and yellow arrows denote the minor fissure.

Automatic lobe segmentation is important for both clinical and technical purposes. In clinical practice, doctors very often base their assessment of a disease severity and the corresponding treatment plan on the affected lung lobe. As such, upon encountering a disease or lesion in the lung, radiologists may navigate through the nearby slices to identify the affected lobe, especially when the fissure lines are not clearly visible in the target slice. An automatic lobe segmentation model can therefore shorten the CT reading session by continually informing the radiologists about their location in the lung anatomy. From the technical perspective, accurate lung lobe segmentation can improve several subsequent clinical tasks, including nodule malignancy prediction (cancers mostly occur in the left or right upper lobes), automatic lobe-aware report generation for each nodule, and assessment and quantification of pulmonary diseases, by narrowing down the search space to the lung lobes most-likely to be affected. However, identifying fissures poses a challenge for both human and machine perception. *First*, fissures are most often incomplete, not extending to the lobar boundaries. Several studies in the literature have confirmed the incompleteness of fissures as a very common phenomenon [1]. *Second*, the visual characteristics of lobar boundaries can change in presence of pathologies. Such morphological changes could also be related to the varying thicknesses, locations, and shapes of the fissures. *Third*, there also exist other fissures in the lungs that can be misinterpreted as the major or minor fissures that separate the lobes (e.g., accessory fissures and azygos fissures).

To address the need for accurate and robust lobe segmentation, we have proposed a fully automatic and reliable deep learning solution via progressive dense V-net (PDV-net). The PDV-net model takes entire CT volume and through three dense feature blocks, generates the segmentation progressively improving at each pathway. Our model generates accurate segmentation of the lung lobes in about 2 s in only a single forward pass of the network, eliminating the need for any user interactions or any prior segmentation of lungs, vessels, or airways, which are common assumptions in the design of existing models.

2   Related Work

Various automatic and semi-automatic approaches have been proposed for lung lobe segmentation. Despite the methodological differences, the existing approaches are similar in that they require either prior segmentation of airways and vessels (e.g., Bragman et al. [2]) or demand previously defined atlases (e.g., van Rikxoort et al. [11] and Ross et al. [13]). Therefore, they suffer from slow execution time, cumbersome process of generating the atlas, and relatively lower performance for pathological cases. A significant shift from this common trend is the work of George et al. [4] wherein a 2D fully convolutional neural network followed by a 3D random walker algorithm is used to segment lobes. However, their method still relied on the random walker algorithm whose optimal parameters could change from one dataset to another. It is most desirable to have an end-to-end solution that does not rely on any subsequent heuristic method.

In the presented work, we mitigate the aforementioned limitations, namely reliance on prior masks, slow runtime, and lack of robustness by an end-to-end, single-pass, deep-learning-based framework that does not rely on any prior airway/vessel segmentation, anatomical knowledge, or atlases.

3   Method

We combine the ideas from dense V-network [5] and progressive holistically nested networks [7] to obtain a new architecture: progressive dense V-network (PDV-net), an end-to-end solution for organ segmentation in 3D volumetric data. Our proposed architecture is illustrated in Fig. 2. As seen, the input to the network is first down-sampled and concatenated with a strided $5 \times 5 \times 5$ convolution of the input with 24 kernels. The concatenation result is then passed to 3 dense feature blocks, each consisting of 5, 10, and 10 densely-wired convolution layers respectively. The growth rates of dense blocks are set to 4, 8, and 16 respectively. All the convolutional layers in a dense block have a kernel size of $3 \times 3 \times 3$ and are followed by batch normalization and parametric rectified linear units (PReLU).

Consecutively, the outputs of the dense feature blocks are utilized in low and high resolution passes via convolutional down-sampling and skip connections. This enables the generation of feature maps at three different resolutions. The outputs of the skip connections of the second and third dense feature blocks are further up-sampled in order to be consistent with the size of the output in the first skip connection. The feature maps from skip1 are passed to a convolutional layer followed by a softmax, which outputs the probability maps. In the second pathway, the feature maps from skip1 and skip2 are merged and the output probability maps are produced by a convolutional layer followed by softmax.

Similarly, we get the final segmentation result from the merged feature maps resulted from the skip2 and skip3 connections. Unlike dense V-net, PDV-net generates the final output by progressively improving the outputs at previous pathways. To train the suggested architecture, we choose to use a dice-based loss function [10] at each stage of the progressive architecture.

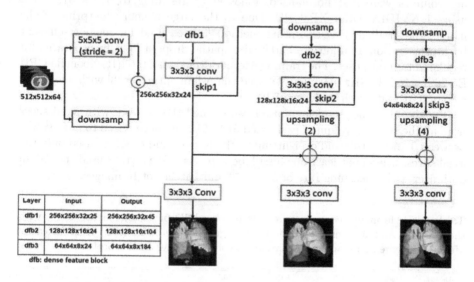

Fig. 2. PDV-net model for the segmentation of lung lobes. Segmentation outputs at different pathways are progressively improved for the final result.

4   Experiments

Datasets: We used 3 public datasets to evaluate our models. **First,** we selected a subset of chest CTs (354 cases) from the publicly available LIDC dataset for annotation. To ensure variability in the data, CT scans were selected such that both challenging and visible fissures are well-represented in the dataset. The ground truth masks were generated in a semi-automatic fashion by multiple observers using 3D Slicer. To mitigate bias in the ground truth, the generated masks were later refined and validated by an expert radiologist. The dataset was split into 270 training and 84 test cases. 10% of the training set was utilized as the validation set. **Second,** we selected 154 CTs from LTRC database. The LTRC dataset includes lobe masks for pathological cases that have clear evidence of COPD or ILD diseases, including emphysema and fibrosis. The LTRC cases allow us to measure the robustness of our model against pathologies in the lungs. **Third,** we used 55 cases of the Lobe and Lung Analysis (LOLA11) challenge [9] and submitted the results to the challenge organizers for evaluation.

Baselines for Comparison: We used a U-Net architecture [12] and a dense V-Net for comparison. The former is used in the most recent published article [4] for lung lobe segmentation and the latter is a strong baseline for comparison, which we use for the first time for lung lobe segmentation.

Implementation Details: For the proposed model and dense V-net, the training volumes were first normalized, followed by rescaling to $512 \times 512 \times 64$, using 1 NVIDIA Titan XP GPU. Due to the large memory footprint of the model, the gradient check-pointing method [3] was used for memory-efficient back-propagation. In addition, batch-wise spatial dropout [5] is incorporated for regularization purposes. The training was performed on a Intel(R) Xeon(R) CPU E5-2697 v4@2.30 GHz machine. We used the Adam optimizer [8] with a learning rate of 0.01 and a weight decay of 10^{-7}.

For the 2D U-net implementation, we trained the network with axial slices from all the training volumes, each sized 512×512 and normalized to have values between 0 and 1. To avoid over-fitting to the background class, we used only the axial slices, wherein at least one lung lobe is present. We further used the Adam optimizer with a learning rate of 5×10^{-5} and batches of 10 images.

Table 1. Performance comparison of the proposed 3D progressive dense V-net with the 2D U-net and 3D dense V-net models in segmenting 84 LIDC and 154 LTRC cases. Mean Dice score and standard deviation for each lobe have been reported.

Dataset	Model	RUL	RML	RLL	LUL	LLL	Overall
LIDC(84)	2D U-Net	0.908 ± 0.049	0.844 ± 0.076	0.940 ± 0.054	0.959 ± 0.042	0.949 ± 0.056	0.920 ± 0.043
	3D DV-Net	0.929 ± 0.036	0.873 ± 0.058	0.951 ± 0.018	0.958 ± 0.020	0.949 ± 0.041	0.932 ± 0.023
	3D PDV-Net	**0.937 ± 0.031**	**0.882 ± 0.057**	**0.956 ± 0.017**	**0.966 ± 0.014**	**0.966 ± 0.037**	**0.939 ± 0.020**
LTRC(154)	2D U-Net	0.914 ± 0.039	0.866 ± 0.054	0.952 ± 0.023	0.961 ± 0.023	0.954 ± 0.021	0.929 ± 0.025
	3D DV-Net	0.949 ± 0.013	0.901 ± 0.021	0.959 ± 0.009	0.961 ± 0.007	0.958 ± 0.012	0.946 ± 0.008
	3D PDV-Net	**0.952 ± 0.011**	**0.908 ± 0.020**	**0.961 ± 0.008**	**0.966 ± 0.006**	**0.960 ± 0.010**	**0.950 ± 0.007**

LIDC Results: Table 1 shows the calculated overall and lobe-wise Dice scores for each of the models. The proposed progressive dense V-net model, with an overall score of 0.939 ± 0.020, significantly outperformed the 2D model, with an overall score of 0.9201 ± 0.0431. As is evident in Table 1, the 3D progressive dense V-net yields consistently larger Dice score for each of the lung lobes against both dense V-net and U-net. Moreover, the lower standard deviation for each lobe indicates that the progressive model is more robust. We have also shown a qualitative comparison between the 3 models in Fig. 3 where the lung fissures are better captured by our progressive dense V-net model than by 2D U-net and dense V-net.

We further used Bland-Altman plots to measure the agreement between our progressive dense V-net and ground truth segmentations of the 84 LIDC cases (Fig. 4). A good agreement was observed between our segmentation model and ground truth in every plot (Lung and LLL being the two best agreements).

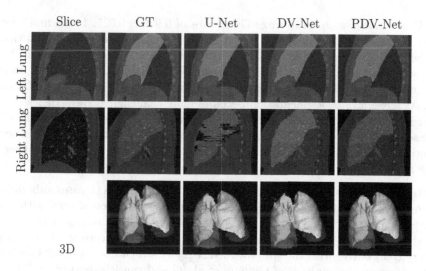

Fig. 3. Qualitative comparison between the proposed 3D progressive dense V-Net (PDV-Net), dense V-Net (DV-Net), and U-net. Note how noisy patches are removed from the final segmentation generated by PDV-Net. Color coding: almond: LUL, blue: LLL, yellow: RUL, cyan: RML, pink: RLL. (Color figure online)

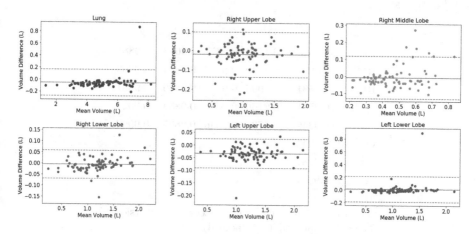

Fig. 4. Bland-Altman plots show the agreement between 3D progressive dense V-net and ground truth.

Pearson correlation showed that all six volume sets in ground truth are strongly correlated with the corresponding six volume sets in the PDV-net segmentation, with $p < 0.001$.

LTRC Results: Table 1 shows that the 3D progressive dense V-net achieves an average Dice score of 0.950 ± 0.007, significantly improving the dense V-net (0.946 ± 0.008). Once again, the progressive dense V-net model outperformed the

2D U-net model with an average Dice score of 0.929 ± 0.025. Individual lobes were segmented better in the proposed 3D progressive dense V-net model than in the 3D dense V-net and the 2D U-net models (Table 1). Note that the LTRC dataset includes many pathological cases where the fissure lines are either invisible, distorted, or absent in presence of pathologies such as emphysema, fibrosis, etc. As a result, lobe segmentation becomes more challenging. Nevertheless, our model performed well in segmenting lobes in pathological cases from the LTRC dataset. Moreover, our model outperformed the model of George et al. [4] in segmenting the LTRC cases both in Dice score (0.941 ± 0.255) and inference speed (4–8 minutes per case).

LOLA11 Results: The segmentation results on the LOLA11 cases submitted online were evaluated as overlap (Jaccard) scores. To be consistent with our previous analyses, we converted the Jaccard scores to Dice scores. The results are shown in Table 2. Our method achieved an overall Dice score of 0.934, which is very competitive with the state-of-the-art [2] with a Dice score of 0.938, while outperforming the methods of Giuliani et al. [6] and van Rikxoort et al. [11].

Table 2. Performance evaluation of 3D PDV-Net models on 55 LOLA cases: showing lobe-wise mean Dice scores, standard deviations, median scores, first quartiles, and third quartiles

Lobe	Mean ± SD	Q_1	Median	Q_3
RUL	0.9518 ± 0.1750	0.9371	0.9688	0.9881
RML	0.8621 ± 0.4149	0.8107	0.9284	0.9663
RLL	0.9581 ± 0.1993	0.9621	0.9829	0.9881
LUL	0.9551 ± 0.2160	0.9644	0.9834	0.9924
LLL	0.9342 ± 0.3733	0.9546	0.9805	0.9902
Overall	0.9345			
[6]	0.9282			
[2]	0.9384			
[11]	0.9195			

*Jaccard score to Dice score conversion: Dice $= 2 \times$ Jaccard$/(1 +$ Jaccard$)$

Robustness Analysis: We further investigated the robustness of our model by grouping the 84 LIDC cases in three ways. For the first grouping, the Dice scores were put in three different Z-spacing buckets: Z-spacing ≤ 1, $1 <$ Z-spacing < 2, and Z-spacing ≥ 2. In the second grouping, the Dice scores were put in four manufacturer buckets: GE, Philips, Siemens, and Toshiba. In the third grouping, the Dice scores were grouped according to the reconstruction kernel into 3 buckets: soft, lung, and bone. The one-way ANOVA analysis confirmed that there were no significant differences between the average Dice scores of the buckets within each grouping, suggesting that our model is robust against the choice of reconstruction kernel, size of reconstruction interval, and different CT scan vendors. Moreover, nodule volume in each of the 84 cases does not affect the lobe segmentation performance. There is no correlation between nodule volume and lobe segmentation accuracy, found from Pearson correlation.

We also studied how the segmentation correlation is affected by lung pathologies. For this purpose, we analyzed the correlation between Dice scores and emphysema index (proportion of the lung affected by emphysema) in LTRC cases. According to the Pearson correlation, it was found that lobe segmentation accuracy is not correlated with emphysema index, indicating the robustness of our proposed model in segmenting lobes from pathological cases.

Speed Analysis: The proposed 3D progressive dense V-net model takes approximately 2 s to segment lung lobes from one CT scan using 1 Nvidia Titan XP GPU, which is six times faster than the 2D U-net model. As per our knowledge from the lung lobe segmentation models available in literature, this is by far the fastest model. Note that no prior published research has yet considered a 3D convolutional model for lung lobe segmentation.

5   Conclusions

Automatic and reliable lung lobe segmentation is a challenging task in the presence of chest pathologies and in the absence of visible, complete fissures. In this paper, we introduced a new 3D segmentation approach, namely, progressive dense V-networks for the automatic, fast, and reliable segmentation of lung lobes from chest CT scans, without any prior segmentation. We evaluated our method using 3 test datasets: 84 cases from LIDC, 154 cases from LTRC, and 55 cases from LOLA11. Our results demonstrated that the suggested model outperforms, or at worst performs comparably to, the state-of-the-art while running at an average speed of 2 s per case. Our analyses further demonstrated the robustness of the suggested method against varying configurations of CT reconstruction, choice of CT vendor, and presence of lung pathologies.

References

1. Aziz, A., Ashizawa, K., Nagaoki, K., Hayashi, K.: High resolution CT anatomy of the pulmonary fissures. J. Thoracic. Imag. **19**(3), 186–191 (2004)
2. Bragman, F.J., McClelland, J.R., Jacob, J., Hurst, J.R., Hawkes, D.J.: Pulmonary lobe segmentation with probabilistic segmentation of the fissures and a groupwise fissure prior. IEEE Tran. Med. Imag. **36**(8), 1650–1663 (2017)
3. Bulatov, Y.: Saving memory using gradient-checkpointing (2018). https://github.com/openai/gradient-checkpointing
4. George, K., Harrison, A.P., Jin, D., Xu, Z., Mollura, D.J.: Pathological pulmonary lobe segmentation from CT images using progressive holistically nested neural networks and random walker. In: Cardoso, M.J. (ed.) DLMIA/ML-CDS -2017. LNCS, vol. 10553, pp. 195–203. Springer, Cham (2017). https://doi.org/10.1007/978-3-319-67558-9_23

5. Gibson, E., et al.: Automatic multi-organ segmentation on abdominal CT with dense v-networks. IEEE Tran. Med. Imag. (2018)

6. Giuliani, N., Payer, C., Pienn, M., Olschewski, H., Urschler, M.: Pulmonary lobe segmentation in ct image using alpha-expansion. In: Proceedings of VISIGRAPP, pp. 387–394 (2018)

7. Harrison, A.P., Xu, Z., George, K., Lu, L., Summers, R.M., Mollura, D.J.: Progressive and multi-path holistically nested neural networks for pathological lung segmentation from CT images. In: Descoteaux, M., Maier-Hein, L., Franz, A., Jannin, P., Collins, D.L., Duchesne, S. (eds.) MICCAI 2017. LNCS, vol. 10435, pp. 621–629. Springer, Cham (2017). https://doi.org/10.1007/978-3-319-66179-7_71

8. Kingma, D.P., Ba, J.: Adam: A method for stochastic optimization. arXiv:1412.6980 (2014)

9. LOLA11: Lobe and lung analysis (2011). http://lola11.com

10. Milletari, F., Navab, N., Ahmadi, S.: V-net: Fully convolutional neural networks for volumetric medical image segmentation. In: Proceedings of 3DV, pp. 565–571. IEEE (2016)

11. van Rikxoort, E., Prokop, M., de Hoop, B., Viergever, M., Pluim, J., van Ginneken, B.: Automatic segmentation of pulmonary lobes robust against incomplete fissures. IEEE Tran. Med. Imag. 29(6), 1286–1296 (2010)

12. Ronneberger, O., Fischer, P., Brox, T.: U-net: convolutional networks for biomedical image segmentation. In: Navab, N., Hornegger, J., Wells, W.M., Frangi, A.F. (eds.) MICCAI 2015. LNCS, vol. 9351, pp. 234–241. Springer, Cham (2015). https://doi.org/10.1007/978-3-319-24574-4_28

13. Ross, J., et al.: Automatic lobe segmentation using particles, thin plate splines, and a maximum a posteriori estimation. Proc. MICCAI **6363**, 163–171 (2010)

Computed Tomography Image Enhancement Using 3D Convolutional Neural Network

Meng Li[1,4(✉)], Shiwen Shen[2], Wen Gao[1], William Hsu[2], and Jason Cong[3,4]

[1] National Engineering Laboratory for Video Technology, Peking University, Beijing, China
mmli@pku.edu.cn
[2] Department of Radiological Sciences, University of California, Los Angeles, USA
[3] Computer Science Department, University of California, Los Angeles, USA
[4] UCLA/PKU Joint Research Institute in Science and Engineering, Los Angeles, USA

Abstract. Computed tomography (CT) is increasingly being used for cancer screening, such as early detection of lung cancer. However, CT studies have varying pixel spacing due to differences in acquisition parameters. Thick slice CTs have lower resolution, hindering tasks such as nodule characterization during computer-aided detection due to partial volume effect. In this study, we propose a novel 3D enhancement convolutional neural network (3DECNN) to improve the spatial resolution of CT studies that were acquired using lower resolution/slice thicknesses to higher resolutions. Using a subset of the LIDC dataset consisting of 20,672 CT slices from 100 scans, we simulated lower resolution/thick section scans then attempted to reconstruct the original images using our 3DECNN network. A significant improvement in PSNR (29.3087dB vs. 28.8769dB, p-value $< 2.2e-16$) and SSIM (0.8529dB vs. 0.8449dB, p-value $< 2.2e-16$) compared to other state-of-art deep learning methods is observed.

Keywords: Super resolution · Computed tomography
Medical imaging · Convolutional neural network
Image enhancement · Deep learning

1   Introduction

Computed tomography (CT) is a widely used screening and diagnostic tool that provides detailed anatomical information on patients. Its ability to resolve small objects, such as nodules that are 1–30 mm in size, makes the modality indispensable in performing tasks such as lung cancer screening and colonography. However, the variation in image resolution of CT screening due to differences in radiation dose and slice thickness hinders the radiologist's ability to discern

D. Stoyanov et al. (Eds.): DLMIA 2018/ML-CDS 2018, LNCS 11045, pp. 291–299, 2018.
https://doi.org/10.1007/978-3-030-00889-5_33

subtle suspicious findings. Thus, it is highly desirable to develop an approach that enhances lower resolution CT scans by increasing the detail and sharpness of borders to mimic higher resolution acquisitions [1].

Super-resolution (SR) is a class of techniques that increase the resolution of an imaging system [2] and has been widely applied on natural images and is increasingly being explored in medical imaging. Traditional SR methods use linear or non-linear functions (e.g., bilinear/bicubic interpolation and example-based methods [3,4]) to estimate and simulate image distributions. These methods, however, produce blurring and jagged edges in images, which introduce artifacts and may negatively impact the ability of computer-aided detection (CAD) systems to detect subtle nodules. Recently, deep learning, especially convolutional neural networks (CNN), has been shown to extract high-dimensional and non-linear information from images that results in a much improved super-resolution output. One example is the super-resolution convolutional neural network (SRCNN) [5]. SRCNN learns an end-to-end mapping from low- to high-resolution images. In [6,7], the authors applied and evaluated the SRCNN method to improve the image quality of magnified images in chest radiographs and CT images. Moreover, [9] introduced an efficient sub-pixel convolution network (ESPCN), which was shown to be more computationally efficient than SRCNN. In [10], the authors proposed a SR method that utilizes a generative adversarial network (GAN), resulting in images have better perceptual quality compared to SRCNN. All these methods were evaluated using 2D images. However, for medical imaging modalities that are volumetric, such as CT, a 2D convolution ignores the correlation between slices. We propose a 3DECNN architecture, which executes a series of 3D convolutions on the volumetric data. We measure performance using two image quality metrics: peak signal-to-noise ratio (PSNR) and structural similarity (SSIM). Our approach achieves significant improvement compared with improved SRCNN approach (FSRCNN) [8,9] on both metrics.

2   Method

2.1   Overview

For each slice in the CT volume, our task is to generate a high-resolution image I^{HR} from a low-resolution image I^{LR}. Our approach can be divided into two phases: model training and inference. In the model training phase, we first down-sample a given image I to obtain the low-resolution image I^{LR}. We then use the original data as the high-resolution images I^{HR} to train our proposed 3DECNN network. In the model inference phase, we use a previously unseen low-resolution CT volume as input to the trained 3DECNN model and generate a super resolution image I^{SR}.

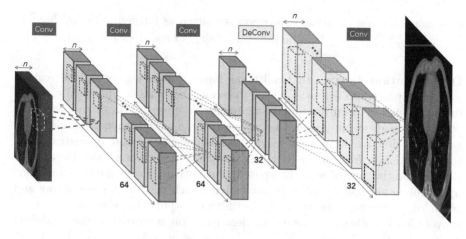

Fig. 1. Proposed 3DECNN architecture

2.2 Formulation

For CT images, spatial correlations exist across three dimensions. As such, the key to generating high-quality SR images is to make full use of available information along all dimensions. Thus, we apply cube-shaped filters on the input CT slices and slides these filters through all three dimensions of the input. Our model architecture is illustrated in Fig. 1. This filtering procedure is repeated in 3 stacked layers. After the 3D filtering process, a 3D deconvolution is used to reconstruct images and up-sample them to larger ones. The output of this 3D deconvolution is a reconstructed SR 3D volume. However, to compare with other SR methods such as SRCNN and ESPCN, which produces 2D outputs, we transform our 3D volume into a 2D output. As such, we add a final convolution layer to smooth pixels into a 2D slice, which is then compared to the outputs of the other methods. In the following paragraphs, we describe mathematical details of our 3DECNN architecture.

3D Convolutional Layers. In this work, we incorporate the feature extraction optimizations into the training/learning procedure of convolution kernels. The original CT images are normalized to values between [0,1]. The first CNN layer takes a normalized CT image (represented as a 3-D tensor) as input and generates multiple 3-D tensors (feature maps) as output by sliding the cube-shaped filters (convolution kernels), which are sized of '$k_1 \times k_2 \times k_3$', across inputs. We define convolution input tensor notations as $\langle N, C_{in}, H, W \rangle$ and output $\langle N, C_{out}, H, W \rangle$, in which C_i stands for the number of 3-D tensors and $\langle N, H, W \rangle$ stands for the feature map block's thickness, height, and width, respectively. Subsequent convolution layers take the previous layer's output feature maps as input, which are in a 4-D tensor. Convolution kernels are in a dimension of $\langle C_{in}, C_{out}, k_1, k_2, k_3 \rangle$. The sliding stride parameter $\langle s \rangle$ defines how many pixels to skip between each adjacent convolution on input feature maps. Its mathematical expression is written as follows: $out[c_o][n][h][w] = \sum_{n=0}^{C_i} \sum_{i=0}^{k_1} \sum_{j=0}^{k_2} \sum_{k=0}^{k_3} W[c_o][c_i][i][j][k] * In[c_i][s*n+i][s*h+j][s*w+k]$.

Deconvolution Layer. In traditional image processing, a reverse feature extraction procedure is typically used to reconstruct images. Specifically, design functions such as linear interpolation, are used to up-scale images and also average overlapped output patches to generate the final SR image. In this work, we utilize deconvolution to achieve image up-sampling and reconstruct feature information from previous layers' outputs at the same time. Deconvolution can be thought of as a transposed convolution. Deconvolution operations up-sample input feature maps by multiplying each pixel with cubic filters and summing up overlap outputs of adjacent filters' output [11]. Following the above convolution's mathematic notations, deconvolution is written as the following: $out[c_o][n][h[w] = \sum_{n=0}^{C_i} \sum_{i=0}^{k_1} \sum_{j=0}^{k_2} \sum_{k=0}^{k_3} W[c_o][c_i][i][j][k] * In[c_i][\frac{n}{s}+k_1-i][\frac{h}{s}+k_2-j][\frac{w}{s}+k_3-k]$. Activation functions are used to apply an element-wise non-linear transformation on the convolution or deconvolution output tensors. In this work, we use ReLU as the activation function.

Hyperparameters. There are four hyperparameters that have an influence on model performance: number of feature layers, feature map depth, number of convolution kernels, and size of kernels. The number of feature extraction layers $\langle l \rangle$ determines the upper-bound complexity in features that the CNN can learn from images. The feature map depth $\langle n \rangle$ is the number of CT slices that are taken in together to generate one SR image. The number of convolution kernels $\langle f \rangle$ decides the number of total feature maps in a layer and thus decides the maximum information that can be represented in the output of this layer. The size of convolution and deconvolution kernels $\langle k \rangle$ decides the visible scope that the filter can see in the input CT image or feature maps. Given the impact of each hyperparameter, we performed a grid search of the hyperparameter space to find the best combination of $\langle n, l, f, k \rangle$ for our 3DECNN model.

Loss Function. Peak signal-to-noise ratio (PSNR) is the most commonly used metric to measure the quality of reconstructed lossy images in all kinds of imaging systems. A higher PSNR generally indicates a higher quality of the reconstruction image. PSNR is defined as the log on the division of the max pixel value over mean squared root. Therefore, we directly use the squared mean error function as our loss function: $J(w, b) = \frac{1}{m} \sum_{i=1}^{m} L(\hat{y}^{(i)}, y^{(i)}) = \frac{1}{m} \sum_{i=1}^{m} ||\hat{y}^{(i)} - y^{(i)}||^2$, where w and b represent *weight* parameters and *bias* parameters. m is the number of training samples. $\hat{y}$ and y refer to the output of the neural network and the target, respectively. In addition, the target loss function is minimized using stochastic gradient descent with the back-propagation algorithm [13].

3   Experiments and Results

In this section, we first introduce the experiment setup, including dataset and data preparation. Then we show the design space of the hyper-parameters, at which time we show how to explore different CNN architectures and find the best model. Subsequently, we compare our method with recent state-of-the-art work and demonstrate the performance improvement. Lastly, we present examples of the generated SR CT images using our proposed method and previous state-of-the-art results.

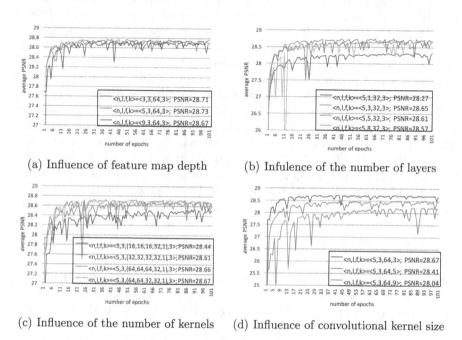

(a) Influence of feature map depth   (b) Infulence of the number of layers

(c) Influence of the number of kernels   (d) Influence of convolutional kernel size

Fig. 2. Design space of hyper-parameters

3.1   Experiment Setup

Dataset. We use the public available Lung Image Database Consortium image collection (LIDC) dataset for this study [12], which consists of low- and diagnostic-dose thoracic CT scans. These scans have a wide range of slice thickness ranging from 0.6 to 5 mm. And the pixel spacing in axial view (x-y direction) ranges from 0.4609 to 0.9766 mm. We randomly select 100 scans out of a total of 1018 cases from the LIDC dataset, result in a total consisting of 20672 slices. The selected CT scans are then randomized into four folds with similar size. Two folds are used for training, and the remaining two folds are used for validation and test, respectively.

Data Preprocessing. For each CT scan, we first downsample it on axial view by the desired scaling factor (set 3 in our experiment) to form the LR images. Then the corresponding HR images are ground truth images.

Hyperparameter Tuning $\langle n, l, f, k \rangle$. We choose the four most influential parameters to explore in our experiment and discuss, which is *feature depth (n), number of layers (l), number of filters (f)* and *filter kernel size (k)*.

The effect of the **feature depth** $\langle n \rangle$ is shown in Fig. 2(a). It presents the training curves of three different 3DECNN architectures, in which their $\langle l, f, s \rangle$ are the same and $\langle n \rangle$ varies in $[3, 5, 9]$. Among the three configurations, $n = 3$ has a better average PSNR than the others. The effect of the **number of layers** $\langle l \rangle$ is shown Fig. 2(b), which demonstrates that a deeper CNN may not always be better. With fixed $\langle n, f, s \rangle$ and varying $l \in [1, 3, 5, 8]$, here l indicate the number of convolutional layers before the deconvolution process. We can observe apparent different performance on the training curves. We determine that $l = 3$ achieves higher average PSNR. The effect of the **number of filters** $\langle f \rangle$ is shown in Fig. 2(c), in which we fix $\langle n, l, k \rangle$ and choose $\langle f \rangle$ in four collections. An apparent drop in PSNR is seen when $\langle f \rangle$ chooses the too small configuration $\langle 16, 16, 16, 32, 1 \rangle$. $\langle 64, 64, 64, 32, 1 \rangle$ and $\langle 64, 64, 32, 32, 1 \rangle$ has approximately the same PSNR (28.66 vs. 28.67) so we choose latter one to save training time. The effect of the **filter kernel size** $\langle k \rangle$ is shown in Fig. 2(d), in which we fix $\langle n, l, f \rangle$ and vary k in the collection of $[3, 5, 9]$. Experiment result proves that $k = 3$ achieves the best PSNR. The PSNR decrease with filter kernel size demonstrate that relatively remote pixels contribute less to feature extraction and bring much signal noise to the final result.

Final Model. For the final design, we set $\langle n, l, (f_1, k_1), (f_2, k_2), (f_3, k_3), (f_4^{deconv}, k_4^{deconv}), (f_5, k_5) \rangle = \langle 5, 3, (64, 3), (64, 3), (32, 3), (32, 3), (1, 3) \rangle$. We set the learning rate α as 10^{-3} for this design and achieve a good convergence. We implemented our 3DECNN model using Pytorch and trained/validated our model on a workstation with a NVIDIA Tesla K40 GPU. The training process took roughly 10 h.

Table 1. PSNR and SSIM results comparison.

		BICUBIC	FSRCNN-s [8]	FSRCNN [8]	ESPCN [9]	proposed
PSNR (bB)	Mean	27.2903	28.4731	28.7681	28.8769	**29.3087**
	Standard deviation (SD)	2.7754	2.8659	2.9197	2.9405	3.0253
SSIM	Mean	0.8190	0.8393	0.8431	0.8449	**0.8529**
	Standard deviation (SD)	0.1135	0.1061	0.1080	0.1071	0.1050

3.2   Results Comparison with T-Test Validation

We compare the proposed model to bicubic interpolation and two existing the-state-of-the-art deep learning methods for super resolution image enhancement: (1) FSRCNN [8] and (2) ESPCN [9]. We reimplemented both methods, retraining and testing them in the manner as our proposed method. Both the FSRCNN-s and the FSRCNN architectures used in [8] are compared here. A paired t-test is adopted to determine whether a statistically significant difference exists in mean measurements of PSNR and SSIM when comparing 3DECNN to bicubic, FSRCNN, and ESPCN. Table 1 shows the mean and standard deviation for the four methods in PSNR and SSIM using 5,168 test slices. The paired t-test results show that the proposed method has significantly higher mean PSNR, and mean differences are 2.0183 dB (p-value $< 2.2e - 16$), 0.8357 dB (p-value $< 2.2e-16$), 0.5406 dB (p-value $< 2.2e-16$), and 0.4318 dB (p-value $< 2.2e-16$) for bicubic, FSRCNN-s, FSRCNN and ESPCN, respectively. It also shows that out model has significantly higher SSIM, and the mean differences are 0.0389 (p-value $< 2.2e - 16$), 0.0136 (p-value $< 2.2e - 16$), 0.0098 (p-value $< 2.2e - 16$), and 0.0080 (p-value $< 2.2e - 16$). To subjectively measure the image perceived quality, we also visualize and compare the enhanced images in Fig. 3. The zoomed areas in the figure are lung nodules. As the figures shown, our approach achieved better perceived quality compared to other methods.

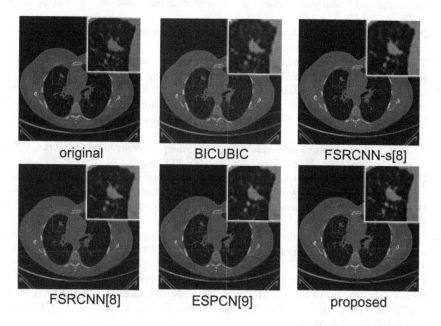

Fig. 3. Comparison with the-state-of-the-art works

4   Discussion and Future Work

We present the results of our proposed 3DECNN approach to improve the image quality of CT studies that are acquired at varying, lower resolutions. Our method achieves a significant improvement compared to existing state-of-art deep learning methods in PSNR (mean improvement of $0.43dB$ and p-value $< 2.2e - 16$) and SSIM (mean improvement of 0.008 and p-value $< 2.2e - 16$). We demonstrate our proposed work by enhancing large slice thickness scans, which can be potentially applied to clinical auxiliary diagnosis of lung cancer. As future work, we explore how our approach can be extended to perform image normalization and enhancement of ultra low-dose CT images (studies that are acquired at 25% or 50% dose compared to current low-dose images) with the goal of producing comparable image quality while reducing radiation exposure to patients.

Acknowledgement. This work is partly supported by National Natural Science Foundation of China (NSFC) Grant 61520106004, the National Institutes for Health under award No. R01CA210360. The authors would also like to thank the UCLA/PKU Joint Research Institute, Chinese Scholarship Council for their support of our research.

References

1. Greenspan, H.: Super-resolution in medical imaging. Comput. J. **52**(1), 43–63 (2008)
2. Park, S.C., Park, M.K., Kang, M.G.: Super-resolution image reconstruction: a technical overview. IEEE Signal Process. Mag. **20**(3), 21–36 (2003)
3. Yang, J., et al.: Image super-resolution via sparse representation. IEEE Trans. Image Process. **19**(11), 2861–2873 (2010)
4. Ota, Junko, et al.: Evaluation of the sparse coding super-resolution method for improving image quality of up-sampled images in computed tomography. In: Medical Imaging 2017: Image Processing, vol. 10133. International Society for Optics and Photonics (2017)
5. Dong, C., et al.: Image super-resolution using deep convolutional networks. IEEE Trans. Pattern Anal. Mach. Intell. **38**(2), 295–307 (2016)
6. Umehara, K., et al.: Super-resolution convolutional neural network for the improvement of the image quality of magnified images in chest radiographs. In: Medical Imaging 2017: Image Processing, vol. 10133. International Society for Optics and Photonics (2017)
7. Umehara, K., Ota, J., Ishida, T.: Application of super-resolution convolutional neural network for enhancing image resolution in chest CT. J. Digit. Imaging, 1–10 (2017)
8. Dong, C., Loy, C.C., Tang, X.: Accelerating the super-resolution convolutional neural network. In: Leibe, B., Matas, J., Sebe, N., Welling, M. (eds.) ECCV 2016. LNCS, vol. 9906, pp. 391–407. Springer, Cham (2016). https://doi.org/10.1007/978-3-319-46475-6_25
9. Shi, W., et al.: Real-time single image and video super-resolution using an efficient sub-pixel convolutional neural network. In: Proceedings of the IEEE Conference on Computer Vision and Pattern Recognition (2016)

10. Mahapatra, D., Bozorgtabar, B., Hewavitharanage, S., Garnavi, R.: Image super resolution using generative adversarial networks and local saliency maps for retinal image analysis. In: Descoteaux, M., Maier-Hein, L., Franz, A., Jannin, P., Collins, D.L., Duchesne, S. (eds.) MICCAI 2017. LNCS, vol. 10435, pp. 382–390. Springer, Cham (2017). https://doi.org/10.1007/978-3-319-66179-7_44
11. Wojna, Z., et al.: The Devil is in the Decoder, arXiv:1707.05847 (2017)
12. Armato, S.G.: The lung image database consortium (LIDC) and image database resource initiative (IDRI): a completed reference database of lung nodules on CT scans. Med. Phys. **38**(2), 915–931 (2011)
13. LeCun, Y., Bottou, L., Bengio, Y.: Gradient-based learning applied to document recognition. Proc. IEEE **86**(11), 2278–2324 (1998)

Paediatric Bone Age Assessment Using Deep Convolutional Neural Networks

Vladimir I. Iglovikov[1], Alexander Rakhlin[2], Alexandr A. Kalinin[3(✉)], and Alexey A. Shvets[4]

[1] ODS.ai, San Francisco, CA 94107, USA
iglovikov@gmail.com
[2] Neuromation OU, 10111 Tallinn, Estonia
rakhlin@neuromation.io
[3] University of Michigan, Ann Arbor, MI 48109, USA
akalinin@umich.edu
[4] Massachusetts Institute of Technology, Cambridge, MA 02142, USA
shvets@mit.edu

Abstract. Skeletal bone age assessment is a common clinical practice to diagnose endocrine and metabolic disorders in child development. In this paper, we describe a deep learning approach to the problem of bone age assessment using data from the 2017 Pediatric Bone Age Challenge organized by the Radiological Society of North America. This dataset consists of 12,600 radiological images. Each radiograph in the dataset is an image of a left hand labeled with bone age and sex of a patient. Our approach introduces a comprehensive preprocessing protocol based on the positive mining technique. We use images of whole hands as well as specific hand parts for both training and prediction. This allows us to measure the importance of specific hand bones for automated bone age analysis. We further evaluate the performance of the suggested methods in the context of skeletal development stages. Our approach outperforms other common methods for bone age assessment.

Keywords: Medical imaging · Computer-aided diagnosis (CAD) · Computer vision · Image recognition · Deep learning

1 Introduction

Clinicians use bone age assessment (BAA) in order to estimate maturity of a child's skeletal system since the difference between assigned bone and chronological ages may indicate a growth problem. BAA methods usually include taking a single X-ray image of the left hand from the wrist to fingertips and comparing it with a standardized reference. Over the past decades, BAA has been performed manually by either comparing the patient's radiograph with an atlas of

D. Stoyanov et al. (Eds.): DLMIA 2018/ML-CDS 2018, LNCS 11045, pp. 300–308, 2018.
https://doi.org/10.1007/978-3-030-00889-5_34

representative ages [4] or using a scoring system that examines specific bones [16]. Only recently software solutions, such as BoneXpert [17], have been developed and approved for the clinical use in Europe. BoneXpert uses a computer vision algorithm to reconstruct the contours of 13 bones of a hand. However, it is sensitive to the image quality and does not utilize carpal bones, despite their suggested importance for BAA in infants and toddlers [3]. Methods based on classical computer vision reduce time needed for evaluating a single radiograph, but they still require substantial feature engineering, doctoral supervision and expertise.

Recently, deep learning-based approaches demonstrated performance improvements over conventional machine learning methods for many tasks in biomedicine [1,6]. In medical image analysis, convolutional neural networks (CNN) have been successfully used, for example, for diabetic retinopathy screening [9], breast cancer detection [10], and other problems [1]. Deep neural network based solutions for BAA were suggested before [7,8,14]. However, most of these studies did not evaluate model performance using different hand bones or different skeletal development stages. Moreover, the performance of deep learning models depends on the quality of training data. Radiographs are obtained from various medical centers, different hardware, and under variable conditions. They also vary in scale, orientation, exposure, and often feature specific markings (Fig. 4).

In this study, we present a deep learning-based method for BAA. One of the key contributions of this work is rigorous preprocessing pipeline. To prevent the model from learning false associations from artifacts in the image, we first remove background by segmenting the hand. Then, we normalize contrast and detect key points. Then, we apply affine transforms to register segmented images in a common coordinate space. Besides improving the quality of data, this step allows us to accurately identify different regions of the hand. We train several deep networks using different parts of hand images to assess how different hand bones contribute to the models' performance across four major skeletal development stages. Finally, we compare regression and classification, sex-specific and sex-agnostic models, and evaluate overall performance of our approach. We validate our method using data from the 2017 Pediatric Bone Age Challenge organized by the Radiological Society of North America (RSNA) [12]. The suggested method is robust and shows superior performance compared to other proposed solutions.

2 Methods

2.1 Preprocessing

First, we extract a hand mask from every image to remove all extraneous objects. Simple background removal methods did not produce satisfactory results, while machine learning-based segmentation typically requires large manually labeled training set. To alleviate labeling costs, we use positive mining, an iterative procedure that combines manual labeling with automatic processing, see Fig. 1. It allows us to quickly obtain accurate masks for the whole training set. For segmentation, we employ slightly modified version of the original U-Net architecture [11] that previously proved itself useful for segmentation problems with limited amounts of data [5], making it a good choice for positive mining.

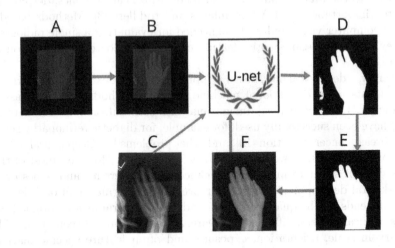

Fig. 1. Iterative procedure of positive mining utilizing U-Net architecture for image segmentation: (A) raw input data; (B) mask manually labeled with the online annotation tool Supervisely [15]; (C) new data; (D) raw prediction; (E) post processed prediction; (F) raw image with mask plotted together for visual inspection.

We train U-Net using a generalized segmentation loss function:

$$L = H - \log J, \tag{1}$$

where H is a binary cross entropy that defined as

$$H = -\frac{1}{n} \sum_{i=1}^{n} (y_i \log \hat{y}_i + (1 - y_i) \log(1 - \hat{y}_i)), \tag{2}$$

where y_i and $\hat{y}_i$ are a binary value (label) and a predicted probability for the pixel i, correspondingly. In the second term of Eq. (1), J is a differentiable generalization of the Jaccard Index

$$J = \frac{1}{n} \sum_{i=1}^{n} \left(\frac{y_i \hat{y}_i}{y_i + \hat{y}_i - y_i \hat{y}_i} \right). \tag{3}$$

By minimizing this loss function, we simultaneously maximize probabilities for correct pixels to be predicted and maximize the intersection between masks and corresponding predictions, which improves overall segmentation performance [5].

First, we manually label 100 hand masks using Supervisely [15]. Then, we train the U-Net model and use it to segment the rest of the training set. For each prediction we only keep the largest connected component. We manually curate all segmented masks to discard those of poor quality and train the model using the expanded training set with good quality masks. We repeat this procedure 6 times to achieve acceptable quality on the whole training set, see Fig. 1. Finally, we manually label approximately 100 images that U-Net fails to segment correctly.

2.2 Key Point Detection Model

Since original atlas-based methods evaluate specific hand bones, we use several hand regions to assess their importance. In order to correctly locate these regions, radiographs need to be registered in a common coordinate space. For registration, we detect coordinates of several key points of a hand and use them to calculate affine transformation parameters (zoom, rotation, translation, and mirror) (Fig. 2). Three specific points on the image are chosen: the tip of the distal phalanx of the third finger, tip of the distal phalanx of the thumb, and the center of the capitate. All images are re-scaled to the same resolution: 2080×1600 and padded with zeros, when necessary. To create training set for key points model, we manually label 800 radiographs. Pixel coordinates of key points serve as training targets for our regression model. Key point detection model is based on a VGG-like architecture [13] with 3 VGG blocks and 3 fully connected layers with dropout Fig. 3. The VGG module consists of 2 convolutional layers with the Exponential Linear Unit (ELU) activation function [2] and max-pooling. The model is trained with Mean Squared Error loss function (MSE). We downscale input images to 130×100 pixels and apply rotation, translation and zoom as augmentations. The model outputs 6 coordinates (2 for every key point) that are used to calculate affine transformations for all radiographs. We register them such that: (1) the tip of the middle finger is aligned horizontally and positioned approximately 100 pixels below the top edge of the image; (2) the capitate is aligned horizontally and positioned approximately 480 pixels above the bottom edge of the image. The key point for the thumb is used to detect mirrored images and adjust them. The results of the segmentation, normalization, and registration are shown in Fig. 4.

2.3 Bone Age Assessment Models

We compare bone age regression and classification using two VGG-style CNNs [13] with 6 convolutional blocks followed by 2 fully connected layers (see Fig. 3). The input size varies depending on the considered region of an image, Fig. 2. Both networks are trained by minimizing Mean Absolute Error (MAE) with augmentations (zoom, rotation shift). The regression network has a single output predicting bone age in month, which is scaled in the range $[-1, 1]$. The classification model (Fig. 3) is similar to the regression one, except for two final layers. First, we assign each bone age a class. As bone ages expressed in months, we assume 240 classes total. The second to the last layer is a softmax layer that outputs vector of probabilities for 240 classes. In the final layer, probabilities are multiplied by a vector of bone ages uniformly distributed over integer values

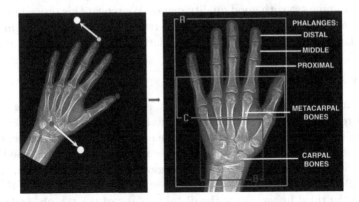

Fig. 2. Image registration. (Left) Key points: the tip of the middle finger (the yellow dot), the center of the capitate (the red dot), the tip of the thumb (the blue dot). Registration positions: for the tip of the middle finger and for the center of the capitate (white dots). (Right) A registered radiograph with three specific regions: (A) a whole hand; (B) carpal bones; (C) metacarpals and proximal phalanges.

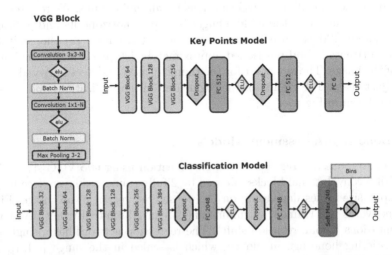

Fig. 3. VGG-style neural network architectures for regression (top) and classification (bottom) tasks.

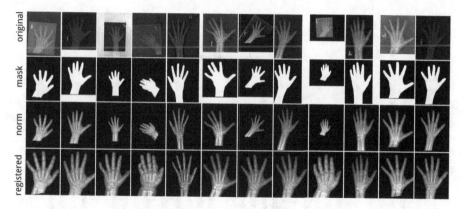

Fig. 4. Preprocessing pipeline: (first row) original images; (second row) binary hand masks that are applied to the original images to remove background; (third row) masked and normalized images; (bottom row) registered images.

[0..239]. The model outputs single value that corresponds to the expectation of the bone age. Training protocol is the same as for the regression model.

According to the features of skeletal development stages described in [3,4,16], we crop three specific regions from registered radiographs, as shown in Fig. 2: (1) whole hand; (2) carpal bones; and (3) metacarpals and proximal phalanges. We split labeled radiographs into training (11,600 images) and validation (1,000 images) sets, preserving sex ratio. We create several models with a breakdown by: (1) prediction type; (2) sex (males, females, both); and (3) a region (A, B, C). Given these conditions, we produce 18 basic models (2 × 3 × 3). Furthermore, we construct several meta-models by averaging different regional models.

3   Results

As shown in Fig. 4, original images varied in quality and often had artifacts. In order to assess the effect of preprocessing on prediction performance, we evaluate the regression network on original images, segmented and normalized images, and segmented, normalized and registered images. Corresponding MAEs of 31.56, 8.76, and 8.08 months accordingly demonstrate performance improvement due to the preprocessing. All further results were obtained on the preprocessed data.

The performance of all models evaluated on validation data set is shown in Fig. 5. The region of metacarpals and proximal phalanges (region C in Fig. 2) shows higher accuracy using both regression and classification models. Classification performs better than regression, while the linear ensemble of three regional models outperforms each separate model. The regional pattern MAE(B) > MAE(C) > MAE(A) > MAE (ensemble) is observed for different model types and patient sexes with few exceptions.

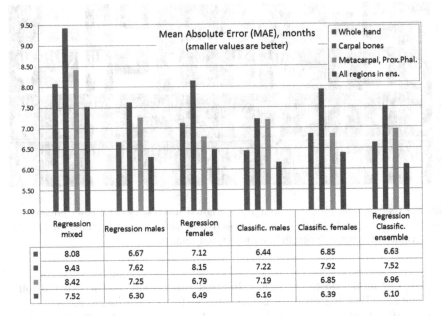

Fig. 5. Mean absolute errors on the validation data set for regression and classification models for different bones and sexes. Colors correspond to different regions. Table: regions are shown in rows, models in columns. There is a total of 15 individual models and 9 ensembles.

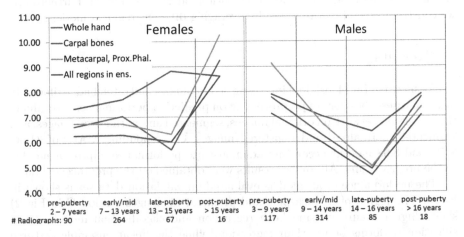

Fig. 6. Mean absolute error in months as a function of skeletal development stages for different sexes. Different colors on the plot correspond to different regions of a radiograph. For males and females the development stages are labelled at the bottom of each plot.

Following [3,8], we also consider four major skeletal development stages: pre-puberty, early-and-mid puberty, late puberty, and post-puberty, see Fig. 6. Infant and toddler categories were excluded due to scarcity of data. Unlike Lee *et al.* [8], we do not observe better results when training on carpal bones compared to other areas. With two exceptions (pre-puberty for males and post-puberty for females), metacarpals and proximal phalanges provide better accuracy than carpals do. Gilsanz and Ratib [3] suggest carpal bones as the best predictor of skeletal maturity only in infants and toddlers. Thus, we find no sound evidence to support the suggestion that carpal bones can be considered the best predictor in pre-puberty. For both sexes the accuracy peaks at late-puberty, the most frequent age in the dataset, showing the influence of the dataset size on the performance.

In the RSNA2017 Pediatric Bone Age Assessement challenge, our solution has been evaluated using the test set consisting of 200 radiographs. Based on organizers' report our method achieves MAE of 4.97 months, higher than local validation, possibly due to the better image or label quality in the test set.

4   Conclusion

In this study, we suggest a deep learning-based approach to the problem of the automatic BAA. Despite the challenging quality of the radiographs, our approach demonstrates robust results and surpasses existing automated models in performance. By using different hand zones, we find that BAA can be done just for carpal bones or for metacarpals and proximal phalanges with around 10–15% increase in error compared to the whole hand. Our approach can be improved by either using more powerful deep networks or increasing the training set size.

References

1. Ching, T., et al.: Opportunities and obstacles for deep learning in biology and medicine. J. R. Soc. Interface **15**(141) (2018)
2. Clevert, D.A., Unterthiner, T., Hochreiter, S.: Fast and accurate deep network learning by exponential linear units (ELUs). arXiv preprint arXiv:1511.07289 (2015)
3. Gilsanz, V., Ratib, O.: Hand Bone Age: A Digital Atlas of Skeletal Maturity. Springer Science & Business Media, Heidelberg (2005). https://doi.org/10.1007/b138568
4. Greulich, W.W., Pyle, S.I.: Radiographic atlas of skeletal development of the hand and wrist. Am. J. Med. Sci. **238**(3), 393 (1959)
5. Iglovikov, V., Shvets, A.: Ternausnet: U-net with vgg11 encoder pre-trained on imagenet for image segmentation. arXiv preprint arXiv:1801.05746 (2018)
6. Kalinin, A.A., et al.: Deep learning in pharmacogenomics: from gene regulation to patient stratification. Pharmacogenomics **19**(7), 629–650 (2018)
7. Larson, D.B., Chen, M.C., Lungren, M.P., Halabi, S.S., Stence, N.V., Langlotz, C.P.: Performance of a deep-learning neural network model in assessing skeletal maturity on pediatric hand radiographs. Radiology, 170236 (2017)

8. Lee, H., et al.: Fully automated deep learning system for bone age assessment. J. Digit. Imaging, 1–15 (2017)

9. Rakhlin, A.: Diabetic retinopathy detection through integration of deep learning classification framework. In: bioRxiv, p. 225508 (2017)

10. Rakhlin, A., Shvets, A., Iglovikov, V., Kalinin, A.A.: Deep convolutional neural networks for breast cancer histology image analysis. In: Campilho, A., Karray, F., ter Haar Romeny, B. (eds.) ICIAR 2018. LNCS, vol. 10882, pp. 737–744. Springer, Cham (2018). https://doi.org/10.1007/978-3-319-93000-8_83

11. Ronneberger, O., Fischer, P., Brox, T.: U-net: convolutional networks for biomedical image segmentation. In: Navab, N., Hornegger, J., Wells, W.M., Frangi, A.F. (eds.) MICCAI 2015. LNCS, vol. 9351, pp. 234–241. Springer, Cham (2015). https://doi.org/10.1007/978-3-319-24574-4_28

12. RSNA Pediatric Bone Age Challenge. http://rsnachallenges.cloudapp.net/competitions/4 (2017). Accessed 16 July 2017

13. Simonyan, K., Zisserman, A.: Very deep convolutional networks for large-scale image recognition. arXiv preprint arXiv:1409.1556 (2014)

14. Spampinato, C., Palazzo, S., Giordano, D., Aldinucci, M., Leonardi, R.: Deep learning for automated skeletal bone age assessment in X-ray images. Med. Image Anal. **36**, 41–51 (2017)

15. Supervisely. https://supervise.ly/. Accessed 16 July 2017

16. Tanner, J., Whitehouse, R., Cameron, N., Marshall, W., Healy, M., Goldstein, H.: Assessment of Skeletal Maturity and Prediction of Adult Height (TW2 Method). Academic Press, London (1983)

17. Thodberg, H.H., Kreiborg, S., Juul, A., Pedersen, K.D.: The BoneXpert method for automated determination of skeletal maturity. IEEE Trans. Med. Imaging **28**(1), 52–66 (2009)

Automatic Myocardial Strain Imaging in Echocardiography Using Deep Learning

Andreas Østvik[1,2,3(✉)], Erik Smistad[1,2,3], Torvald Espeland[1,2,4],
Erik Andreas Rye Berg[1,2,4], and Lasse Lovstakken[1,2]

[1] Centre for Innovative Ultrasound Solutions, NTNU, Trondheim, Norway
andreas.ostvik@ntnu.no
[2] Department of Circulation and Medical Imaging, NTNU, Trondheim, Norway
[3] Department of Health, SINTEF Digital, Trondheim, Norway
[4] Clinic of Cardiology, St. Olavs Hospital, Trondheim, Norway

Abstract. Recent studies in the field of deep learning suggest that motion estimation can be treated as a learnable problem. In this paper we propose a pipeline for functional imaging in echocardiography consisting of four central components, (i) classification of cardiac view, (ii) semantic partitioning of the left ventricle (LV) myocardium, (iii) regional motion estimates and (iv) fusion of measurements. A U-Net type of convolutional neural network (CNN) was developed to classify muscle tissue, and partitioned into a semantic measurement kernel based on LV length and ventricular orientation. Dense tissue motion was predicted using stacked U-Net architectures with image warping of intermediate flow, designed to tackle variable displacements. Training was performed on a mixture of real and synthetic data. The resulting segmentation and motion estimates was fused in a Kalman filter and used as basis for measuring global longitudinal strain. For reference, 2D ultrasound images from 21 subjects were acquired using a GE Vivid system. Data was analyzed by two specialists using a semi-automatic tool for longitudinal function estimates in a commercial system, and further compared to output of the proposed method. Qualitative assessment showed comparable deformation trends as the clinical analysis software. The average deviation for the global longitudinal strain was $(-0.6 \pm 1.6)\%$ for apical four-chamber view. The system was implemented with Tensorflow, and working in an end-to-end fashion without any ad-hoc tuning. Using a modern graphics processing unit, the average inference time is estimated to (115 ± 3) ms per frame.

Keywords: Deep learning · Echocardiography · Functional imaging

1 Introduction

Recent years have shown that quantitative assessment of cardiac function has become indispensable in echocardiography. Evaluation of the hearts contractile apparatus has traditionally been limited to geometric measures such as ejection

D. Stoyanov et al. (Eds.): DLMIA 2018/ML-CDS 2018, LNCS 11045, pp. 309–316, 2018.
https://doi.org/10.1007/978-3-030-00889-5_35

fraction (EF) and visual estimation (eyeballing) of myocardial morphophysiology [3]. Despite being a central part of standard protocol examinations at the outpatient clinic, the methods tend to have poor inter- and intravariability. With tissue doppler imaging (TDI) and speckle tracking(ST), the quantification tools have moved beyond these measures, and enabled new methods for assessing the myocardial deformation pattern [12]. Myocardial deformation imaging, e.g. strain and strain rate, derived from TDI and ST, have high sensitivity, and can allow an earlier detection of cardiac dysfunction. However, these methods also have several limitations. For instance, TDI is dependent on insonation angle, i.e. measurements are along the ultrasound beam. A poor parallel alignment with the myocardium can thus influence the results. Speckle tracking is less angle dependant (typically dependant on the lateral resolution), but has suffered from poor temporal resolution and ad-hoc setups. Recent work in the field of deep learning (DL) suggest that motion estimation can be treated as a learnable problem [7]. Herein, we investigate this approach in combination with cardiac view classification and segmentation to achieve fully automatic functional imaging.

1.1   Relevant Work and Perspective

Automatic view classification and segmentation of relevant cardiac structures in echocardiography has been a topic of great interest and research [2,9]. For segmentation, work has mainly been conducted on 3D echocardiography, but 2D approaches are also proposed [13]. To the authors' knowledge, no published study have utilized motion estimation from deep learning in echocardiography. These methods claim to be more robust in terms of noise and small displacements [7] than traditional optical flow methods, thus appealing for ultrasound and myocardial motion estimation. Combining the components could potentially allow fast and fully automated pipelines for calculating clinically relevant parameters, with feasibility of on-site analysis. In this study, the goal is to address this, and measure the global longitudinal strain (GLS) from the four-chamber view in an end-to-end fashion.

Variability of global longitudinal strain has been discussed in several papers. Recently, a head-to-head comparison between speckle tracking based GLS measurements of nine commercial vendors [5] was conducted. Results show that the reproducibility compared to other clinical measurements such as EF is good, but the intervendor variation is significant. The same expert obtaining GLS in the apical four-chamber view of 63 patients on nine different systems, gave average results in the range of -17.9% to -21.4%. The commercial system used as reference in this study had an offset of -1.7%, i.e. overestimating, from the mean measurement. The inter- and intraobserver relative mean error was 7.8% and 8.3% respectively.

2   Method

Our proposed pipeline is comprised of four steps, (i) classification of cardiac view, (ii) segmentation of the left ventricle (LV) myocardium, (iii) regional motion estimates and (iv) fusion of measurements. An illustration of the system after view classification is illustrated in Fig. 1. Step (i)–(iii) utilizes convolutional neural networks (CNNs), while the last step uses a traditional Kalman filter method.

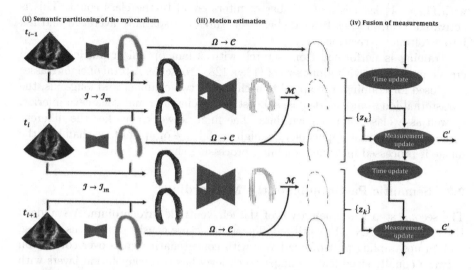

Fig. 1. Visualization of the measurement pipeline. US images are forwarded through a segmentation network, and the resulting masks are used to extract the centerline and relevant parts of the image. The masked US data is further processed through the motion estimation network yielding a map of velocities. The centerline position and velocities of the myocard are used in the measurement update step of a Kalman filter. The updated results are used as a basis for strain measurements.

2.1   Cardiac View Classification

The view classification is the first essential step in the automatic pipeline, and is used to quality assure and sort incoming data. We employ a feed-forward CNN composed of inception blocks and a dense connectivity pattern [6,14]. Initially, input is propagated through two component blocks with (3×3) convolution kernels followed by max pooling. The first and second convolution layer has 16 and 32 filters respectively. We use pooling with size (2×2) and equal strides. After the second pooling layer, data is processed through an inception module with three parallel routes. Each route consist of a bottleneck, two of which were followed by blocks with larger convolution kernels, i.e. (3×3) and (5×5) respectively. The input of the inception module is concatenated with the output and processed into a transition module with bottleneck and max pooling. This step is repeated three times, and we double the amount of filters before every new pooling layer. The dense connectivity pattern alleviates the vanishing gradient problem, and can enhance feature propagation and reusability. After the third transition, the data is processed through two inception blocks with constant amount of filters and no pooling. The route with (5×5) convolution kernels is omitted in these modules, and dropout regularization was used between them. The final classification block consists of a compressing convolution layer with (1×1) kernels and number of filters equal to the class count. This is activated with another PReLU, before features are spatially averaged and fed into a softmax activation.

Training is performed from scratch with Adam optimizer and categorical cross entropy loss, with input size of (128×128) greyscale. A total of eight classes were used for training, the apical four chamber, two chamber and long-axis, the parasternal long- and short-axis, subcostal four-chamber and vena cava inferior, as well as a class for unknown data. The final network classifies the different cardiac views, and if applicable, i.e. high confidence of apical four-chamber, the image is processed into the remaining processing chain.

2.2   Semantic Partitioning of the Myocardium

The second step is segmentation of the left ventricle myocardium. A standard U-Net type of CNN [11] is utilized. The architecture consist of a downsampling, and an upsampling part of five levels with concatenating cross-over connection between equally sized feature maps. Each level has two convolution layers with the same amount of filters ranging from 32 to 128 from top to bottom respectively. All filters have a size of (3×3). Max pooling with size (2×2) and equal strides was used for downsampling and nearest neighbour for upsampling. Training was performed with Adam optimizer and Dice loss, and the size of the input image was set to (256×256) greyscale. The output of the network is a segmentation mask Ω.

The segmentation is used a basis for two different tasks, masking the input of the motion estimation network $\mathcal{I}_m$ and centerline extraction. We mask the US image $\mathcal{I}$ to remove redundant input signal. The contour of the segmentation Ω was used to define the endo- and epicardial borders, and further the centerline $\mathcal{C} = \{(x,y)_1, ..., (x,y)_N\}$ was sampled between with $N = 120$ equally spaced points along the myocard. The latter is passed to the Kalman filter.

2.3   Motion Estimation Using Deep Learning

The motion estimation is based on the work done by Ilg *et al.* [7], and the networks referred to as FlowNets. The design involves stacking of multiple U-Net architectures with image warping of intermediate flow and propagation of brightness error. Two parallel routes are created to tackle large and small displacements separately. The prior is solved by stacking three U-Net architectures, the first which includes explicit correlation of feature maps, while the two succeeding are standard U-Net architectures without custom layers. For small displacement, only one U-Net is used, but compared to the networks for large displacements, the kernel size and stride of the first layer is reduced. At the end, the two routes are fused together with a simple CNN. The networks are trained separately, in a schedule consisting of different synthetic datasets with a wide range of motion vector representations. The small displacement network is fine-tuned on a dataset modified for subpixel motion. Adam optimizer and endpoint error loss is used while training for all the networks. The input size of the network was kept the same as the original implementation, i.e. (512×384).

The output prediction of the network is dense tissue motion vectors in the masked US area. The centerline $\mathcal{C}$ of the current segmentation is used to extract the corresponding set of motion vectors $\mathcal{M} = \{(v_x, v_y)_1, ..., (v_x, v_y)_N\}$.

2.4   Fusion of Measurements

Fusion of measurements was performed employing an ordinary Kalman filter with a constant acceleration model [8] with measurement input $z_k = [x, y, v_x, v_y]_k^T$ for every point-velocity component $k \in \{\mathcal{C}, \mathcal{M}\}$. Essentially, this serves as a simple method for incorporating the temporal domain, which is natural in the context of echocardiography. It adds temporal smoothing, reducing potential pierce noise detectable in image-to-image measurements. The updated centerline $\mathcal{C}' \subseteq \Omega$ is used to calculate the longitudinal ventricular length ι, i.e. the arc length, for each timestep t. Further, this is used to estimate the global longitudinal strain $\epsilon(t) = (\iota(t) - \iota_0)/\iota_0$ along the center of the myocard.

3   Datasets for Training and Validation

Anonymous echocardiography data for training the view classification and segmentation models was acquired from various patient studies with Research Ethics Board (REB) approval. The echocardiography data used are obtained at various outpatient clinics with a GE Vivid E9/95 ultrasound system (GE Vingmed Ultrasound, Horten, Norway), and consist of data from over 250 patients. The health status of subjects is unknown, but representative for a standard outpatient clinic. The data includes manual expert annotation of views, and the epi- and endocard borders of the left ventricle. The view classification and segmentation networks are trained separately on this data, with a significant fraction left out for testing. The motion estimation network was trained on three synthetic datasets, namely FlyingChairs [4], FlyingThings3D [10] and ChairsSDHom [7]. Disregarding the fundamentals of motion, the datasets have no resemblance to echocardiography. However, they can be modified to have representations covering both sub- and superpixel motion, which is necessary to reproduce motion from the whole cardiac cycle.

For validation of GLS, 21 subjects called for evaluation of cardiac disease in two clinical studies were included. Both are REB approved, and informed consent was given. Two specialists in cardiology performed standard strain measurements using a semi-automatic method implemented in GE EchoPAC[1]. The method uses speckle tracking to estimate myocardial deformation, but the methodology is unknown. The results were used as a reference for evaluating the implemented pipeline.

---

[1] http://www3.gehealthcare.com/en/products/categories/ultrasound/vivid/echopac.

4   Results

GLS was obtained successfully in all patients. The results for apical four-chamber views are displayed in Fig. 2, together with the GLS curves of the average and worst case subjects. The average deviation of the systolic GLS between the two methods was $(-0.6\pm1.6)\%$. The average strain on all subjects was $(-17.9\pm2.3)\%$ and $(-17.3\pm2.5)\%$, for the reference and proposed method respectively.

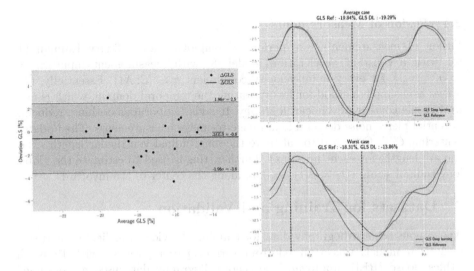

Fig. 2. Bland-Altman plot of global longitudinal strain from all subjects. The estimated GLS traces of the average and worst case, together with the corresponding reference, are displayed to the right.

The view classification achieved an image-wise F_1 score of 97.9% on four-chamber data of 260 patients, and the segmentation a dice score of (0.87 ± 0.03) on 50 patients, all unknown and independent from the training set. The system was implemented as a Tensorflow dataflow graph [1], enabling easy deployment and optimized inference. Using a modern laptop with a Nvidia GTX 1070 GPU, the average inference time was estimated to (115 ± 1) ms per frame, where flow prediction accounts for approximately 70% of the runtime.

5   Discussion

Compared to reference, the measurements from the proposed pipeline were slightly underestimated. The reference method is not a gold standard for GLS and might not necessarily yield correct results for all cases. Speckle tracking can fail where noise hampers the echogenicity. We could identify poor tracking in the apical area due to noise for some subjects, and this would in turn result in larger strain. Further, the vendor comparison study [5] shows that the commercial system used in this study on average overestimates the mean of all vendors by 1.7%. This in mind, we note that the results from the current implementations are in the expected range. For individual cases, the deformation have overlapping and synchronized trends, as is prevalent from Fig. 2.

The proposed pipeline involves several sources of error, especially the segmentation and motion networks being the fundamental building blocks of the measurements. Using the segmentation mask to remove redundant signal in the US image seems feasible and useful for removing some noise in the motion network. However, it is not essential when measuring the components of the centerline, as they are far from the borders of the myocard, where the effect is noticable.

Future work will include the addition of multiple views, e.g. apical two- and long-axis, allowing average GLS. This is considered a more robust metric, less prone to regional noise. Also, fusion of models are currently naive, and we expect results to improve inducing models with more relevance to cardiac motion. The same holds for the motion estimation, i.e. the network could benefit from training on more relevant data. Further, we wish to do this for regional strain measurements. For clinical validation, we need to systematically include the subject condition and a larger test material.

6   Conclusion

In this paper we present a novel pipeline for functional assessment of cardiac function using deep learning. We show that motion estimation with convolutional neural networks is generic, and applicable in echocardiography, despite training on synthetic data. Together with cardiac view classification and myocard segmentation, this is incorporated in an automatic pipeline for calculating global longitudinal strain. Results coincide well with relevant work. The methods and validation are still at a preliminary stage in terms of clinical use, and some limitations and future work are briefly mentioned.

References

1. Abadi, M., et al.: Tensorflow: a system for large-scale machine learning. OSDI **16**, 265–283 (2016)
2. Bernard, O., et al.: Standardized evaluation system for left ventricular segmentation algorithms in 3D echocardiography. IEEE Trans. Med. Imaging **35**(4), 967–977 (2016). https://doi.org/10.1109/TMI.2015.2503890
3. Dalen, H., et al.: Segmental and global longitudinal strain and strain rate based on echocardiography of 1266 healthy individuals: the hunt study in Norway. Eur. J. Echocardiogr. **11**(2), 176–183 (2009)
4. Dosovitskiy, A., et al.: FlowNet: learning optical flow with convolutional networks. In: Proceedings of the IEEE International Conference on Computer Vision, pp. 2758–2766 (2015)

5. Farsalinos, K.E., Daraban, A.M., Ünlü, S., Thomas, J.D., Badano, L.P., Voigt, J.U.: Head-to-head comparison of global longitudinal strain measurements among nine different vendors: the EACVI/ASE inter-vendor comparison study. J. Am. Soc. Echocardiogr. **28**(10), 1171–1181 (2015)
6. Huang, G., Liu, Z., van der Maaten, L., Weinberger, K.Q.: Densely connected convolutional networks. In: Proceedings of the IEEE Conference on Computer Vision and Pattern Recognition (2017)
7. Ilg, E., Mayer, N., Saikia, T., Keuper, M., Dosovitskiy, A., Brox, T.: FlowNet 2.0: evolution of optical flow estimation with deep networks. In: IEEE Conference on Computer Vision and Pattern Recognition (CVPR), July 2017. http://lmb. informatik.uni-freiburg.de//Publications/2017/IMKDB17
8. Kalman, R.E.: A new approach to linear filtering and prediction problems. J. Basic Eng. **82**(1), 35–45 (1960)
9. Madani, A., Arnaout, R., Mofrad, M., Arnaout, R.: Fast and accurate view classification of echocardiograms using deep learning. npj Digit. Med. **1**(1), 6 (2018)
10. Mayer, N., et al.: A large dataset to train convolutional networks for disparity, optical flow, and scene flow estimation. In: Proceedings of the IEEE Conference on Computer Vision and Pattern Recognition, pp. 4040–4048 (2016)
11. Ronneberger, O., Fischer, P., Brox, T.: U-net: convolutional networks for biomedical image segmentation. In: Navab, N., Hornegger, J., Wells, W.M., Frangi, A.F. (eds.) MICCAI 2015. LNCS, vol. 9351, pp. 234–241. Springer, Cham (2015). https://doi.org/10.1007/978-3-319-24574-4_28
12. Smiseth, O.A., Torp, H., Opdahl, A., Haugaa, K.H., Urheim, S.: Myocardial strain imaging: how useful is it in clinical decision making? Eur. Heart J. **37**(15), 1196–1207 (2016). https://doi.org/10.1093/eurheartj/ehv529
13. Smistad, E., Østvik, A., Haugen, B.O., Lovstakken, L.: 2D left ventricle segmentation using deep learning. In: 2017 IEEE International Ultrasonics Symposium (IUS), pp. 1–4. IEEE (2017)
14. Szegedy, C., Vanhoucke, V., Ioffe, S., Shlens, J., Wojna, Z.: Rethinking the inception architecture for computer vision. In: Proceedings of the IEEE Conference on Computer Vision and Pattern Recognition, pp. 2818–2826 (2016)

Reinforced Auto-Zoom Net: Towards Accurate and Fast Breast Cancer Segmentation in Whole-Slide Images

Nanqing Dong[1,2]([✉]), Michael Kampffmeyer[3], Xiaodan Liang[4], Zeya Wang[1], Wei Dai[1], and Eric Xing[1]

[1] Petuum, Inc., Pittsburgh, USA
nd367@cornell.edu
[2] Cornell University, Ithaca, USA
[3] UiT The Arctic University of Norway, Tromsø, Norway
[4] Carnegie Mellon University, Pittsburgh, USA

Abstract. Convolutional neural networks have led to significant breakthroughs in the domain of medical image analysis. However, the task of breast cancer segmentation in whole-slide images (WSIs) is still underexplored. WSIs are large histopathological images with extremely high resolution. Constrained by the hardware and field of view, using high-magnification patches can slow down the inference process and using low-magnification patches can cause the loss of information. In this paper, we aim to achieve two seemingly conflicting goals for breast cancer segmentation: accurate and fast prediction. We propose a simple yet efficient framework Reinforced Auto-Zoom Net (RAZN) to tackle this task. Motivated by the zoom-in operation of a pathologist using a digital microscope, RAZN learns a policy network to decide whether zooming is required in a given region of interest. Because the zoom-in action is selective, RAZN is robust to unbalanced and noisy ground truth labels and can efficiently reduce overfitting. We evaluate our method on a public breast cancer dataset. RAZN outperforms both single-scale and multi-scale baseline approaches, achieving better accuracy at low inference cost.

Keywords: Breast cancer · Deep reinforcement learning Medical image segmentation · Whole-slide images

1 Introduction

Breast cancer is one of the most common causes of mortality in the female population in the world [2]. It accounts for around 25% of all the cancers diagnosed in women [3]. For traditional diagnostic tools like mammography, even experienced radiologists can miss $10 - 30\%$ of breast cancers during routine screenings [7].

© Springer Nature Switzerland AG 2018
D. Stoyanov et al. (Eds.): DLMIA 2018/ML-CDS 2018, LNCS 11045, pp. 317–325, 2018.
https://doi.org/10.1007/978-3-030-00889-5_36

With the advent of digital imaging, whole-slide imaging has gained attention from the clinicians and pathologists because of its reliability. Whole-slide images (WSIs) have been permitted for diagnostic use in the USA [1]. They are the high-resolution scans of conventional glass slides with Hematoxylin and Eosin (H&E) stained tissue. There are four types of tissue in breast biopsy: *normal*, *benign*, *in situ carcinoma*, and *invasive carcinoma*. Figure 1 shows examples of the four types of breast tissue. In clinical testing, the pathologists diagnose breast cancer based on (1) the percentage of tubule formation, (2) the degree of nuclear pleomorphism, and (3) the mitotic cell count [8].

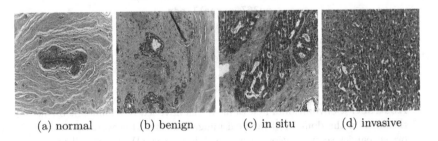

(a) normal   (b) benign   (c) in situ   (d) invasive

Fig. 1. Examples of different types of tissue. The microscopy images (patches of WSIs at 200× magnification) are labeled according to the predominant tissue type in each image.

Convolutional Neural Networks (CNNs) can be trained in an end-to-end manner to distinguish the different types of cancer, by extracting high-level information from images through stacking convolutional layers. Breast cancer classification has been fundamentally improved by the development of CNN models [16]. However, breast cancer segmentation in WSIs is still underexplored. WSIs are RGB images with high resolution (e.g. 80000 × 60000). Constrained by the memory, WSIs cannot be directly fed into the network. One solution is to crop the WSIs to small patches for patch-wise training [4]. Given a fixed input size, however, there is a trade-off between accuracy and the inference speed. One can efficiently reduce the inference cost by cropping the WSIs to larger patches and rescaling the patches to a smaller input size, but this results in a loss of detail and sacrifices accuracy. In WSIs, the suspicious cancer areas our regions of interest (ROIs), are sparse, since most regions are normal tissue or the glass slide. The four classes are therefore highly imbalanced. Further, the pixel-wise annotation of breast cancer segmentation requires domain knowledge and extensive human labor and the ground truth labels are often noisy at the pixel-level. Training on patches with a small field of view can therefore easily lead to overfitting.

In this paper, we propose a semantic segmentation framework, Reinforced Auto-Zoom Net (RAZN). When a pathologist examines the WSIs with a digital microscope, the suspicious areas are zoomed in for details and the non-suspicious areas are browsed quickly (See Fig. 2 for an intuition.). RAZN is motivated by this attentive zoom-in mechanism. We learn a policy network to decide the zoom-in action through the policy gradient method [14]. By skipping the non-suspicious areas (normal tissue), noisy information (glass background) can be ignored and the WSIs can be processed more quickly. By zooming in the suspicious areas (abnormal tissue), the data imbalance is alleviated locally (in the zoomed-in regions) and more local information is considered. Combining these two can efficiently reduce overfitting for the normal tissue, which is caused by the imbalanced data, and lead to improved accuracy. However, since the zoom-in action is selective, the inference can at the same time be fast.

The previous studies on zoom-in mechanism focus on utilizing multi-scale training to improve prediction performance. The Hierarchical Auto-Zoom Net HAZN [19] uses sub-networks to detect human and object parts at different scales hierarchically and merges the prediction at different scales, which can be considered as a kind of ensemble learning. Zoom-in-Net [17] zooms in suspicious areas generated by attention maps to classify diabetic retinopathy. In both HAZN and Zoom-in-Net, the zoom-in actions are deterministic. So in the training phase, the patches will be upsampled and trained even if it may not decrease the loss. In RAZN, the zoom-in actions are stochastic, and a policy is learned to decide if the zoom-in action can improve the performance.

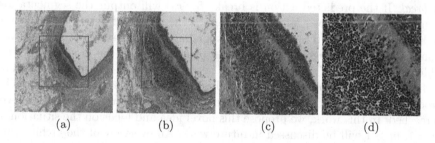

(a)	(b)	(c)	(d)

Fig. 2. Zoom-in process. The regions bounded by the red boxes are zoomed in sequentially with zoom-in rate 2. All zoomed-in regions are resized to the same resolution for visualization. The white regions in (a), (b) and (c) are the background glass slide.

This paper makes the following contributions: (1) we propose an innovative framework for semantic segmentation for images with high resolution by leveraging both accuracy and speed; (2) we are the first to apply reinforcement learning to breast cancer segmentation; (3) we compare our framework empirically with multi-scale techniques used in the domain of computer vision and discuss the influence of multi-scale models for breast cancer segmentation.

2   Reinforced Auto-Zoom Net

In clinical practice, it is impossible for a clinician to go through each region of a WSI at the original resolution, due to the huge image size. The clinician views regions with simple patterns or high confidence quickly at coarse resolution and zooms in for the suspicious or uncertain regions to study the cells at high resolution. The proposed RANZ simulates the examining process of a clinician diagnosing breast cancer on a WSI. Another motivation of RAZN is that the characteristics of the cancer cells have different representations at different field of view. For semantic segmentation tasks on common objects, the objects in the same category share discriminative features and attributes. For example, we can differentiate a cat from a dog based on the head, without viewing the whole body. However, in cancer segmentation, the basic unit is the cell, which consists of nucleus and cytoplasm. The difference between the cells is not obvious. Instead of checking only a single cell, the diagnosis is based on the features of a group of cells, such as the density, the clustering and the interaction with the environment. RANZ is designed to learn this high-level information.

RAZN consists of two types of sub-networks, policy networks $\{f_\theta\}$ and segmentation networks $\{g_\phi\}$. Assume the zoom-in actions can be performed at most m times and the zoom-in rate is r. There is one base segmentation network f_{θ_0} at the coarsest resolution. At the ith zoom-in level, there is one policy network g_{ϕ_i} and one segmentation network, f_{θ_i}. In the inference time, with fixed field of view and magnification level, we have a cropped patch x_0 with shape $[H, W, 3]$, like Fig. 2 (a). Then g_{ϕ_1} will take x_0 as an input and predict the action, $zoom\text{-}in$ or $break$. If the predicted action is break, $f_{\theta_0}(x_0)$ will output the segmentation results and the diagnosis for x_0 is finished. If the predicted action is zoom-in, a high-magnification patch $\bar{x}_0$ with corresponding zoom-in rate will be retrieved from the original image. $\bar{x}_0$, with shape $[rH, rW, 3]$, will be cropped into x_1, which is r^2 patches of shape $[H, W, 3]$. Then each patch of x_1 will be treated as x_0 for the next level of zoom-in action. Figure 2 (b) is a central crop of x_1. The process is repeated recursively until a pre-defined maximum magnification level is reached. In this work, we propose this novel idea and focus on the situation of $m = 1$. $m > 1$ will be discussed in future work. An overview of the architecture is illustrated in Fig. 3.

The segmentation networks are Fully Convolutional Networks (FCNs) [12] and share the same architecture. However, unlike parameter sharing in the common multi-scale training in semantic segmentation [5], each network is parameterized by independent f_θ, where $f_{\theta_i} : \mathbb{R}^{H \times W \times 3} \to \mathbb{R}^{H \times W \times C}$ and C is the number of classes. The reason for choosing independent networks for each zoom-in level is that CNNs are not scale-invariant [9]. Each FCN can thus learn high-level information at a specific magnification level. Given input image x and segmentation annotation y, the training objective for each FCN is to minimize

$$J_{\theta_i}(x, y) = -\frac{1}{HW} \sum_j \sum_c y_{j,c} \log f_{\theta_i}(x)_{j,c}, \tag{1}$$

where j ranges over all the $H \times W$ spatial positions and $c \in \{0, ..., 3\}$ represents the semantic classes (cancer type).

At $m = 1$, the framework is a single-step Markov Decision Process (MDP) and the problem can be formulated by the REINFORCE rule [18]. The policy network projects an image to a single scalar, $g_{\phi_1} : \mathbb{R}^{H \times W \times 3} \to \mathbb{R}$. Given the

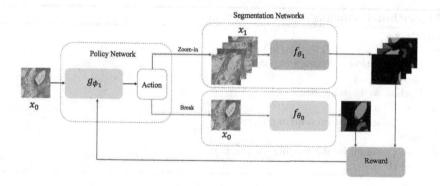

Fig. 3. Illustration of the proposed framework when $m = 1$ and $r = 2$. In the inference phase, given a cropped image x_0, the policy network outputs the action, zoom-in (red arrows) or break (blue arrows). In the training phase, the policy network will be optimized to maximize the reward (purple arrows), which is determined by the segmentation prediction.

state x_0, the policy network defines a policy $\pi_{\phi_1}(x_0)$. The policy samples an action $a \in \{0, 1\}$, which represents break and zoom-in, respectively. We have

$$p = \sigma(g_{\phi_1}(x_0)), \tag{2}$$

$$\pi_{\phi_1}(x_0) = p^a(1 - p)^{1-a}, \tag{3}$$

where $\sigma(\cdot)$ is the sigmoid function and $\pi_{\phi_1}(x_0)$ is essentially a Bernoulli distribution. The motivation of RAZN is to improve the segmentation performance and it is therefore natural to define the reward such that it minimizes the segmentation loss. Based on Eq. 1, we have $J_{\theta_0}(x_0, y_0)$, $J_{\theta_1}(x_1, y_1)$, where x_1 is the transformed x_0 after zoom-in and cropping operations. It is practical in reinforcement learning training to utilize the advantage function to reduce variance [13] and we therefore define the reward as

$$R(a) = a \frac{J_{\theta_1}(x_1, y_1) - J_{\theta_0}(x_0, y_0)}{J_{\theta_0}(x_0, y_0)}. \tag{4}$$

So when $a = 1$, the reward is positive if $J_{\theta_1}(x_1, y_1) > J_{\theta_0}(x_0, y_0)$, and the reward is negative if $J_{\theta_1}(x_1, y_1) < J_{\theta_0}(x_0, y_0)$. The denominator in Eq. 4 functions as a normalizer to prevent reward explosion. To prevent p from saturating at the beginning, we adopt the bounded Bernoulli distribution

$$\tilde{p} = \alpha p + (1 - \alpha)(1 - p). \tag{5}$$

We have $\tilde{p} \in [1 - \alpha, \alpha]$. The training objective is to maximize the expected reward or to minimize the negative expected reward

$$J_{\phi_1}(x_0) = -\mathbb{E}_{a \sim \pi_{\phi_1}(x_0)}[R(a)]. \tag{6}$$

Algorithm 1 Training of RAZN when $m = 1$

Input: x_0
1: Get $J_{\theta_0}(x_0, y_0)$ and $J_{\theta_1}(x_1, y_1)$
2: Sample action a through $\pi_{\phi_1}(x_0)$
3: Get $R(a)(x_0)$
4: Update ϕ_1 by minimizing $J_{\phi_1}(x_0)$
5: **if** $a = 1$ **then**
6:     Update θ_1 by minimizing $J_{\theta_1}(x_1, y_1)$
7: **else**
8:     Update θ_0 by minimizing $J_{\theta_0}(x_0, y_0)$
9: **end if**

The optimization of the policy network is implemented through policy gradient methods [14, 15, 18], where the expected gradients are

$$\frac{\partial}{\partial \phi_1} J_{\phi_1}(x_0) = -\mathbb{E}_{a \sim \pi_{\phi_1}(x_0)}[R(a)\frac{\partial}{\partial \phi_1}\log(a\tilde{p} + (1-a)(1-\tilde{p}))] \tag{7}$$

We adopt an alternating training strategy to update both networks. The training procedure of RAZN is illustrated in Algorithm 1.

3   Experiments

Dataset. The dataset used in this study is provided by Grand Challenge on Breast Cancer Histology Images [1]. The dataset contains 10 high-resolution WSIs with various image size. WSIs are scanned with Leica SCN400 at $\times 40$ magnification. The annotation was performed by two medical experts. As annotation of WSIs requires a large amount of human labor and medical domain knowledge, only sparse region-level labels are provided and annotations contain pixel-level errors. In this dataset, the white background (glass slide) is labeled as *normal* by the annotators. The dataset is unbalanced for the four cancer types.

Implementation. Experiments are conducted on a single NVIDIA GTX Titan X GPU. In this study, $m = 1$, $r = 2$ and $\alpha = 0.8$. The backbone of f_{θ_i} is ResNet18 [10], with no downsampling performed in conv3_1 and conv4_1. g_{ϕ_1} is also based on the ResNet18 architecture. However, each block (consisting of 2 residual blocks [10]) is replaced by a 3×3 convolution followed by batch normalization and ReLU non-linearity. The computational cost for the policy network is 7.1% of the segmentation networks. The input size to the segmentation networks and the policy network is fixed to 256×256. We use the Adam optimizer [11] for both the policy network and segmentation networks and use a stepwise learning rate policy with decay rate 0.1 every 50000 iterations. The initial learning rate is 0.01.

Multi-scale. Given a 256×256 patch, we consider two resolutions in order to simulate the zoom-in process. A coarse resolution (Scale 1), where the patch is

---

[1] https://iciar2018-challenge.grand-challenge.org/dataset.

downsampled to 64×64 and a fine resolution patch (Scale 2), where the patch is downsampled to 128×128. The patches are then resized back to 256×256 using bilinear interpolation. To evaluate the efficiency of the proposed framework, we compare our model with two multi-scale models. The first multi-scale model is the segmentation network f_θ with multi-scale training [5], denoted as MS. We only consider two scales in this experiment (Scale 1 and Scale 2). Similarly, another multi-scale model is the multi-scale fusion with attention [6], which is denoted as Attention. The training details of all models are the same. All models are trained with 200000 batches.

Table 1. Comparison of the performance. Non-carcinoma includes *normal* and *beign*. Carcinoma includes *in situ carcinoma* and *invasive carcinoma*.

	Non-carcinoma	Carcinoma	mIOU	Weighted IOU	Relative inference time
Scale 1	0.45	0.32	0.38	0.07	1.00
Scale 2	0.46	0.31	0.39	0.07	4.01
MS [5]	0.32	0.04	0.18	0.01	5.06
Attention [6]	0.43	0.29	0.36	0.06	5.16
RAZN	0.49	0.49	0.49	0.11	2.71 ± 0.57

Performance. We compare two key indicators of the performance, which are the segmentation performance and the inference speed. We use intersection over union (IOU) as the metric for segmentation performance. We report mean IOU, which is just the average IOU among four classes. Due to the imbalanced data, we also report weighted IOU, where the weight is proportional to the inverse of the frequency of the labels of each class. Further, we report relative inference time for the proposed RAZN and the baseline methods compared to the inference time for the model that only considers Scale 1. We report the average relative inference time over 100 patches. Lower values of relative inference time represent faster inference speed. The results are presented in Table 1. Note, we report the mean and the standard deviation for RAZN, as the inference time will vary depending on whether zooming is required for a given patch or not. It can be shown that RAZN actually performs better than the single scale and the multi-scale baselines. MS's performance is the worst of our benchmarks. MS exaggerates the imbalance problem by augmenting the data, which can confuse the network. We also hypothesize that the cell size is not the critical factor that influences the segmentation of cancer and that MS, therefore, aims to model unnecessary information on this task. Similarly, attention models memorize the scale of the object by fusing the results from different scales. However, when the object is not well-defined at certain scales, like in our task the cancer (group of dense cells), the network may learn to fit noise. Our results illustrate that RAZN instead is more robust when data is noisy and imbalanced, providing an overall accuracy improvement at low inference time.

4 Discussion and Conclusions

We proposed RAZN, a novel deep learning framework for breast cancer segmentation in WSI, that uses reinforcement learning to selectively zoom in on regions of interest. The results show that the proposed model can achieve improved performance, while at the same time reduce inference speed compared to previous multi-scale approaches. We also discuss the use of multi-scale approaches for breast cancer segmentation. We conclude that cancer cells are different from general objects due to their relative small and fixed size. Multi-scale approaches may not work for a noisy and imbalanced data. In future work, we aim to extend the model to study the multiple zoom-in actions situation ($m > 1$) and will investigate the potential of more complex segmentation backbone models to improve overall performance.

References

1. FDA allows marketing of first whole slide imaging system for digital pathology. https://www.fda.gov/NewsEvents/Newsroom/PressAnnouncements/ucm552742.htm
2. American Cancer Society.: Breast cancer facts & figures 2017–2018 (2017)
3. Alshanbari, H., Amin, S., Shuttleworth, J., Slman, K., Muslam, S.: Automatic segmentation in breast cancer using watershed algorithm. Int. J. Biomed. Eng. Sci. 2(2), 648–663 (2015)
4. Bándi, P., et al.: Comparison of different methods for tissue segmentation in histopathological whole-slide images. In: ISBI, pp. 591–595. IEEE (2017)
5. Chen, L.C., Papandreou, G., Kokkinos, I., Murphy, K., Yuille, A.L.: DeepLab: semantic image segmentation with deep convolutional nets, atrous convolution, and fully connected crfs. IEEE TPAMI 40(4), 834–848 (2018)
6. Chen, L.C., Yang, Y., Wang, J., Xu, W., Yuille, A.L.: Attention to scale: Scale-aware semantic image segmentation. In: CVPR, pp. 3640–3649 (2016)
7. Cheng, H.D., Cai, X., Chen, X., Hu, L., Lou, X.: Computer-aided detection and classification of microcalcifications in mammograms: a survey. Pattern Recogn. 36(12), 2967–2991 (2003)
8. Elston, C.W., Ellis, I.O.: Pathological prognostic factors in breast cancer. i. the value of histological grade in breast cancer: experience from a large study with long-term follow-up. Histopathology 19(5), 403–410 (1991)
9. Goodfellow, I., Bengio, Y., Courville, A.: Deep Learning, vol. 1 (2016)
10. He, K., Zhang, X., Ren, S., Sun, J.: Deep residual learning for image recognition. In: CVPR, pp. 770–778 (2016)
11. Kingma, D.P., Ba, J.: Adam: a method for stochastic optimization. In: ICLR (2015)
12. Long, J., Shelhamer, E., Darrell, T.: Fully convolutional networks for semantic segmentation. In: CVPR, pp. 3431–3440 (2015)
13. Rennie, S.J., Marcheret, E., Mroueh, Y., Ross, J., Goel, V.: Self-critical sequence training for image captioning. In: CVPR, pp. 7008–7024 (2017)
14. Sutton, R.S., Barto, A.G.: Reinforcement Learning: An Introduction. MIT Press, Cambridge (1998)
15. Sutton, R.S., McAllester, D.A., Singh, S.P., Mansour, Y.: Policy gradient methods for reinforcement learning with function approximation. In: NIPS. pp. 1057–1063 (2000)

16. Wang, Z., Dong, N., Dai, W., Rosario, S.D., Xing, E.P.: Classification of breast cancer histopathological images using convolutional neural networks with hierarchical loss and global pooling. In: Campilho, A., Karray, F., ter Haar Romeny, B. (eds.) ICIAR 2018. LNCS, vol. 10882, pp. 745–753. Springer, Cham (2018). https://doi.org/10.1007/978-3-319-93000-8_84
17. Wang, Z., et al.: Zoom-in-Net: deep mining lesions for diabetic retinopathy detection. In: Descoteaux, M., Maier-Hein, L., Franz, A., Jannin, P., Collins, D.L., Duchesne, S. (eds.) MICCAI 2017. LNCS, vol. 10435, pp. 267–275. Springer, Cham (2017). https://doi.org/10.1007/978-3-319-66179-7_31
18. Williams, R.J.: Simple statistical gradient-following algorithms for connectionist reinforcement learning. Mach. Learn. **8**, 229–256 (1992)
19. Xia, F., Wang, P., Chen, L.-C., Yuille, A.L.: Zoom better to see clearer: human and object parsing with hierarchical auto-zoom net. In: Leibe, B., Matas, J., Sebe, N., Welling, M. (eds.) ECCV 2016. LNCS, vol. 9909, pp. 648–663. Springer, Cham (2016). https://doi.org/10.1007/978-3-319-46454-1_39

Longitudinal Detection of Radiological Abnormalities with Time-Modulated LSTM

Ruggiero Santeramo[1,2], Samuel Withey[3], and Giovanni Montana[1,2(✉)]

[1] Department of Biomedical Engineering, King's College London, London, UK
{ruggiero.santeramo,giovanni.montana}@kcl.ac.uk
[2] WMG, University of Warwick, Coventry, UK
{ruggiero.santeramo,G.montana}@warwick.ac.uk
[3] Department of Radiology, Guy's and St Thomas' NHS Foundation Trust, London, UK

Abstract. Convolutional neural networks (CNNs) have been successfully employed in recent years for the detection of radiological abnormalities in medical images such as plain x-rays. To date, most studies use CNNs on individual examinations in isolation and discard previously available clinical information. In this study we set out to explore whether Long-Short-Term-Memory networks (LSTMs) can be used to improve classification performance when modelling the entire sequence of radiographs that may be available for a given patient, including their reports. A limitation of traditional LSTMs, though, is that they implicitly assume equally-spaced observations, whereas the radiological exams are event-based, and therefore irregularly sampled. Using both a simulated dataset and a large-scale chest x-ray dataset, we demonstrate that a simple modification of the LSTM architecture, which explicitly takes into account the time lag between consecutive observations, can boost classification performance. Our empirical results demonstrate improved detection of commonly reported abnormalities on chest x-rays such as cardiomegaly, consolidation, pleural effusion and hiatus hernia.

Keywords: Deep learning · CNN · LSTM · Time-modulated LSTM
Medical imaging · X-rays

1 Introduction

Deep learning approaches have exhibited impressive performance in medical imaging applications in recent years [2,7,19]. For instance, convolutional neural networks (CNNs) have had some success in detecting and classifying radiological abnormalities on chest x-rays, a particularly complex task [2,12,15,21]. The

Electronic supplementary material The online version of this chapter (https://doi.org/10.1007/978-3-030-00889-5_37) contains supplementary material, which is available to authorized users.

© Springer Nature Switzerland AG 2018
D. Stoyanov et al. (Eds.): DLMIA 2018/ML-CDS 2018, LNCS 11045, pp. 326–333, 2018.
https://doi.org/10.1007/978-3-030-00889-5_37

majority of these studies have been designed for cross-sectional analyses, viewing a single image in isolation, and discard the fact that a patient may have had previous medical imaging examinations for which the radiological reports are also available. It is standard practice for radiologists to take clinical history into account to add context to their report by using comparison to previous imaging. Some abnormalities will be long-standing, but others may change over time, with varying clinical relevance. Often in elderly patients or those with a history of smoking, the baseline x-ray appearances, i.e. when that patient is "well", can still be abnormal. If individual films are viewed in isolation, it can be challenging to tell with certainty if there are acute findings. If previous imaging is available, it is possible to determine if there has been interval change, for example, acute consolidation (indicating infection). As with humans, it is expected that a neural network can learn from previous patient-specific information, in this case all prior chest radiographs for that patient and their corresponding reports.

The motivation for this work is to assess the potential of recurrent neural networks (RNNs) for the real-time detection of radiological abnormalities when modelling the entire series of past exams that are available for any given patient. In particular, we set out to explore the performance of Long Short-Term Memory (LSTM) networks [8,10], which have lately become the method of choice in sequential modelling, especially when used in combination with CNNs for visual feature extraction [6,20]. The technical challenge faced in our context is that sequential medical exams are event-based observations. As such, they are collected at times of clinical need, i.e. they are not equally spaced, and the number of historical exams available for each patient can vary greatly. Figure 1 shows four longitudinal chest x-rays acquired on the same patient over a certain period of time. This figure also illustrates other challenges faced when modelling this type of longitudinal data: the images may be aquired using different x-ray devices (resulting in different image quality, i.e. resolution, brightness, etc.), there may be differences in patient positioning (i.e. supine, erect, rotated, degree of inspiration), differences in projection (postero-anterior and antero-posterior), and not all images are equally centred (i.e. there can be rotations, translations, etc.).

As LSTMs are typically applied on regularly-sampled data [9,16,17], they are ill-suited to work with irregular time gaps between consecutive observations, as previously noted [3,13]. This is a particularly important limitation in our context as certain radiological abnormalities tend to be observed for longer periods of time whereas others are short-lived. In this article we demonstrate that an architecture combining a CNN with a simple modification of the standard LSTM is able to handle irregularly-sampled data and learn the temporal dynamics of certain visual features resulting in improved pattern detection. Using both simulated and real x-ray datasets, we demonstrate that this capability yields improved image classification performance over an LSTM baseline.

2 Motivating Dataset and Problem Formulation

The dataset used in this study was collected from the historical archives of the PACS (Picture Archiving and Communication System) at Guy's and St.

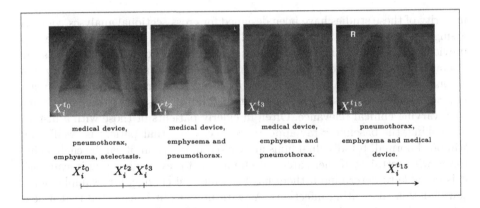

Fig. 1. Example of longitudinal x-rays for a given patient.

Thomas' NHS Foundation Trust, in London, during the period from January 2005 to March 2016. The dataset has been previously used for the detection of lung nodules [14] and for multi-label metric learning [1]. It consists of 745 480 chest radiographs representative of an adult population and acquired using 40 different x-ray systems. Each associated radiological report was parsed using a natural language processing system for the automated extraction of radiological labels [5,14]. For this study, we extracted a subset of 80 737 patients having a history of at least two exams, which resulted in 337 575 images (with 232 610 used for training and 104 965 for testing). Each image was scaled to a standard format of 299×299 pixels. The resulting dataset has an average of 4.18 examinations per patient with an average of 180.29 days between consecutive exams per patient.

In what follows, each individual sequence of longitudinal chest x-rays along with its associated vector of radiological labels is denoted as $\{X_i^t, l_i^t\}$, where $i = 1, \ldots, N$ is the patient index and $t = 1, \ldots, T_i$ is the time index. Typical chest x-ray datasets are characterised by relatively few examinations per patient (e.g. T_i is around 4–5) and highly-irregular sampling rates. Our task is to predict the vector of image labels $l_i^{T_i}$ given the entire history of exams up to time $T_i - 1$ plus the current image, i.e. $X_i^{T_i}$.

3   Time-Modulated LSTM

LSTMs are a particular type of RNNs able to classify, process and predict time series [8,10]. The internal state of an LSTM (a.k.a. the cell state or memory) gives the architecture its ability to 'remember'. A standard LSTM contains memory blocks, and blocks contain memory cells. A typical memory block is made of three main components: an input gate controlling the flow of input activations into the memory cell, an output gate controlling the output flow of cell activations, and a forget gate for scaling the internal state of the cell. The forget gate modulates how much information is used from the internal state of the previous time-step. However, standard LSTMs are ill-suited for our task where the time between consecutive exams is variable, because they have no mechanism for explicitly modelling the arrival time of each observation. In fact, it has been shown that LSTMs, and more generally RNNs, underperform with irregularly sampled data or time series with missing values [4,13]. Previous attempts to adapt LSTMs for use with irregularly sampled datapoints have mostly focused on speeding up the converge of the algorithm in settings with high-resolution sampled data [13] or to discount short-term memory [3].

To address these issues, we introduce two simple modifications of the standard LSTM architecture, called time-modulated LSTM (tLSTM), both making explicit use of the time indexes associated to the inputs. In the proposed architecture, all the images for a given patient are initially processed by a CNN architecture, which extracts a set of imaging features, denoted by $\widehat{X}_i^t$, at each time step. The LSTM takes as inputs l_i^{t-1}, i.e. the radiological labels describing the images acquired at the previous time-step, the current image features, $\widehat{X}_i^t$, and the time lapse between X_i^{t-1} and X_i^t, which we denote as δ_i^t. For the last image in the sequence, the LSTM predicts the image labels, l_i^t, called y_i^t. Figure 2 provides a high-level overview of this model and the equations below define the tLSTM unit:

$$
\begin{aligned}
f_t &= \sigma(W_{fl} * l^{t-1} + W_{fx} * \widehat{X}^t + W_{fj} * \delta^t + b_f), \\
i_t &= \sigma(W_{il} * l^{t-1} + W_{ix} * \widehat{X}^t + W_{ij} * \delta^t + b_i), \\
o_t &= \sigma(W_{ol} * l^{t-1} + W_{ox} * \widehat{X}^t + W_{oj} * \delta^t + b_o), \\
c_t &= \tanh(W_{cl} * l^{t-1} + W_{cx} * \widehat{X}^t + W_{cj} * \delta^t + b_c), \\
h_t &= f_t * h_{t-1} + i_t * c_t, \\
y^t &= o_t * \tanh(h_t)
\end{aligned}
\tag{1}
$$

Here, h_t defines the internal state at time-step t, while f_t, i_t and o_t refer to the forget, input and output gates at time-step t, respectively. These are all computed as linear combinations of the vectors l^{t-1}, $\widehat{X}^t$ and the scalar δ^t, and then transformed by a sigmoid function, $\sigma(\cdot)$. The matrices denoted by W contain learnable weights indexed by two letters (e.g. W_{fl} contains the weights of the forget gate f for labels l, and so on). At time $t = 1$, we initialise $l_i^{t-1} = <0 \ldots 0>$ (an array of zeros) and $\delta_i^t = 0$. The time lapses, δ_i^t, linearly modulate the information inside the internal cell state as well as the output, forget and input gates.

A different variation of the previous model (tLSTMv2) uses the time lapse only to modulate the internal state, h_t. In this case, each δ_i^t actively contributes to updating h_t directly and, implicitly, to estimating the label vector y^t, i.e.

$$
\begin{aligned}
h_t &= f_t * h_{t-1} + i_t * c_t + W_{tj} * \delta^t \\
y^t &= o_t * \tanh(h_t).
\end{aligned}
\tag{2}
$$

The form of the other updating equations, i.e. f_g, i_t, o_t and c_t, is similar to those in Eq. (1), without the $Ws \times \delta^t$ elements.

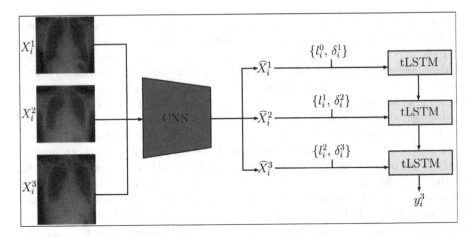

Fig. 2. An overview of the proposed architecture for image label prediction leveraging all historical exams.

4   Simulated Data

In order to better assess the potential advantages introduced by the time-modulated LSTM in settings where observations are event-driven and the underlying patterns to be detected are time-varying, we generated simulated data as an alternative to the real chest x-ray dataset of Sect. 2. Simulating images enables us to precisely control the sampling frequency at which the relevant visual patterns appear and disappear over time as well as the signal to noise ratio. For this study, we simulated a population of image sequences of varying lengths. Within a sequence, each image consisted of a noisy background image containing one or more randomly placed digits drawn from the set $\{0, 3, 6, 8, 9\}$. We simulated three kinds of patterns inspired by the radiological patterns seen in real medical images: (i) *rare patterns* consisting of digits appearing with low probability; (ii) *common patterns* consisting of rapidly appearing and resolving digits; (iii) *persistent labels*, consisting of digits observed for extended periods of time. In analogy to medical images, each digit in our simulation represents a radiological abnormality to be detected, hence multiple (and possibly overlapping) digits are allowed to coexist within an image. The time lapse δ^t was modelled as a uniform random variable taking value in the interval $[1, 10]$. An example of simulated images can be found in the Supplementary Material.

5   Experimental Results

In our experiments with the real x-ray dataset, the CNN component in our architecture conists of a pre-trained Inception v3 [18] without the classification layer. The imaging features $\hat{X}_i^t$ (an array 2048 elements) from the CNN are as used as inputs for the LSTM component along with the image labels. We considered

Table 1. Results on real data*

	Labels				
	cardio.	consol.	pleu. eff.	hernia	avg.
Inception v3					
PPV	0.5477	0.4111	0.6149	0.5204	0.5235
NPV	0.9565	0.9002	0.9106	0.9958	0.9407
F-measure	0.6143	0.5151	0.6575	0.5193	0.5765
LSTM					
PPV	0.6914	0.5841	0.7105	0.5369	0.6307
NPV	0.9406	0.8440	0.8895	0.9969	0.9177
F-measure	0.6199	0.4337	0.6531	0.5755	0.5705
tLSTMv1					
PPV	0.5929	0.4831	0.6358	0,5821	0.5734
NPV	0.9565	0.9000	0.9251	0.9968	0.9445
F-measure	0.6399	0.5552	0.6891	0.5932	0.6193
tLSTMv2					
PPV	0.5980	0.4876	0.6350	0.5461	0.5667
NPV	0.9572	0.8931	0.9120	0.9968	0.9397
F-measure	0.6447	0.5479	0.6696	0.5704	0.6081

*Classification performance (PPV, NPP and F-measure) of a baseline classifier (Inception v3) using only a single image as input and three LSTM architectures using the full sequence of longitudinal observations. tLSTMv1 and tLSTMv2 are the proposed time-modulated LSTM architectures that explitely model time lapses.

four possible radiological labels: cardiomegaly, consolidation, pleural effusion and hiatus hernia. The performance of the time-modulated LSTM models is assessed by the PPV (Positive Predictive Value) and NPV (Negative Predictive Value) along with F-score, i.e the harmonic mean of precision and recall.

We compared the performance of four models: the baseline CNN classifier (Inceptionv3) that only uses each current image to predict the labels, but does not exploit the historical exams for a given patient, and three variations of the architecture illustrated in Fig. 2: one using the standard LSTM and the two versions of time-modulated LSTM model introduced in Sect. 3. Both tLSTM versions introduced noticeable performance improvements; see Table 1. In particular, tLSTMv1 yields an increase of ~7% in F-measure over the baseline and ~8% over a standard LSTM. Moreover, tLSTMv1 achieves a ~9% improvement in PPV over the baseline. Overall, tLSTM achieves improved performance over the standard LSTM due to its ability to handle irregularly sampled data.

For the simulated dataset, we used a pre-trained AlexNet [11] as feature extractor in combination with three versions of the LSTM for modelling sequences of images. A full table with results can be found in the Supplementary Material. We purposely introduced a sufficiently high level of noise in the visual patterns so as to make the classification problem with individual images particularly difficult; accordingly, the single-image classifier did not achieve acceptable classification results. Likewise, the architecture using a standard LSTM did not introduce significant improvements due to the irregularly sampled observations. On the other hand, larger classification improvements were achieved using the time-modulated LSTM units as those were able to decode the sequential patterns by explicitly taking into account the time gaps between consecutive observations.

6   Conclusions

Our experimental results suggest that the modified LSTM architectures, combined with CNNs, are suitable for modelling sequences of event-based imaging observations. By explicitly modelling the individual time lapses between consecutive events, these architectures are able to better capture the evolution of visual patterns over time, which has a boosting effect on the classification performance. The full potential of these models is best demonstrated using simulated datasets whereby we have control over the exact nature of the temporal patterns and the image labels are perfectly known. In real radiological datasets, there are often errors in some of the image labels due to typographical errors, interpretive errors, ambiguous language and, in some cases, long-standing findings not being mentioned. This can cause problems both in CNN training and testing. Despite these challenges, we have demonstrated that improved classification results can also be achieved by the time-modulated LSTM components on a large chest x-ray dataset. Thus we empirically proved that a patient's imaging history can be used to improve automated radiological reporting. In future work, we plan more extensive testing of a system trained end-to-end on a much larger number of radiological classes. The code with the networks used for our experiment can be found online: https://github.com/WMGDataScience/tLSTM.

References

1. Annarumma, M., Montana, G.: Deep metric learning for multi-labelled radiographs. In: 33rd Annual ACM SAC 2018, pp. 34–37. ACM (2018)
2. Bar, Y., Diamant, I., Wolf, L., Lieberman, S., Konen, E., Greenspan, H.: Chest pathology detection using deep learning with non-medical training. In: 2015 IEEE 12th International Symposium on Biomedical Imaging (ISBI), 294–297, 07 2015
3. Baytas, I.M., Xiao, C., Zhang, X., Wang, F., Jain, A.K., Zhou, J.: Patient subtyping via time-aware LSTM networks. In: 23rd ACM SIGKDD (2017)
4. Che, Z., Purushotham, S., Cho, K., Sontag, D., Liu, Y.: Recurrent neural networks for multivariate time series with missing values. Scientific reports (2018)
5. Cornegruta, S., Bakewell, R., Withey, S., Montana, G.: Modelling radiological language with bidirectional long short-term memory networks. In: 7th Workshop on Health Text Mining and Information Analysis (2016)

6. Donahue, J., et al.: Long-term Recurrent Convolutional Networks for Visual Recognition and Description. ArXiv e-prints, November 2014
7. Esteva, A., et al.: Dermatologist-level classification of skin cancer with deep neural networks. Nature **542**, 115 (2017)
8. Gers, F.A., Schmidhuber, J., Cummins, F.: Learning to forget: continual prediction with LSTM. Neural Comput. **12**, 2451–2471 (1999)
9. Graves, A., Mohamed, A., Hinton, G.E.: Speech recognition with deep recurrent neural networks. CoRR (2013)
10. Hochreiter, S., Schmidhuber, J.: Long short-term memory. Neural Comput. **9**(8), 1735–1780 (1997)
11. Krizhevsky, A., Sutskever, I., Hinton, G.E.: Imagenet classification with deep convolutional neural networks. In: Advances in Neural Information Processing Systems, vol. 25, pp. 1097–1105. Curran Associates Inc (2012)
12. Litjens, G., et al.: A Survey on Deep Learning in Medical Image Analysis. ArXiv e-prints, February 2017
13. Neil, D., Pfeiffer, M., Liu, S.-C.: Phased LSTM: accelerating recurrent network training for long or event-based sequences. ArXiv e-prints, October 2016
14. Pesce, E., Ypsilantis, P.-P., Withey, S., Bakewell, R., Goh, V., Montana, G.: Learning to detect chest radiographs containing lung nodules using visual attention networks. ArXiv e-prints, December 2017
15. Rajpurkar, P., et al.: CheXNet: radiologist-level pneumonia detection on Chest X-rays with deep learning. ArXiv e-prints, November 2017
16. Shi, X., Chen, Z., Wang, H., Yeung, D., Wong, W., Woo, W.: Convolutional LSTM network: a machine learning approach for precipitation nowcasting. In: Cortes, C., Lawrence, N.D., Lee, D.D., Sugiyama, M., Garnett, R. (eds.) Advances in Neural Information Processing Systems, vol. 28, pp. 802–810. Curran Associates Inc (2015)
17. Srivastava, N., Mansimov, E., Salakhutdinov R.: Unsupervised learning of video representations using LSTMs. CoRR, abs/1502.04681 (2015)
18. Szegedy, C., Vanhoucke, V., Ioffe, S., Shlens, J., Wojna, Z.: Rethinking the inception architecture for computer vision. In: Proceedings of the IEEE Conference on Computer Vision and Pattern Recognition (2016)
19. Gulshan, V., Peng, L., Coram, M., et al.: Development and validation of a deep learning algorithm for detection of diabetic retinopathy in retinal fundus photographs. JAMA **316**(22), 2402–2410 (2016)
20. Vinyals, O., Toshev, A., Bengio, S., Erhan, D.: Show and tell: a neural image caption generator. In: 2015 IEEE Conference on Computer Vision and Pattern Recognition, pp. 3156–3164. IEEE (2015)
21. Wang, X., Peng, Y., Lu, L., Lu, Z., Bagheri, M., Summers, R.M.: ChestX-ray8: Hospital-scale Chest X-ray Database and Benchmarks on Weakly-Supervised Classification and Localization of Common Thorax Diseases. ArXiv e-prints, May 2017

Iterative Segmentation from Limited Training Data: Applications to Congenital Heart Disease

Danielle F. Pace[1](✉), Adrian V. Dalca[1,2,3], Tom Brosch[4], Tal Geva[5,6], Andrew J. Powell[5,6], Jürgen Weese[4], Mehdi H. Moghari[5,6], and Polina Golland[1]

[1] Computer Science and Artificial Intelligence Lab, MIT, Cambridge, USA
dfpace@mit.edu
[2] Martinos Center for Biomedical Imaging, Massachusetts General Hospital, HMS, Boston, USA
[3] School of Electrical and Computer Engineering, Cornell University, Ithaca, USA
[4] Philips Research Laboratories, Hamburg, Germany
[5] Department of Cardiology, Boston Children's Hospital, Boston, USA
[6] Department of Pediatrics, Harvard Medical School, Boston, USA

Abstract. We propose a new iterative segmentation model which can be accurately learned from a small dataset. A common approach is to train a model to directly segment an image, requiring a large collection of manually annotated images to capture the anatomical variability in a cohort. In contrast, we develop a segmentation model that recursively evolves a segmentation in several steps, and implement it as a recurrent neural network. We learn model parameters by optimizing the intermediate steps of the evolution in addition to the final segmentation. To this end, we train our segmentation propagation model by presenting incomplete and/or inaccurate input segmentations paired with a recommended next step. Our work aims to alleviate challenges in segmenting heart structures from cardiac MRI for patients with congenital heart disease (CHD), which encompasses a range of morphological deformations and topological changes. We demonstrate the advantages of this approach on a dataset of 20 images from CHD patients, learning a model that accurately segments individual heart chambers and great vessels. Compared to direct segmentation, the iterative method yields more accurate segmentation for patients with the most severe CHD malformations.

1 Introduction

We aim to provide whole heart segmentation in cardiac MRI for patients with congenital heart disease (CHD). This involves delineating the heart chambers and great vessels [1], and promises to enable patient-specific heart models for surgical planning in CHD [2]. CHD encompasses a vast range of cardiac malformations and topological changes. Defects can include holes in the heart walls

© Springer Nature Switzerland AG 2018
D. Stoyanov et al. (Eds.): DLMIA 2018/ML-CDS 2018, LNCS 11045, pp. 334–342, 2018.
https://doi.org/10.1007/978-3-030-00889-5_38

(septal defects), great vessels connected to the wrong chamber (e.g., double outlet right ventricle; DORV), dextrocardia (left-right flip), duplication of a great vessel, a single ventricle, and/or prior surgeries creating additional atypical connections. In MRI, different chambers and great vessels locally appear very similar to each other, and there is little or no contrast at the valves and thin walls separating neighboring structures. Finally, labeled training data is very limited. This precludes modeling each CHD subtype separately in an attempt to reduce variability. Moreover, patients with unique combinations of defects and prior surgeries defy categorization. Beyond our application, limited training data is to be expected for new applications of medical imaging not yet in widespread clinical practice. This necessitates development of methods that generalize well from small, imbalanced datasets, possibly also incorporating user interaction.

State-of-the-art methods use a convolutional neural network (CNN) to directly outline all chambers and vessels in one step [3,4]. However, CNNs for CHD have largely been limited to segmenting the blood pool and myocardium [5,6]. Direct co-segmentation of all major cardiac structures works well when applied to adult-onset heart disease, which induces much less severe shape changes compared to CHD. However, it fails completely on held-out subjects with severe CHD malformations after training with our small dataset of CHD patients.

We develop an iterative segmentation approach that evolves a segmentation over several steps in a prescribed way and automatically estimates when to stop, beginning from a single seed for each structure placed by the user. An iterative method can operate more locally, better maintain each structure's connectivity, and propagate information from distant landmarks, similar to traditional snakes, level sets and particle filters [7]. We employ a recurrent neural network (RNN) [8], which uses context to grow the segmentation appropriately even in areas of low contrast. Deep learning research has indeed focused on segmenting a single image iteratively. Examples include recursive refinement of the entire segmentation map [9,10], sequential completion of different instances, regions or fields of view [11–13], slice-by-slice analysis [14] and networks modeling level set evolution [15]. These methods condition on a previous partial solution to make progress towards the final output. This simplified task may enable training from smaller datasets.

We train the model by minimizing a loss over a training dataset of example segmentation *trajectories*. Maximizing the likelihood of observed sequences is known as teacher forcing [8,16]. For example, we may require vessel segmentation to proceed at a constant rate along the vessel centerline, or a heart chamber segmentation to dilate outwards. Even if the stopping prediction is incorrect, since the segmentation evolution follows a prescribed pattern it is likely that one of the intermediate segmentations will be accurate. In contrast, using the final segmentation alone could lead to unpredictable growth patterns. Teacher forcing also leads to a simplified optimization over decoupled time steps, avoiding back-propagation through time.

We focus on segmenting the aorta (a representative great vessel) and the left ventricle (a representative cardiac chamber). We validate our iterative segmentation approach using a dataset of 20 CHD patients, and compare it to direct segmentation methods which we have developed for this problem.

2 Iterative Segmentation Model

Given an input image $\mathbf{x}$ defined on the domain Ω, we seek a segmentation label map $\mathbf{y}$ that assigns one of L anatomical labels to each voxel in $\mathbf{x}$.

Generative Model: We model the segmentation $\mathbf{y}$ as the endpoint of a sequence of segmentations $\mathbf{y}_0, \ldots, \mathbf{y}_T$, where $\mathbf{y}_t : \Omega \to \{1, \ldots, L\}$ for time steps $t = 0, \ldots, T$. The intermediate segmentations $\mathbf{y}_t$ capture a growing part of the anatomy of interest. In practice, the initial segmentation map $\mathbf{y}_0$ is created by centering a small sphere around an initial seed point placed by the user.

The number of iterations required to achieve an accurate segmentation depends on the shape and size of the object being segmented. To capture this, we introduce a sequence of indicator variables $s_0, \ldots, s_T$, where $s_t \in \{0, 1\}$ specifies whether the segmentation is completed at time step t. If $s_t = 1$, then $\mathbf{y}_t$ is deemed the final segmentation and we set $\mathbf{y}_i = \mathbf{y}_{i-1}$ and $s_i = 1$ for all $i > t$.

Given an image and an initial segmentation, the inference task is to compute $p(\mathbf{y}_T, s_T | \mathbf{x}, \mathbf{y}_0, s_0 = 0)$. We assume that the segmentations $\{\mathbf{y}_t\}$ and stopping indicators $\{s_t\}$ follow a first order Markov chain given the input image:

$$p(\mathbf{y}_t, s_t | \mathbf{x}, \mathbf{y}_0, \ldots, \mathbf{y}_{t-1}, s_0, \ldots, s_{t-1}) = p(\mathbf{y}_t, s_t | \mathbf{x}, \mathbf{y}_{t-1}, s_{t-1}), \tag{1}$$

$$p(\mathbf{y}_t, s_t | \mathbf{x}, \mathbf{y}_0, s_0) = \sum_{\mathbf{y}_{t-1}} \sum_{s_{t-1}} p(\mathbf{y}_t, s_t | \mathbf{x}, \mathbf{y}_{t-1}, s_{t-1}) \cdot p(\mathbf{y}_{t-1}, s_{t-1} | \mathbf{x}, \mathbf{y}_0, s_0). \tag{2}$$

Transition Probability Model: We must define the transition probability $p(\mathbf{y}_t, s_t | \mathbf{x}, \mathbf{y}_{t-1}, s_{t-1})$ to complete the recursion in Eq. (2). There are two possible cases: $s_{t-1} = 1$ and $s_{t-1} = 0$. Based on the definition of s_{t-1}, we obtain

$$p(\mathbf{y}_t, s_t | \mathbf{x}, \mathbf{y}_{t-1}, s_{t-1} = 1) = \mathbb{1}(\mathbf{y}_t = \mathbf{y}_{t-1}) \cdot \mathbb{1}(s_t = 1), \tag{3}$$

where $\mathbb{1}(\cdot)$ denotes the indicator function. To compute $p(\mathbf{y}_t, s_t | \mathbf{x}, \mathbf{y}_{t-1}, s_{t-1} = 0)$, we introduce a latent representation $\mathbf{h}_t = h(\mathbf{x}, \mathbf{y}_{t-1})$ that jointly captures all of the necessary information from image $\mathbf{x}$ and previous segmentation $\mathbf{y}_{t-1}$. Intuitively, predicting whether the segmentation $\mathbf{y}_t$ is complete given $\mathbf{x}$ can be performed by examining whether $\mathbf{y}_{t-1}$ is "almost" complete. Therefore, the segmentation $\mathbf{y}_t$ and stopping indicator s_t are conditionally independent given $\mathbf{h}_t$:

$$p(\mathbf{y}_t, s_t | \mathbf{x}, \mathbf{y}_{t-1}, s_{t-1} = 0) = p(\mathbf{y}_t, s_t | \mathbf{h}_t) = p(\mathbf{y}_t | \mathbf{h}_t) \cdot p(s_t | \mathbf{h}_t). \tag{4}$$

We model the function $h(\mathbf{x}, \mathbf{y}_{t-1})$ and distributions $p(\mathbf{y}_t | \mathbf{h}_t)$ and $p(s_t | \mathbf{h}_t)$ as stationary; they do not depend on the time step t.

Learning: We learn a representation of $p(\mathbf{y}_t, s_t | \mathbf{x}, \mathbf{y}_{t-1}, s_{t-1} = 0)$ given a training dataset of example desired trajectories of segmentations. Specifically, we consider a training dataset $\mathcal{D}$ of N images $\{\mathbf{x}^i\}_{i=1}^N$, each of which has a corresponding sequence of segmentations $\mathbf{y}_0^i, \ldots, \mathbf{y}_{T_i}^i$ and of stopping indicators $s_0^i, \ldots, s_{T_i}^i$, where $s_0^i = \ldots = s_{T_i-1}^i = 0$ and $s_{T_i}^i = 1$. The parameter values to be determined are $\boldsymbol{\theta} = \{\boldsymbol{\theta}_h, \boldsymbol{\theta}_y, \boldsymbol{\theta}_s\}$ corresponding to $h(\mathbf{x}, \mathbf{y}_{t-1}; \boldsymbol{\theta}_h)$, $p(\mathbf{y}_t|\mathbf{h}_t; \boldsymbol{\theta}_y)$, and $p(s_t|\mathbf{h}_t; \boldsymbol{\theta}_s)$, respectively. We seek the parameter values that minimize the expected negative log-likelihood of the output segmentation and stopping indicator sequences given the image and initial conditions, i.e., $\boldsymbol{\theta}^* = \operatorname{argmin}_{\boldsymbol{\theta}} \mathcal{L}(\boldsymbol{\theta})$,

$$\mathcal{L}(\boldsymbol{\theta}) = \mathbb{E}_{\mathbf{x}, \mathbf{y}_0, \ldots, \mathbf{y}_T, s_0, \ldots, s_T \sim \mathcal{D}}\Big[-\log p(\mathbf{y}_1, \ldots, \mathbf{y}_T, s_1, \ldots, s_T | \mathbf{x}, \mathbf{y}_0, s_0; \boldsymbol{\theta}) \Big]$$

$$= -\mathbb{E}\Big[\sum_{t=1}^T \log p(\mathbf{y}_t | h(\mathbf{x}, \mathbf{y}_{t-1}; \boldsymbol{\theta}_h); \boldsymbol{\theta}_y) + \log p(s_t | h(\mathbf{x}, \mathbf{y}_{t-1}; \boldsymbol{\theta}_h); \boldsymbol{\theta}_s) \Big]. \quad (5)$$

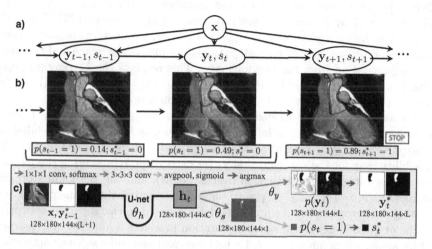

Fig. 1. Iterative segmentation as an RNN. (a) Generative model. (b) The RNN uses the same augmented U-net at each step to predict the next segmentation and stopping indicator. (c) Architecture details (conditioning dropped for clarity).

Note that teacher forcing has lead to decoupled time steps. The first and second terms in the likelihood above penalize differences for the segmentations and the stopping indicators, respectively, between the predicted probabilities and the ground truth. In practice, we perform class rebalancing for both terms, and further supplement the segmentation loss by more strongly weighting pixels on the boundaries of the ground truth segmentation.

Inference: Computing $p(\mathbf{y}_T, s_T | \mathbf{x}, \mathbf{y}_0, s_0 = 0)$ via the recursion in Eq. (2) is intractable due to the summation over all possible segmentations $\mathbf{y}_{t-1}$. To approximate, we follow a widely accepted practice of using the most likely segmentation $\mathbf{y}_{t-1}^*$ and stopping indicator s_{t-1}^* as input to the subsequent computation:

$$p(\mathbf{y}_t, s_t | \mathbf{x}, \mathbf{y}_0, s_0 = 0; \boldsymbol{\theta}) \approx p(\mathbf{y}_t, s_t | \mathbf{x}, \mathbf{y}_{t-1}^*, s_{t-1}^*; \boldsymbol{\theta}),$$
$$\text{where } \mathbf{y}_{t-1}^*, s_{t-1}^* = \underset{\mathbf{y}_{t-1}, s_{t-1}}{\operatorname{argmax}} \, p(\mathbf{y}_{t-1}, s_{t-1} | \mathbf{x}, \mathbf{y}_0, s_0 = 0; \boldsymbol{\theta}). \tag{6}$$

The segmentation is fully automatic given the initial seed. If the stopping indicator is predicted incorrectly, a user can manually override it by asking for more iterations or by choosing a segmentation from a previous step.

RNN: We implement our iterative segmentation model as an RNN (Fig. 1), which is formed by connecting identical copies of an augmented 3D U-net [17] trained to estimate $p(\mathbf{y}_t, s_t | \mathbf{x}, \mathbf{y}_{t-1}, s_{t-1} = 0)$. Thus, parameters are shared both spatially and temporally. At each step, the U-net inputs the image and the most likely segmentation from the previous step. This respects the Markov property in Eq. (1), unlike if any hidden layers were connected between successive steps. If the stopping indicator $s_t^* = 1$, the segmentation propagation halts.

Our augmented U-net modeling $p(\mathbf{y}_t, s_t | \mathbf{x}, \mathbf{y}_{t-1}, s_{t-1} = 0)$ has $L + 1$ input channels, containing the input image and a binary map for each of the L labels in the segmentation $\mathbf{y}_{t-1}$ (including the background). There are two outputs: the probability map for the segmentation $\mathbf{y}_t$ (at each voxel, representing the parameters of the categorical distribution over L labels), and the Bernoulli stopping parameter $p(s_t = 1 | \mathbf{x}, \mathbf{y}_{t-1}, s_{t-1} = 0)$. Jointly predicting the segmentation and stopping indicator enables a smaller model compared to two separate networks.

The original U-net for image segmentation produces a final set of C learned feature maps, which undergo $C \cdot L$ $1 \times 1 \times 1$ convolutions and a softmax activation to give the output segmentation probabilities. We use these C learned feature maps as the latent joint representation $\mathbf{h}_t = h(\mathbf{x}, \mathbf{y}_{t-1}; \boldsymbol{\theta}_h)$. The U-net parameters can therefore be split into two sets. The parameters for the final $1 \times 1 \times 1$ convolutions are $\boldsymbol{\theta}_y$ of $p(\mathbf{y}_t | \mathbf{h}_t; \boldsymbol{\theta}_y)$, and the remainder are $\boldsymbol{\theta}_h$ of $h(\mathbf{x}, \mathbf{y}_{t-1}; \boldsymbol{\theta}_h)$. The probability $p(s_t = 1 | \mathbf{h}_t; \boldsymbol{\theta}_s)$ is computed by applying C additional $3 \times 3 \times 3$ convolutions with parameters $\boldsymbol{\theta}_s$ to the feature maps in $\mathbf{h}_t$, followed by a global average and sigmoid activation to yield a scalar in $\{0, 1\}$.

Generating Segmentation Trajectories: Our training dataset of images and segmentation trajectories is derived from a collection of paired images and complete segmentations. Several acceptable trajectories exist for each pair, e.g., starting from different initial seeds. To this end, at the beginning of each epoch a random tuple $(\mathbf{y}_{t-1}, \mathbf{y}_t, s_t)$ is generated for each image. These tuples all follow the same principle that we want the network to learn.

As a concrete example, the trajectories used in our experiments are as follows. For the *aorta*, the segmentation grows from the seed along the vessel centerline, by a random distance to form $\mathbf{y}_{t-1}$ and an additional 10 pixels for $\mathbf{y}_t$. The seed is placed in the descending aorta, and the endpoint is at the valve where the aorta connects to a left or right ventricle. This seed could be automatically detected in the future, and the lack of contrast at the valve provides a challenging test case for our automatic stopping. For the *left ventricle*, we randomly place the seed in the center region of the chamber, and perform a random number of dilations to form $\mathbf{y}_{t-1}$, and 3 more dilations to form $\mathbf{y}_t$.

Data Augmentation: Data augmentation is essential to prevent overfitting on a small training dataset. We mimic the diversity of heart shapes and sizes, global intensity changes caused by inhomogeneity artifacts, and noise induced by elevated heart rates or arrhythmias. We apply random rigid and nonrigid transformations, random constant intensity shifts, and random additive Gaussian noise. We also investigate including random left-right (L-R) and anterior-posterior (A-P) flips, to better handle dextrocardia or other cardiac malpositions, since in these cases the left ventricle may lie on the right side of the body.

If the augmented U-net for $p(\mathbf{y}_t, s_t | \mathbf{x}, \mathbf{y}_{t-1}, s_{t-1} = 0)$ is trained solely using error-free segmentations $\mathbf{y}_{t-1}$, then it may not operate well on its own imperfect intermediate results at test time. We increase robustness by performing additional data augmentation on the input segmentations $\mathbf{y}_{t-1}$. We corrupt these segmentations by applying random nonrigid deformations, and by inserting random blob-like structures that vary in number, location and size and are attached to the segmentation foreground or free-floating. Since the target segmentation $\mathbf{y}_t$ remains unchanged, the model learns to correct mistakes in its input.

3   Experimental Validation

We evaluate our iterative segmentation and tailored direct segmentation methods, focusing on segmenting the aorta and left ventricle (LV) of CHD patients.

Data: We use the HVSMR dataset of 20 MRI scans from patients with a variety of congenital heart defects [18]. Each high-resolution ($\approx 0.9\,\text{mm}^3$) 3D image was acquired on a 1.5 T scanner (Philips Achieva), without contrast agent and using a free-breathing SSFP sequence with ECG and respiratory navigator gating. The HVSMR dataset includes blood pool and myocardium segmentations only. A trained rater manually separated all of the heart chambers and great vessels. The 20 images were categorized after visually assessing any gross morphological malformations: 4/20 severe (prior major reconstructive surgery, single ventricle, dextrocardia), 5/20 moderate (DORV, VSD, abnormal chamber shapes), and 11/20 mild (ASD, stenosis, etc.). The dataset was randomly split into 4 folds for cross-validation (15 training, 5 testing), with an equal number of mild, moderate and severe cases in each. Input images were resized to $\approx 128 \times 180 \times 144$.

Experiments: In our tests, binary segmentation of each structure outperformed co-segmenting all of the heart chambers and vessels. We trained several models aimed at segmenting the aorta and left ventricle of CHD patients. **DIR** uses a single U-net to perform direct binary segmentation. **DIR-DIST** includes the Euclidean distance to the initial seed as an additional input channel. **ITER (stop)**

is iterative segmentation using our RNN with automatic stopping, and **ITER (max)** simulates a user by choosing the segmentation with the best Dice coefficient after 30 iterations of our RNN. Finally, **ITER-SEG-ABL** is an ablation study with no data augmentation on the input segmentations. We tuned the architectural parameters for each experiment separately, nevertheless resulting in similar networks. All U-nets had 3 levels, 24 feature maps at the first level, and $\approx$870,000 parameters. The best network for direct segmentation of the aorta used $2 \times 2 \times 2$ max pooling (receptive field $= 40^3$), while all others used $3 \times 3 \times 3$ max pooling (receptive field $= 68^3$). For training, optimization using adadelta ran for 2000 epochs with a batch size of 1. For iterative segmentation, the argmax in Eq. (6) is computed per voxel, by assuming that the segmentation of each voxel is conditionally independent of all other voxels given $\mathbf{h}_t$. Segmentations were post-processed to keep only the largest island or the island containing the initial seed, for experiments in which this improves overall accuracy. Aorta segmentations were not penalized for descending aortas longer than in the gold-standard.

Results: Figures 2 and 3 report the results. There was no notable difference in accuracy between the mild and moderate groups. DIR-DIST was the best direct segmentation method, demonstrating the advantage of leveraging user interaction. For all methods, incorporating L-R and A-P flips in the data augmentation improved performance for severe subjects. Iterative segmentation stopped automatically after 18 ± 3 steps for both the aorta and the LV, requiring $\approx$15 s. The potential benefits of our iterative segmentation approach are demonstrated by the performance of ITER (max), which shows improvement for all of the severe cases while maintaining accuracy for the others. The stopping prediction is not

Method	AO mild/mod.	AO severe	LV mild/mod.	LV severe
DIR	92.5±6.5	81.2±16.3	94.1±3.5	68.6±25.5
DIR-DIST	92.3±8.6	89.7±2.9	94.1±2.2	83.0±6.2
ITER (stop)	91.5±7.0	91.8±4.6	91.2±4.4	83.3±9.0
ITER (max)	93.3±6.3	93.6±1.5	93.7±2.3	87.8±3.5
ITER-SEG-ABL (stop)	65.9±24.1	45.0±33.4	62.2±24.9	49.2±31.3
ITER-SEG-ABL (max)	66.3±24.4	45.8±37.4	64.4±22.4	52.7±25.1

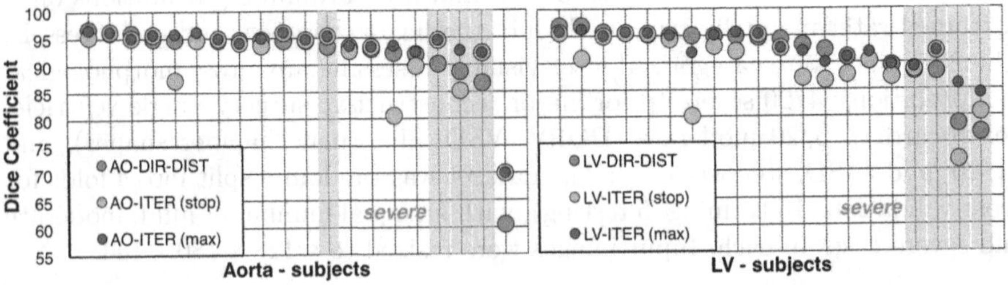

Fig. 2. Aorta (AO) and LV segmentation validation. DIR-DIST is the best direct segmentation method, but iterative segmentation generalizes better to severe subjects. Top: Dice coefficients for all methods. Bottom: Results for all 20 subjects, sorted by DIR-DIST score and with severe subjects highlighted in green. (Color figure online)

perfect at test time: the number of iterations separating the automatic stopping point from the best segmentation in a sequence was 0.8 ± 1.0 iterations for the aorta and 3.0 ± 2.5 iterations for the LV. The sole aorta containing a stent was poorly segmented by all methods (Fig. 3e). The stent caused a strong inhomogeneity artifact that the iterative segmentation could not grow past, and the stopping criterion was never triggered.

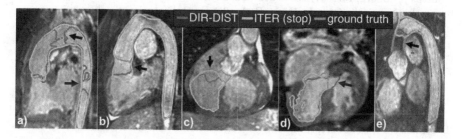

Fig. 3. Representative aorta and LV segmentations in held-out subjects with severe CHD. Arrows illustrate both the benefits and failure cases of iterative segmentation with automatic stopping, where it (a) successfully segments a difficult case, (b) stops too late, (c) correctly stops near a valve, (d) avoids growing through a septal defect, (e) cannot grow through a dark region caused by a stent.

4   Conclusions

We presented an iterative segmentation model and its RNN implementation. We showed that for whole heart segmentation, the iterative approach was more robust to the cardiac malformations of severe CHD. Future work will investigate the potential general applicability of iterative segmentation when one is restricted to a small training dataset despite wide anatomical variability.

Acknowledgements. NSERC CGS-D, Phillips Inc., Wistron Corporation, BCH Translational Research Program and Office of Faculty Development, Harvard Catalyst, Charles H. Hood Foundation and American Heart Association.

References

1. Zhuang, X.: Challenges and methodologies of fully automatic whole heart segmentation: a review. J. Healthc. Eng. 4(3), 371–408 (2013)
2. Pace, D.F., Dalca, A.V., Geva, T., Powell, A.J., Moghari, M.H., Golland, P.: Interactive whole-heart segmentation in congenital heart disease. In: Navab, N., Hornegger, J., Wells, W.M., Frangi, A.F. (eds.) MICCAI 2015. LNCS, vol. 9351, pp. 80–88. Springer, Cham (2015). https://doi.org/10.1007/978-3-319-24574-4_10
3. Payer, C., Štern, D., Bischof, H., Urschler, M.: Multi-label whole heart segmentation using CNNs and anatomical label configurations. In: Pop, M., et al. (eds.) STACOM 2017. LNCS, vol. 10663, pp. 190–198. Springer, Cham (2018). https://doi.org/10.1007/978-3-319-75541-0_20

4. Wang, C., Smedby, Ö.: Automatic whole heart segmentation using deep learning and shape context. In: Pop, M., et al. (eds.) STACOM 2017. LNCS, vol. 10663, pp. 242–249. Springer, Cham (2018). https://doi.org/10.1007/978-3-319-75541-0_26

5. Wolterink, J.M., Leiner, T., Viergever, M.A., Išgum, I.: Dilated convolutional neural networks for cardiovascular MR segmentation in congenital heart disease. In: Zuluaga, M.A., Bhatia, K., Kainz, B., Moghari, M.H., Pace, D.F. (eds.) RAMBO/HVSMR -2016. LNCS, vol. 10129, pp. 95–102. Springer, Cham (2017). https://doi.org/10.1007/978-3-319-52280-7_9

6. Yu, L., Yang, X., Qin, J., Heng, P.-A.: 3D FractalNet: dense volumetric segmentation for cardiovascular MRI volumes. In: Zuluaga, M.A., Bhatia, K., Kainz, B., Moghari, M.H., Pace, D.F. (eds.) RAMBO/HVSMR -2016. LNCS, vol. 10129, pp. 103–110. Springer, Cham (2017). https://doi.org/10.1007/978-3-319-52280-7_10

7. Sonka, M., Hlavac, V., Boyle, R.: Image Processing, Analysis and Machine Vision. Thompson, Toronto (2008)

8. Goodfellow, I., Bengio, Y., Courville, A.: Deep Learning. MIT Press, Cambridge (2016)

9. Pinheiro, P., Collobert, R.: Recurrent convolutional neural networks for scene labeling. In: ICML pp. I-82–I-90 (2014)

10. Zhou, Y., Xie, L., Shen, W., Wang, Y., Fishman, E.K., Yuille, A.L.: A fixed-point model for pancreas segmentation in abdominal CT scans. In: Descoteaux, M., Maier-Hein, L., Franz, A., Jannin, P., Collins, D.L., Duchesne, S. (eds.) MICCAI 2017. LNCS, vol. 10433, pp. 693–701. Springer, Cham (2017). https://doi.org/10.1007/978-3-319-66182-7_79

11. Ren, M., Zemel, R.: End-to-end instance segmentation with recurrent attention. In: CVPR, pp. 6656–6664 (2017)

12. Banica, D., Sminchisescu, C.: Second-order constrained parametric proposals and sequential search-based structured prediction for semantic segmentation in RGB-D images. In: CVPR, pp. 3517–3526 (2015)

13. Januszewski, M., et al.: High-precision automated reconstruction of neurons with flood-filling networks. Nat Methods, Preprint (2018)

14. Zheng, Q., Delingette, H., Duchateau, N., Ayache, N.: 3D consistent and robust segmentation of cardiac images by deep learning with spatial propagation. IEEE Trans. Med. Imaging, Preprint (2018)

15. Chakravarty, A., Sivaswamy, J.: RACE-net: a recurrent neural network for biomedical image segmentation. IEEE J. Biomed. Health Inform., Preprint (2018)

16. Williams, R., Zipser, D.: A learning algorithm for continually running fully recurrent neural networks. Neural Comput. 1(2), 270–280 (1989)

17. Ronneberger, O., Fischer, P., Brox, T.: U-Net: convolutional networks for biomedical image segmentation. In: Navab, N., Hornegger, J., Wells, W.M., Frangi, A.F. (eds.) MICCAI 2015. LNCS, vol. 9351, pp. 234–241. Springer, Cham (2015). https://doi.org/10.1007/978-3-319-24574-4_28

18. HVSMR Challenge, MICCAI (2016). axial-cropped, http://segchd.csail.mit.edu

ScarGAN: Chained Generative Adversarial Networks to Simulate Pathological Tissue on Cardiovascular MR Scans

Felix Lau[1]($\boxtimes$), Tom Hendriks[1,2], Jesse Lieman-Sifry[1], Sean Sall[1], and Dan Golden[1]

[1] Arterys Inc., 51 Federal Street, San Francisco, CA 94107, USA
{felix,tom.hendriks,jesse,sean,dan}@arterys.com
[2] Department of Cardiology, University of Groningen, University Medical Center Groningen, Hanzeplein 1, 9713 GZ Groningen, The Netherlands
t.hendriks@umcg.nl

Abstract. We consider the problem of segmenting the left ventricular (LV) myocardium on late gadolinium enhancement (LGE) cardiovascular magnetic resonance (CMR) scans of which only some of the scans have scar tissue. We propose ScarGAN to simulate scar tissue on healthy myocardium using chained generative adversarial networks (GAN). Our novel approach factorizes the simulation process into 3 steps: (1) a mask generator to simulate the shape of the scar tissue; (2) a domain-specific heuristic to produce the initial simulated scar tissue from the mask; (3) a refining generator to add details to the simulated scar tissue. Unlike other approaches that generate samples from scratch, we simulate scar tissue on normal scans resulting in highly realistic samples. We show that experienced radiologists are unable to distinguish between real and simulated scar tissue. Training a U-Net with additional scans with scar tissue simulated by ScarGAN increases the percentage of scar pixels in LV myocardium prediction from 75.9% to 80.5%.

1 Introduction

Recently, deep learning has shown promising results to automate many tasks in radiology such as skin lesion classification [2]. The performance of these deep convolutional neural networks (DCNNs) is sometimes on par with clinicians but usually requires a large amount of training images and labels. Training a DCNN that performs equally well across different patients is challenging because some pathologies are rare.

Automated Myocardium Segmentation of LGE Scans. LGE imaging is an established method to detect myocardial scarring and measure the infarct size using a gadolinium-based contrast but not all LGE scans have visible scar tissue [11]. Contrast accumulates in regions of the myocardium that contain a

© Springer Nature Switzerland AG 2018
D. Stoyanov et al. (Eds.): DLMIA 2018/ML-CDS 2018, LNCS 11045, pp. 343–350, 2018.
https://doi.org/10.1007/978-3-030-00889-5_39

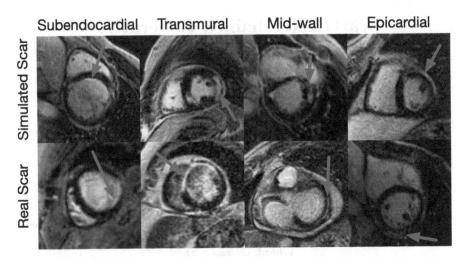

Fig. 1. Samples of real and simulated scar tissue on LGE scans categorized by enhancement patterns. Red arrows indicate the location of real or simulated scar tissue. (Color figure online)

high proportion of fibrosis (scar tissue) which results in a hyperenhancement on the acquired images.

We apply a U-Net segmentation network [9] to segment the LV myocardium but it does not perform well on patients with scar tissue. The subtle differences between scar tissue and blood pool are extremely challenging for DCNNs and even physicians to delineate.

ScarGAN. We propose ScarGAN, an approach utilizing chained generative adversarial networks (GANs) to simulate scar tissue in the LV myocardium on LGE scans of healthy patients as data augmentation. Figure 1 shows examples of simulated scar tissue grouped by their enhancement patterns. Overview of the ScarGAN architecture can be seen in Fig. 2.

The main contributions of this work are:

- We present ScarGAN to simulate scar tissue in healthy myocardium on LGE CMR scans;
- We factorize the simulation process into multiple steps and allow domain-specific heuristics to be added to reduce the difficulty of training GANs;
- We present qualitative and quantitative results to demonstrate that scar tissue simulated by ScarGAN is highly realistic and cannot be distinguished from real scar tissue by radiologists;
- We demonstrate that simulated scar tissue can improve myocardium segmentation network without collecting more scans and annotations of a specific pathology.

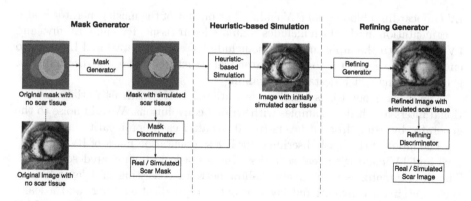

Fig. 2. Overview of ScarGAN. A mask generator simulates the shape of scar tissue segmentation mask (LV endo is light blue; LV myo is green; LV endo is orange; scar tissue is red); a heuristic-based method provides an initial simulated scar tissue using the simulated shape; a refining generator add details of scar tissue to the image. (Color figure online)

2   Related Work

The GAN framework was first proposed by Goodfellow et al. [4] and consists of 2 networks: a generative network $G(z)$ that transforms a noise vector z into realistic samples, and a discriminator network $D(x)$ that classifies samples as real or fake. In pix2pix [5], a fully convolutional U-Net in the generator performs image translation; the generative network receives an image in one domain and outputs the corresponding image of another domain. Both of the GANs in ScarGAN are based on pix2pix.

Previous works [12,13] have used GANs to refine the results of a simulator and are structurally similar to our method. However, the "simulator" in Scar-GAN is also a GAN and no manual modeling of scar tissue is required.

GANs have been also used in medical imaging for data augmentation. Synthetic training samples (such as skin lesions [1] and liver lesions [3]) are generated by GANs to increase dataset size. Salehinejad et al. [10] use DCGAN to synthesize X-ray chest scans with under-represented diseases and to classify lung diseases. The motivation of the work from Salehinejad et al. is most similar to ours but instead of generating images from scratch, ScarGAN simulates diseases on scans of healthy patients.

3   ScarGAN

Mask Generator. In the first stage, ScarGAN uses a mask generator to simulate the shape of the scar tissue in the myocardium on an LGE SAX image. The input of the mask generator is a segmentation mask which includes right ventricular endocardium blood pool (RV endo), LV myocardium (LV myo) and

LV endocardium blood pool (LV endo). The output of the mask generator is also a segmentation mask which includes simulated scar tissue, RV endo, LV myo and LV endo. Both the input and output include RV endo, LV myo and LV endo to encourage the generator to learn anatomical structures before the discriminator gets too strong which destabilizes training.

The mask generator is a fully convolutional U-Net with 64 initial convolutional filters and it downsamples with strided convolutions. We add noise to the generator by using dropout layers (p = 0.25) after each nonlinearity layer.

The input of the mask discriminator is a segmentation mask of RV endo, LV myo and LV endo with real scar tissue or a mask with simulated scar tissue. The discriminator is a relatively shallow network consisting of 4 layer blocks, each contains a convolutional layer, a batch normalization layer, and a leaky ReLU nonlinearity layer ($\alpha = 0.2$). Unlike pix2pix, we do not follow PatchGAN in which the discriminator classifies patches of the images, and instead classify the whole image as real or simulated.

Following LSGAN [7], we use squared error as the main loss function and add multi-class cross-entropy between the input and output segmentation masks for regularization. We train the mask discriminator for 2 gradient steps for every gradient step performed on the mask generator.

To prevent mode collapse, half of the simulated masks are stored in a buffer for "experience replay" [8] and half of the training batches are randomly drawn from this buffer. The previously simulated samples stabilize training for both the discriminator and generator and prevent the generator from exploiting the discriminator by generating scar tissue of one specific shape which the discriminator has "forgotten."

Heuristic-based Simulation. In the second stage, we apply the shape of the simulated scar tissue from the mask to the image using a heuristic-based method, leveraging the domain-specific knowledge that scar tissue is hyperintense and has a similar signal intensity to the LV blood pool. We replace the corresponding pixels within generated scar tissue with the 10th percentile intensity of the LV endo pixels. However this causes the intensities within the scar tissue to become uniform, which is not characteristic of real scar tissue.

Although this approach does not produce photorealistic simulation of the scar tissue, it provides a good starting point for another GAN to refine the initial simulation.

Refining Generator. In the final stage, ScarGAN uses a refining network to add details to the initial simulation from the heuristic-based method above. This stage is inspired by SimGAN [12] but the refining generator in ScarGAN refines results from another GAN instead of a simulator. The input to the refining generator is an image with heuristic-based simulated scars and its output is a refined image with simulated scars. The network architectures of the refining generator and refining discriminator are the same as those described in the mask generator section. We do not need to increase the capacity of the generator given that the initial simulation provides a good starting point.

Similar to the mask generator, we follow LSGAN [7] and use squared error as the main loss function. We add absolute error between the input and the refined image for regularization so that the generator is encouraged to modify small regions of the image. We train the discriminator for 3 gradient steps for every 1 gradient weight update to the refining generator.

4   Results and Evaluation

Dataset. Our dataset consists of 159 LGE CMR SAX scans of which only 33.6% of the SAX images have some visible scar tissue. The LGE scans are acquired by multiple types of scanners across multiple regions and countries.

Ground truth RV endo, LV myo, and LV endo segmentation masks are collected from 3 physicians with extensive experience analyzing CMR scans. Ground truth scar tissue masks are collected using the Full-Width-at-Half-Maximum (FWHM) method in accordance to the Society of Cardiovascular Magnetic Resonance imaging (SCMR) guidelines [11].

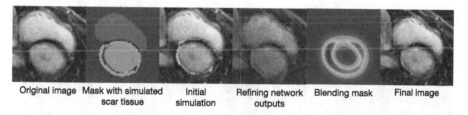

Original image   Mask with simulated   Initial   Refining network   Blending mask   Final image
scar tissue   simulation   outputs

Fig. 3. ScarGAN simulation pipeline. From left to right: original image with no scar tissue; mask with RV endo (light blue), LV myo (green), and LV endo (orange) and simulated scar tissue (red); heuristic-based simulation; output from refining network; blending mask; final image with simulated scar tissue (Color figure online)

Generating Diverse Simulated Scar Tissue. We augment the LGE dataset by simulating scar tissue on healthy myocardium to train a segmentation network to segment RV endo, LV myo and LV endo. The full augmentation pipeline is visualized in Fig. 3. Although it is possible to train a network to directly segment scar tissue, analyzing LGE scans using scar tissue segmentation is not part of the guideline recommendations [11].

Despite using an experience replay buffer, we still sometimes observe mode collapse in the mask generator. To obtain diverse scar tissue, we try to condition the input by a noise vector or inject noise using dropout at inference time. However neither of these methods yield significantly different shapes. We note that this phenomenon is consistent with the findings in pix2pix [5].

Instead, we snapshot the weights of mask generator for every 10,000 training steps. We pick 5 of these snapshots by visually inspecting the shape of some of the simulated scar tissue. These weight snapshots are selected if simulated scar tissue is of relatively diverse shapes within the training set and across the snapshots.

As a final post-processing step, we create a blending mask to combine the refined image and the original image to remove any artifacts outside the myocardium. We initialize the blending mask as the myocardium mask and then apply Gaussian blur with a kernel size of 5px because the boundary between LV blood pool and LV myocardium is not clear-cut. The final image is created by computing a per-pixel weighted average between the refined image and the original image.

Quantitative Evaluation of Simulated Scar Tissue. We ask 3 physicians, including 2 radiologists with more than 10 years of experience, to classify whether the scar tissue on 30 LGE SAX images is simulated or not. 50% have real scar tissue and 50% of the images have scar tissue simulated by ScarGAN. These images are shown in random order and are randomly drawn from a hold-out set. We do not impose any time limit for the annotator to classify the images. The classification accuracy of the physicians is 60%, 47% and 50%. The results demonstrate that experienced physicians are unable to identify simulated scar tissue better than chance and that scar tissue simulated by ScarGAN is highly realistic (Fig. 1).

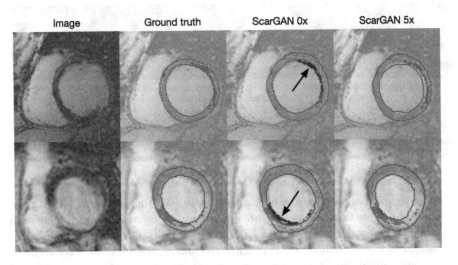

Fig. 4. Comparison of predicted and ground truth contours on the LGE SAX images from 2 unique patients. Light red mask is scar tissue correctly included in myocardium; dark red mask is scar tissue erroneously included in blood pool (also indicated by black arrows). The green and blue lines show the predicted LV epi and LV endo contours, respectively. (Color figure online)

Segmenting LGE Scans. We evaluate the effectiveness of ScarGAN as a data augmentation technique by training a segmentation network that predicts LV endo and LV myo masks on LGE scans. The segmentation network is U-Net-based DeepVentricle [6] and is fine-tuned on the 159 LGE CMR scans dataset described above. We apply traditional data augmentation to all models such as translation, scale, rotation and elastic deformation.

We note that scar tissue is not visible in standard SSFP scans as no contrast agents have been administered, so the network must learn all knowledge about scar tissue from the LGE dataset. We find that the fine-tuned U-Net is unable to discriminate between blood pool and scar tissue, which have similar intensities. To address this failure mode, we modify the loss function to put stronger emphasis on scar tissue such that a higher weighting is assigned to the corresponding pixels within scar tissue. We note that this weighting is an important hyperparameter – if it is too high, the network will overestimate the percentage of scar tissue pixels by erroneously including blood pool as part of the myocardium; if it is too low, the percentage of scar tissue pixels will be underestimated by erroneously excluding scar tissue from the myocardium.

We evaluate the model on the percentage of scar tissue pixels erroneously included in LV endo and the percentage of scar tissue pixels correctly included in LV myo in each scan. We perform 4-fold cross-validation on the segmentation network and ScarGAN networks. The dataset is split using anonymized patient IDs such that all scans of one patient are assigned to a single fold. We keep the validation set intact and no scans with simulated scar tissue are added to the validation set.

Table 1. Evaluation metrics of model trained on LGE scans with and without simulated scars

Dataset subset	Training data (number of scans with real scars / no scars / simulated scars)	% of scar in LV myo	% of scar in LV endo
ScarGAN 0x	69 / 0 / 0	75.9	10.7
ScarGAN 0x+	69 / 90/ 0	71.8	14.1
ScarGAN 1x	69 / 0 / 90	79.7	7.6
ScarGAN 3x	69 / 0 / 270	79.2	8.4
ScarGAN 5x	69 / 0 / 450	**80.5**	**7.5**

As shown in Table 1, we train the segmentation models on different subsets of the dataset: (1) ScarGAN 0x: only scans with scar tissue, (2) ScarGAN 0x+: all scans with and without scar tissue, (3) ScarGAN kx: scans with real and simulated scar tissue where k is the number of mask generator weight snapshots we used to simulate scar tissue. We notice that adding scans without scar tissue is detrimental to the network's ability to distinguish scar tissue. In contrast, adding simulated scar tissue reduces the average percentage of scar tissue pixels erroneously included in LV endo from 10.66% to 7.55%, and increases the average percentage of scar tissue pixels correctly included in LV myo from 75.9% to 80.5%. The mean LV endo and LV epi contour dice coefficients are 0.869 and 0.906. Figure 4 shows predicted and ground truth LV endo and LV epi contours in the test set. This indicates that it is possible to improve model performance on patients with pathologies by collecting scans without any pathologies and use ScarGAN to simulated those pathologies.

5   Conclusion and Future Work

We propose ScarGAN, an approach using chained GANs to simulate scar tissue on healthy myocardium and to reduce the need to collect scans from patients with diseases. The use of chained GANs reduces training difficulty and allows domain-specific knowledge to be applied. We find that simulated scar tissues cannot be distinguished by physicians and can improve segmentation performance.

In the future, we can evaluate ScarGAN with other pathologies and on classification tasks. We can also train both the mask generator and refining generator end-to-end.

References

1. Baur, C., Albarqouni, S., Navab, N.: MelanoGANs: high resolution skin lesion synthesis with GANs. arXiv preprint arXiv:1804.04338 (2018)
2. Esteva, A., Kuprel, B., Novoa, R.A., Ko, J., Swetter, S.M., Blau, H.M., Thrun, S.: Dermatologist-level classification of skin cancer with deep neural networks. Nature **542**(7639), 115 (2017)
3. Frid-Adar, M., Diamant, I., Klang, E., Amitai, M., Goldberger, J., Greenspan, H.: GAN-based synthetic medical image augmentation for increased CNN performance in liver lesion classification. arXiv preprint arXiv:1803.01229 (2018)
4. Goodfellow, I.J., et al.: Generative adversarial nets. In: Advances in Neural Information Processing Systems, pp. 2672–2680) (2014)
5. Isola, P., Zhu, J.Y., Zhou, T., Efros, A.A.: Image-to-Image translation with conditional adversarial networks. arXiv preprint arXiv:1611.07004 (2016)
6. Lieman-Sifry, J., Le, M., Lau, F., Sall, S., Golden, D.: FastVentricle: cardiac segmentation with ENet. In: International Conference on Functional Imaging and Modeling of the Heart, pp. 127–138. Springer, Cham, June 2017
7. Mao, X., Li, Q., Xie, H., Lau, R.Y., Wang, Z., Smolley, S.P.: Least squares generative adversarial networks. In: 2017 IEEE International Conference on Computer Vision (ICCV), pp. 2813–2821. IEEE, October 2017
8. Pfau, D., Vinyals, O.: Connecting generative adversarial networks and Actor-Critic methods. arXiv preprint arXiv:1610.01945 (2016)
9. Ronneberger, O., Fischer, P., Brox, T.: U-Net: Convolutional Networks for Biomedical Image Segmentation. In: Navab, N., Hornegger, J., Wells, W.M., Frangi, A.F. (eds.) MICCAI 2015. LNCS, vol. 9351, pp. 234–241. Springer, Cham (2015). https://doi.org/10.1007/978-3-319-24574-4_28
10. Salehinejad, H., Valaee, S., Dowdell, T., Colak, E., Barfett, J.: Generalization of deep neural networks for chest pathology classification in X-Rays using generative adversarial networks. arXiv preprint arXiv:1712.01636 (2017)
11. Schulz-Menger, J., Bluemke, D.A., Bremerich, J., Flamm, S.D., Fogel, M.A., Friedrich, M.G., Kim, R.J., von Knobelsdorff-Brenkenhoff, F., Kramer, C.M., Pennell, D.J., Plein, S., Nagel, E.: Standardized image interpretation and post processing in cardiovascular magnetic resonance: society for cardiovascular magnetic resonance (SCMR) board of trustees task force on standardized post processing. J. Cardiovasc. Magn. Reson. **15**(1), 35 (2013)
12. Shrivastava, A., Pfister, T., Tuzel, O., Susskind, J., Wang, W., Webb, R.: Learning from simulated and unsupervised images through adversarial training. In: CVPR, vol. 2, no. 4, p. 5. July 2017
13. Sixt, L., Wild, B., Landgraf, T.: RenderGAN: Generating realistic labeled data. Front. Robot. AI **5**, 66 (2016)

8th International Workshop on Multimodal Learning for Clinical Decision Support, ML-CDS 2018

A Multi-scale Multiple Sclerosis Lesion Change Detection in a Multi-sequence MRI

Myra Cheng[1], Alfiia Galimzianova[1(✉)], Žiga Lesjak[2], Žiga Špiclin[2], Christopher B. Lock[1], and Daniel L. Rubin[1]

[1] Stanford University, Stanford, CA 94305, USA
alfiia@stanford.edu
[2] University of Ljubljana, 1000 Ljubljana, Slovenia

Abstract. Multiple sclerosis (MS) is a disease characterized by demyelinating lesions in the brain and spinal cord. Quantification of the amount of change in MS lesions in magnetic resonance imaging (MRI) over time is important for evaluation of drug effectiveness in clinical trials. Manual analysis of such longitudinal datasets is time- and cost prohibitive, and also prone to intra- and inter-rater variability. Accurate automated change detection methods would be highly desirable. We propose a new MS lesion change detection method that integrates a voxel's multi-sequence MR intensity with its immediate neighborhood context and the texture of the extended neighborhood in a machine learning framework. On our dataset of 15 patients, the proposed method had higher performance (median AUC-ROC $= 0.97$, AUC-PR $= 0.43$, Wilcoxon's signed rank test, $p < 0.001$) than implemented baseline methods. As such, the proposed method has potential clinical applications as an efficient, low-cost algorithm to capture and quantify local lesion change and growth.

Keywords: Multiple sclerosis · Change detection
Multi-scale image descriptors

1 Introduction

Multiple sclerosis (MS) is a disease of the central nervous system (CNS) that affects over 400,000 people in the U.S. and 2.5 million people worldwide. It is one of the leading causes of non-traumatic disability among young and middle-aged adults [1]. Currently, MS has no cure, although there is an ongoing research in search for improved treatment and management of the disease. The success of such research depends on clinical trials, in which the response to treatment and change in disease status must be quantified in an accurate and consistent manner.

Multi-sequence magnetic resonance imaging (MRI) is the standard imaging exam performed to analyze the white-matter lesions for diagnosis and follow-up evaluation of MS. Quantitative evaluation of the changes in the MS lesions

© Springer Nature Switzerland AG 2018
D. Stoyanov et al. (Eds.): DLMIA 2018/ML-CDS 2018, LNCS 11045, pp. 353–360, 2018.
https://doi.org/10.1007/978-3-030-00889-5_40

appearance requires annotation of the corresponding areas in the brain, which when done manually is time-consuming and subjective. To address these challenges, reliable automated methods are needed.

The strategies for automated change detection can be categorized as longitudinal volumetric analysis, deformable image registration, and longitudinal analysis of MR intensity [5]. Longitudinal volumetric analysis relies on segmentation of MS lesions at each imaging timepoint independently and can only provide global measures of the lesion change, such as the count of new lesions and the total lesion volume difference. Deformable image registration relies on deformation fields obtained during non-rigid alignment of the MR images at two timepoints and can quantify local changes through analysis of enlarging and shrinking lesions, while detection of new or disappearing lesions is limited. The longitudinal analysis can address the issues of the previous two strategies through rigid of affine registration being followed by intensity analysis at matching anatomical sites, thus allowing for local quantification of all types of lesion change [4]. The computational core of such analysis is detection of lesion change for each voxel of the brain MR image set from two imaging timepoints. Although single-timepoint MS lesion segmentation approaches have incorporated multiple scales of spatial information for context [6], longitudinal MS lesion analysis has been limited to change detection using voxel intensities independently [4]. Texture descriptors specifically can aid in a compact representation of a local context of the multi-sequence MR images and, moreover, have been successfully applied to MS lesion segmentation [11].

In this work, we propose a change detection method that incorporates the local context of the multi-sequence MR images at three scales. The multi-scale descriptors are extracted from the intensity information of the voxels immediate neighborhood, and the intensity and texture information of a larger surrounding image patch. Our experiments demonstrated that incorporating the contextual information to change detection improved the performance at each scale and the proposed method statistically significantly outperformed the baseline state-of-the-art approach [8].

2   Materials and Methods

2.1   Dataset

We used anonymized imaging data from 15 MS patients with two imaging exams, each with three MRI sequences: T1-weighted (T1), T2-weighted (T2), and fluid-attenuated inversion recovery (FLAIR), acquired at 1.5T. Pre-processing included resampling to the common spatial resolution of $1 \times 1 \times 3 \, mm^3$, inhomogeneity correction on all sequences using N4 bias correction [10], registration of all sequences at both timepoints to a common space [2], and intracranial volume extraction from the T1 sequences using BET 2 [7]. The reference lesion change labels were acquired as a consensus segmentation of the corresponding regions by two neuroradiologists.

2.2   MS Lesion Change Detection

For each patient, we consider six three-dimensional volumes: T1, T2, and FLAIR at two time points. We denote intensity of a voxel v from the intracranial volume mask for patient i, from the imaging study conducted at time t_j $(j = 1, 2)$ by $M_{iv}^{t_j}$, where $M \in \{T1, T2, FLAIR\}$. For common interpretations of voxel intensities, each volume was normalized by computing the z-scores of the intracranial volume intensities:

$$\widetilde{M}_{iv}^{t_j} = \frac{M_{iv}^{t_j} - \mu_{i,M}^{t_j}}{\sigma_{i,M}^{t_j}}$$

where the mean $\mu_{i,M}^{t_j}$ and standard deviation $\sigma_{i,M}^{t_j}$ are computed as sample statistics across the voxels in the intracranial volume mask for patient i at time t_j. For each patient, dissimilarity maps were extracted by voxel-wise subtraction of the normalized image between two time points for each imaging sequence M as $\Delta M_{iv} = \widetilde{M}_{iv}^{t_2} - \widetilde{M}_{iv}^{t_1}$.

Lesion Change Model and Voxel-Level Descriptors. We model the presence of change in a set of preregistered multi-sequence MR images as a function of descriptors extracted from $\widetilde{M}_{iv}^{t_1}$ and ΔM_{iv} for each imaging sequence M. With the voxel-level lesion change represented by a random variable R, the probabilities for each test patient i at voxel v are modeled as a logistic regression:

$$logit[P\{R_{iv} = 1\}] = \alpha_0 + \Sigma_{x=1}^6 \alpha_x I_{iv}^x \tag{1}$$

where $I^x \in \{\widetilde{FLAIR}^{t_1}, \Delta FLAIR, \widetilde{T1}^{t_1}, \Delta T1, \widetilde{T2}^{t_1}, \Delta T2\}$ constitute the six input image volumes for patient i.

Incorporating Neighborhood Information. The first scale of the context we incorporate into the model in Eq. (1) is the immediate neighborhood of a voxel in the form of $\Delta FLAIR$ values over a $K \times K$ neighborhood of each considered voxel. With x representing the indices of the neighborhood voxels, and these values were used as additional descriptors to learn additional coefficients β:

$$logit[P\{R_{iv} = 1\}] = \alpha_0 + \Sigma_{x=1}^6 \alpha_x I_{iv}^x + \Sigma_{x=1}^8 \beta_x \Delta FLAIR_{iv}^x \tag{2}$$

Incorporating Local Texture Descriptors. To incorporate a wider context, we extracted texture descriptors from a larger $L \times L$ neighborhood of a voxel on a $\Delta FLAIR$ sequence. From voxel intensities within the brain mask, descriptors representing intensity statistics, such as mean, standard deviation, and kurtosis, were generated. Texture-based descriptors were extracted from the gray-level co-occurrence matrix (GLCM) of each patch using Haralick descriptors [3] and the gray-length run-length matrix (GLRLM) descriptors [9]. This resulted in 31-dimensional vectors, which were normalized to their z-scores to obtain T_{iv}^x, $x = 1, \ldots, 31$ for each selected voxel v. The logit model using these 31 descriptors is denoted as:

$$logit[P\{R_{iv} = 1\}] = \gamma_0 + \Sigma_{x=1}^{31} \gamma_x T_{iv}^x \tag{3}$$

Table 1. Median $\pm$ median absolute deviation values for patient-level AUC-ROC and AUC-PR generated across 45 independent three-fold cross-validated trials.

Metric	Baseline 1	Baseline 2	Baseline 3	Proposed
AUC-ROC	0.94 ± 0.04	0.94 ± 0.04	0.93 ± 0.04	0.97 ± 0.01
AUC-PR	0.14 ± 0.19	0.17 ± 0.18	0.29 ± 0.13	0.43 ± 0.16

Multi-scale Method. The joint multi-scale model combines the multi-sequence voxel intensities with the immediate neighborhood and the local texture descriptors. This descriptor was used as input to fit the logistic regression function:

$$logit[P\{R_{iv} = 1\}] = \alpha_0 + \Sigma_{x=1}^{6}\alpha_x I_{iv}^x + \Sigma_{x=1}^{8}\beta_x \Delta FLAIR_{iv}^x + \Sigma_{x=1}^{31}\gamma_x T_{iv}^x \quad (4)$$

The logistic regression model was first learned using the balanced dataset over a selection mask, computed at voxel v for patient i as:

$$S_{iv} = \begin{cases} 1 & \Delta FLAIR_{iv} > \sigma_{\Delta} FLAIR_i \\ 0 & \text{otherwise} \end{cases}.$$

In testing, the learned set of coefficients $\alpha_0, \dots \alpha_6, \beta_1, \dots \beta_8, \gamma_1, \dots \gamma_{31}$ was applied to infer the lesion change probability maps for the whole intracranial volume of a test subject.

3   Experiments and Results

The proposed method (Eq. (4)) was compared to an implementation of the existing state-of-the-art method [8] that considers only the multi-sequence voxel intensities (Eq. (1), referred here as Baseline 1); a method using the intensities as well as the immediate neighborhood context information from a 3×3 neighborhood (Eq. (2), referred to as Baseline 2); and a method using texture-based descriptors (Eq. (3), referred to as Baseline 3).

A three-fold cross-validation scheme was used. To minimize the effect of random variation on training and testing subsets within folds, each three-fold experiment was run three times, resulting in 45 patient-level ROC and PR curves for each method. Table 1 and Fig. 2 depict comparisons of AUC-ROC and AUC-PR for the four methods. The higher performance of the Multi-Scale Method compared to other methods was statistically significant ($p < 0.001$) both in terms of AUC-ROC and AUC-PR.

3.1   Importance of Texture-Based Descriptors

Comparing Baseline 2 and the Multi-Scale Method, texture-based radiomic features clearly contribute to the latters higher performance. Here we investigate the discriminative power of the set of texture descriptors. Figure 3 shows the differences in descriptor values between voxels with lesion change and voxels with

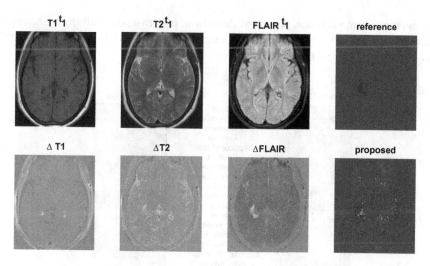

Fig. 1. A sample of the input images, manually annotated reference labels for lesion change, and the lesion change probability map generated by the proposed method.

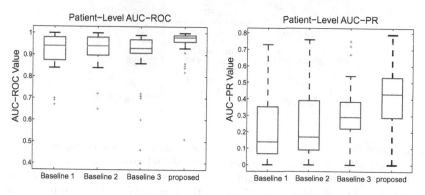

Fig. 2. Distributions of patient-level AUC-ROC (left) and AUC-PR (right) values generated across 45 3-fold cross-validated trials on test patients.

no change. Since the descriptors were normalized for each patients data, the learned coefficients γ_x as in Eq. (4) indicate the significance of the corresponding descriptors in differentiating lesion change detection. Coefficients in Eq. (4) that are consistently large in magnitude suggest that they are especially important to generating the output lesion change probability map.

To study the importance of specific texture-based descriptors, a large set of coefficients were generated using a Monte-Carlo simulation. With repeated random sampling of image data from ten patients, 32 sets of coefficients were generated. A one-sample Wilcoxon signed-rank test was used to evaluate which coefficients consistently differ most from zero (null hypothesis that the median value is zero). The top ten descriptors ($p < 0.01$) were found to be homogeneity, sum average, sum variance, standard deviation, contrast, dissimilarity, difference variance, difference entropy, short run-length emphasis (RE), and long run high gray-level emphasis (GE).

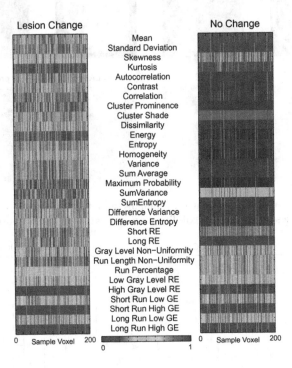

Fig. 3. Normalized descriptor values for sample voxels with lesion change (left) and with no change (right). The voxels were randomly selected from a sample patient, and all voxels are within the intracranial volume mask and voxel selection mask. Note the differences in descriptor values between the two classes, which are indicative of discriminative potential of these radiomic descriptors. In the descriptor index, GE stands for gray-level emphasis and RE stands for run-length emphasis.

4   Discussion

We proposed a multi-scale MS lesion change detection method, which had the highest performance when compared to three baseline methods that employed the multi-sequence MR images at fewer scales. The proposed method differs from others by extracting descriptors from not only the voxel itself, as in Ref. [8], which corresponded to Baseline 1, but also at two additional spatial scales, i.e. at immediate and extended neighborhoods. Since a radiologist annotates image voxels not in isolation but in the context of its surrounding voxels, it is intuitive that multi-scale context information improves lesion change detection.

Comparing Baseline 2 and the Multi-Scale Method, texture descriptors clearly contribute to the latter's higher performance. The Multi-Scale Method and Base-line 3 had higher AUC-PR than Baseline 1 and 2, suggesting that texture-based descriptors improve the algorithms performance in the task of differentiating lesion change areas from non-lesion change areas. The top ten descriptors reported in the Results section (e.g. homogeneity, sum average) were especially critical in distinguishing between areas with and without lesion change, since their learned weights differ most from a median value of zero across multiple experiments. Extracting only these descriptors resulted in comparable performance (median AUC-ROC = 0.97, AUC-PR = 0.40) to using all 31 texture-based descriptors (median AUC-ROC = 0.97, AUC-PR = 0.43), which suggests that they may be sufficient for less computationally expensive use in a clinical setting.

While radiomic descriptors have made progress in tumor detection and segmentation for other diseases, this work is one of the first to use these descriptors in MS lesion change detection and highlights the importance of specific descriptors for this purpose. As expected, despite the significant contributions of texture descriptors, the intensities of the central voxel and its immediate neighborhood nonetheless contributed significantly to the performance. As per our experiments, the proposed Multi-Scale Method outperformed Baseline 3 due to these additional descriptors. This once again emphasizes the importance of a multi-scale approach. As a reference point, we also evaluated the coefficients directly provided by Ref. [8]. It resulted in a median AUC-ROC of 0.82, which was significantly lower than the results from training on our dataset as presented in Table 1, but the result is high enough to confirm the generalizability of such an approach, which can be attributed to the standard image preprocessing routines applied in both studies.

Quantitative longitudinal MS lesion analysis could provide insight into disease progression that occurs subtler and earlier than clinical markers like deterioration of physical movement. In the current clinical practice, lesion analysis is limited to recording lesion count and location. Manual annotation of the MS lesion change is challenging due to the number of sequences (T1, T2 and FLAIR in our study) that need to be taken into account when performing the labeling of each potential new lesion area. Moreover, the task becomes even more time and cost expensive in a setting of a large-scale clinical trials, where, due to the larger number of imaging timepoints of interests, it is crucial to have a consistent annotation in order to reliably evaluate the effectiveness of the tested treatment. Reliable automated methods such as our approach can be used to expedite and assist the radiologists daunting task of labeling lesion change for many patients and provide objective evaluations in a consistent and efficient manner.

To conclude, we proposed a multi-scale MS lesion change detection method, which incorporates not only information at voxel level, but also information from neighborhood and texture-based descriptors from the larger patch surrounding each voxel. The method statistically significantly improved over the state-of-the-art method. We also showed the importance of texture-based descriptors to effective lesion change detection, which to the best of our knowledge has not been explored in previous works.

Acknowledgments. This material is based upon work supported by Philips Healthcare.

References

1. NIH fact sheets - multiple sclerosis. https://report.nih.gov/nihfactsheets/ViewFactSheet.aspx?csid=103
2. Avants, B.B., Tustison, N.J., Stauffer, M., Song, G., Wu, B., Gee, J.C.: The insight ToolKit image registration framework. Front. Neuroinformatics **8**, 44 (2014). https://doi.org/10.3389/fninf.2014.00044
3. Haralick, R.M.: Statistical and structural approaches to texture. Proc. IEEE **67**(5), 786–804 (1979). https://doi.org/10.1109/PROC.1979.11328
4. Lesjak, Ž., Pernuš, F., Likar, B., Špiclin, Ž.: Validation of white-matter lesion change detection methods on a novel publicly available MRI image database. Neuroinformatics **14**(4), 403–420 (2016). https://doi.org/10.1007/s12021-016-9301-1
5. Lladó, X., et al.: Automated detection of multiple sclerosis lesions in serial brain MRI. Neuroradiology **54**(8), 787–807 (2012). https://doi.org/10.1007/s00234-011-0992-6
6. Mechrez, R., Goldberger, J., Greenspan, H.: Patch-based segmentation with spatial consistency: Application to MS lesions in brain MRI. https://doi.org/10.1155/2016/7952541
7. Smith, S.M.: Fast robust automated brain extraction. Hum. Brain Mapp. **17**(3), 143–155 (2002). https://doi.org/10.1002/hbm.10062
8. Sweeney, E.M., Shinohara, R.T., Shea, C.D., Reich, D.S., Crainiceanu, C.M.: Automatic lesion incidence estimation and detection in multiple sclerosis using multisequence longitudinal MRI. Am. J. Neuroradiol. **34**(1), 68–73 (2012). https://doi.org/10.3174/ajnr.A3172
9. Tang, X.: Texture information in run-length matrices. IEEE Trans. Image Process. **7**(11), 1602–1609 (1998). https://doi.org/10.1109/83.725367
10. Tustison, N.J., et al.: N4itk: improved n3 bias correction. IEEE Trans. Med. Imaging **29**(6), 1310–1320 (2010). https://doi.org/10.1109/TMI.2010.2046908
11. Zhang, Y.: MRI texture analysis in multiple sclerosis. https://doi.org/10.1155/2012/762804

Multi-task Sparse Low-Rank Learning
for Multi-classification of Parkinson's Disease

Haijun Lei[1(✉)], Yujia Zhao[1], and Baiying Lei[2]

[1] College of Computer Science and Software Engineering,
Guangdong Province Key Laboratory of Popular High-Performance Computers,
Shenzhen University, Shenzhen, China
leiby@szu.edu.cn

[2] National-Regional Key Technology Engineering Laboratory for Medical
Ultrasound, Guangdong Key Laboratory for Biomedical Measurements
and Ultrasound Imaging, School of Biomedical Engineering,
Health Science Center, Shenzhen University, Shenzhen, China

Abstract. Identifying prodromal stages of Parkinson's disease (PD) draws
increasing recognition as non-motor symptoms may appear before classical
clinical diagnosis based on motor signs. To effectively develop a computer-
aided diagnosis for multiple disease progression stages, neuroimaging has been
widely applied for its convenience of revealing the intricate brain structure.
However, the high dimensional neuroimaging features and limited sample size
bring the main challenges for the diagnosis task. To handle it, a multi-task sparse
low-rank learning framework is proposed to unveil the underlying relationships
between input data and output targets by building a matrix-regularized feature
network. Inductions of multiple tasks are simultaneously performed to capture
intrinsic feature relatedness with multi-task learning. By discarding the irrelevant features and preserving the discriminative structured features, our proposed
method can select the most relevant features and identify different stages of PD
with different multi-classification models. Extensive experimental results on the
Parkinson's progression markers initiative (PPMI) dataset demonstrate that the
proposed method achieves promising classification performance and outperforms the conventional algorithms.

Keywords: Multi-task learning · Low-rank · Sparse learning
Parkinson's disease

1 Introduction

PD has gained increasing attention as the growing aging problem of the population.
The chronic progression nature and imperceptible neuro-diminishment of PD make the
treatment comparatively difficult [1]. There is suggestive evidence that olfaction
changes, sleep behavior disorder, subtle cognitive changes and depression can be
present at early PD stages, suggesting high potential of having PD [2]. Before the
occurrence of motor symptoms permits the clinical diagnosis of PD, about or above
50% of the dopaminergic neurons of the substantia nigra have degenerated. The time
span between the onset of neurodegeneration and manifestation of the typical motor

© Springer Nature Switzerland AG 2018
D. Stoyanov et al. (Eds.): DLMIA 2018/ML-CDS 2018, LNCS 11045, pp. 361–368, 2018.
https://doi.org/10.1007/978-3-030-00889-5_41

symptoms is referred as prodromal phase of PD (PROD) [3]. The term SWEDD (scans without evidence for dopaminergic deficit) refers to the absence of an imaging abnormality in patients clinically presumed to have PD [4]. PROD and SWEDD are different disorders of PD, whose patients require targeted treatment. Therefore, early PD diagnosis offers timely prevention treatment of the patients.

Using the rich information of neuroimaging techniques, we can monitor the minor neuro changes, which are not easy to perceive in normal clinical symptom-based diagnosis. Common neuroimaging techniques include magnetic resonance imaging (MRI), diffusion-weighted tensor imaging (DTI). Recently, many machine learning methods have been applied to utilize the neuroimages in the computer-aided diagnosis of neurodegenerative disease. A robust feature-sample selection scheme was developed for PD diagnosis [5]. Due to the challenges of high dimensionality and limited sample size, the overfitting problem could be occurred in the data analysis. Recent studies have demonstrated that feature selection is capable of overcoming this issue. A l_1-regularizer (i.e., a sparse term) is introduced in the estimation model for feature selection when the sample size is significantly smaller than the feature dimension [6]. However, sparsity regularization is insufficient in multi-classification application since there are four progressive classification targets: normal control (NC), SWEDD, PROD and PD.

In fact, the relationship between input data (i.e., MRI images) and output targets (i.e., prediction results) have more to explore. Inspired by the fact that the brain is organized with modular structures, we intend to find the most representative features to train our multi-class classifiers by extracting the low-rank structure of the matrix-regularized feature network as well as its sparseness.

On the other hand, gray matter (GM), white matter (WM), and cerebrospinal fluid (CSF) are the most significant biomarkers in the brain which are later used as features. The conventional feature extraction methods apply a simple linear combination to use the three matters without considering their own contributing factor. We model this problem as a multi-task learning framework by proposing a model that efficiently leverages the multi-modal data [7]. Our model considers the multi-classification of disease stages using each modal as one task. We assume that these tasks are related and can benefit each other for the classification purpose. Then we perform the three tasks simultaneously to capture their intrinsic relatedness to achieve better classification performance.

Moreover, clinical symptoms have been considered as a vital indicator of PD diagnosis. The judgement results of clinicians are reflected on the clinical assessment scores for each potential PD patient. The combination of constructive information with the neuroimaging information provides sufficient information for computer-aided analytical diagnosis. For this reason, we propose a multi-task sparse low-rank learning (MSLRL) framework for multi-classification of PD. The proposed MSLRL framework combines the sparsity and low-rank constraints together for each task to select the most PD related features. To the best of our knowledge, this is the first work to introduce multi-task sparse low-rank learning to PD diagnosis using neuroimages. Experimental results demonstrate the prominent performance of our proposed method on the PPMI dataset.

2 Method

The proposed method intends to find a subset of features that are most related to PD. The multi-task sparse low-rank learning framework is shown in Fig. 1. We extract our feature input data from MRI images. In order to predict the accurate labels, we add a low-rank and sparse constraint to the matrix-regularized feature network and extract the respective weighted significance by clustering for each task. Each task applies the same feature selection method in a jointly multi-task framework. The shared weight matrix leads to the selected features with reduced dimensions to train a support vector machine (SVM) based classifiers.

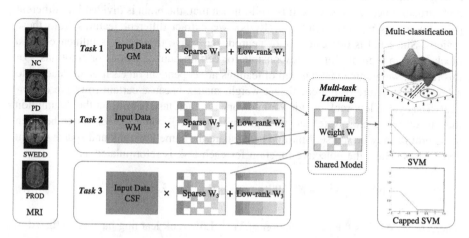

Fig. 1. Flowchart of our proposed MSLRL method. The shared model is learned from the multi-task learning by considering each tissue modal as task.

Supposing that we have m subjects and each has n features belong to k tasks. In the linear regression model $\mathbf{Y}^{(i)} = \mathbf{X}^{(i)}\mathbf{W}^{(i)}$, $\mathbf{Y}^{(i)} \in \mathbb{R}^{m \times 1}$ is the ground truth label vector of i-th task, $\mathbf{X}^{(i)} \in \mathbb{R}^{m \times n}$ is the input data matrix of i-th task, and $\mathbf{W}^{(i)} \in \mathbb{R}^{n \times 1}$ is the weight coefficient matrix for each feature of i-th task. We can get $\mathbf{W}^{(i)}$ by solving the following objective function:

$$\min_{\mathbf{W}^{(i)}} \left\| \mathbf{Y}^{(i)} - \mathbf{X}^{(i)}\mathbf{W}^{(i)} \right\|_F^2, \tag{1}$$

where $\|\mathbf{A}\|_F$ is the Frobenius norm (F-norm) of $\mathbf{A}$ which is defined as $\|\mathbf{A}\|_F = \sqrt{\sum_i \|\mathbf{A}_i\|_2^2}$, where $\mathbf{A}_i$ is the row vector. F-norm also known as the l_2-norm or the l_2-regularizer. Equation (1) is a simple and straightforward linear regression model without constraint on any variable. However, it does not consider the properties of weight matrix, which result in inferior performance. In most machine learning applications, over-fitting is a common problem when the data matrix is unbalanced. Especially in the field of neuroimaging-aided diagnosis, the brain images are rare, and yet they provide extensive information, leading to high dimensionality. A sparse term like l_1-regularizer is generally adopted to regulate the weight matrix by setting certain entries to zero for sparseness. Let $\|\mathbf{A}\|_1$ be the l_1-norm of $\mathbf{A}$ and is defined as $\|\mathbf{A}\|_1 = \sum_{i=1}^{N} |\mathbf{A}_i|$, we can formulate the objective function using sparse representation as:

$$\min_{\mathbf{W}^{(i)}} \left\| \mathbf{Y}^{(i)} - \mathbf{X}^{(i)} \mathbf{W}^{(i)} \right\|_F^2 + \lambda \left\| \mathbf{W}^{(i)} \right\|_1, \tag{2}$$

Equation (2) selects the most representative features under the assumption of sparsity of $\mathbf{W}^{(i)}$ and constraint of the first data-fitting term. In the model, we aim to find a weight matrix that represents the feature significance. We further explore the low-rank structure between features. It is well-known that, the brain is divided into different parts known as regions of interest (ROIs), we extract different features from these regions. Since PD is one category of neurodegenerative disease, it is influenced by a block of brain regions that are responsible for certain human actions or emotions. For this reason, we assume that a group of features are dependent on each other, leading to a low-rank structure of the coefficient weight matrix because certain rows are dependent. The sparse low-rank learning framework for each task is built on the assumption that, features are closely related with group of features while the relevance between these groups may be sparse. Multiple tasks share the same low-rank and sparse weight coefficients. Thus, the objective function for each task is reformulated as:

$$\min_{\mathbf{W}^{(i)}} \left\| \mathbf{Y}^{(i)} - \mathbf{X}^{(i)} \mathbf{W}^{(i)} \right\|_F^2 + \lambda_1 \left\| \mathbf{W}^{(i)} \right\|_1 + \lambda_2 rank\left(\mathbf{W}^{(i)} \right), \tag{3}$$

where $rank(\mathbf{W}^{(i)})$ is the rank function of $\mathbf{W}^{(i)}$. Low-rank learning has been utilized in matrix recovery and network modeling. The weight matrix $\mathbf{W}^{(i)}$ in Eq. (3) has dimension of n rows representing the respective feature significance. The rank minimization of $\mathbf{W}^{(i)}$ explores the low-rank structure among features to obtain the intrinsic relationship. However, it is difficult to solve $\mathbf{W}^{(i)}$ since the *rank* function is non-convex and the rank minimization is a NP-hard problem. Recently, researchers have proved that trace norm function is the convex envelop of the *rank* function over the domain $\|\mathbf{W}^{(i)}\|_2 \leq 1$, which provides the lowest bounds of the rank function *rank* [11]. The trace norm $\|\mathbf{W}\|_*$ is defined as:

$$\|\mathbf{W}\|_* = \sum_{i=1}^{\min\{n,k\}} \sigma_i = Tr\left((\mathbf{W}^T \mathbf{W})^{\frac{1}{2}} \right), \tag{4}$$

where σ_i is the i-th singular value of $\mathbf{W}$ and can be obtained by singular value decomposition (SVD). Thus, we can establish the final objective function with a l_1-norm $\|\mathbf{W}\|_1$ and a trace norm $\|\mathbf{W}\|_*$ as:

$$\min_{\mathbf{W}} \sum_{i=1}^{k} \left\| \mathbf{Y}^{(i)} - \mathbf{W}^{(i)} \mathbf{X}^{(i)} \right\|_F^2 + \alpha \|\mathbf{W}\|_1 + \beta \|\mathbf{W}\|_*, \tag{5}$$

where α and β are the parameters controlling the sparse degree and the low-rank degree, respectively. When $\alpha = 0$, Eq. (5) has only the low-rank constraint. When we add a l_2-norm $\|\mathbf{W}\|_2$ to Eq. (2), we can get the standard elastic net formulation. Moreover, if we change the l_1-norm $\|\mathbf{W}\|_1$ in Eq. (2) to $l_{2,1}$-norm $\|\mathbf{W}\|_{2,1}$, we can get the classic least absolute shrinkage and selection (LASSO).

For optimization for Eq. (5), we notice that, the l_1-norm and trace norm are non-differentiable. Thus, we solve $\mathbf{W}$ using the proximal gradient descent method due to its effectiveness in solving l_1-norm involved equations. Since we have three terms in Eq. (5), we update $\mathbf{W}$ by the value of each term. First, we find the proximal operator of $\alpha\|\mathbf{W}\|_1$ according to:

$$prox_{\alpha\|\cdot\|_1}(\mathbf{W}) = \left[sign(w_{ij}) \cdot \max\{|w_{ij}| - \alpha, 0\}\right]_{n \times k}, \qquad (6)$$

where $prox()$ denotes the proximal operator and $sign()$ is the sign function. Similarly, we can obtain the proximal operator of $\beta\|\mathbf{W}\|_*$ using:

$$prox_{\beta\|\cdot\|_*}(\mathbf{W}) = \mathrm{U}diag(\max\{\widehat{\sigma}_1, 0\}, \cdots, \max\{\widehat{\sigma}_l, 0\})\mathrm{V}^\mathrm{T}, \qquad (7)$$

where U is the unitary matrix in the SVD of $\mathbf{W}$ so that $\mathbf{W} = \mathrm{U}diag(\sigma_1, \cdots, \sigma_l)\mathrm{V}^\mathrm{T}$ with $\widehat{\sigma}_i = \sigma_i - \beta$ and $l = \min\{n, k\}$. Then, we consider the first data-fitting term $\left\|\mathbf{Y}^{(i)} - \mathbf{W}^{(i)}\mathbf{X}^{(i)}\right\|_F^2$. Given $f_1\left(\mathbf{W}^{(i)}\right) = \left\|\mathbf{Y}^{(i)} - \mathbf{W}^{(i)}\mathbf{X}^{(i)}\right\|_F^2$, we can get the derivative of $\mathbf{W}^{(i)}$ as $\nabla f\left(\mathbf{W}^{(i)}\right) = \mathbf{X}^{(i)\mathrm{T}}\mathbf{X}^{(i)}\mathbf{W}^{(i)} - \mathbf{X}^{(i)\mathrm{T}}\mathbf{Y}^{(i)}$. Consequently, we can solve $\mathbf{W}$ by iteratively updating the values until convergence.

3 Experiments

3.1 Experimental Settings

We validate our method by classifying different stages of PD subjects. We choose SVM classifiers to construct a multi-class classification model for its efficiency in separating different class samples with the maximum margin [8]. Another classifier we apply is the capped l_p-norm SVM [9]. This upgraded classifier can deal with both light and heavy outliers, boosting classification performance. The main parameters used are α and β in Eq. (5), where α controls the sparse term $\|\mathbf{W}\|_1$ and β controls the low-rank term $\|\mathbf{W}\|_*$, respectively. The initial values are set as $\alpha \in \{2^{-5}, \ldots, 2^5\}$, $\beta \in \{2^{-5}, \ldots, 2^5\}$. The fine-tuned parameter values are specified by a 5-fold cross-validation strategy. The results are evaluated using: accuracy (ACC), sensitivity (SEN), specificity (SPEC), and area under the receiver operating characteristic curve (AUC). For fair evaluation, the classification performance of the proposed method is evaluated via a 10-fold cross-validation strategy.

3.2   Data Preprocessing

The data used in this experiment are MRI images from the PPMI dataset. All the original images are preprocessed by the anterior commissure-posterior commissure correction and skull-stripping for later operation. Then we segment the images into GM, WM, and CSF using Statistical Parametric Mapping (SPM) [10]. Following the automated anatomical labeling atlas which parcel brain into 116 regions, we compute the mean tissue density value of each region as features. In this work, we collect 643 subjects (127 NC, 380 PD, 56 SWEDD and 34 PROD). For each subject, the feature dimension is 116 for each tissue modal (116 GM, 116 WM, 116 CSF). Apart from these features, we also collect four clinical scores, namely, sleep scores, olfaction scores, depression scores, and Montreal cognitive assessment scores as features. Theses clinical scores are the clinical assessment results from the clinicians' experience and diagnosis. With the guidance of these clinical scores as features, we can build a more reliable classification model.

3.3   Classification Performance

To further validate the effectiveness of our MSLRL method, we compare the method with other similar methods. Apart from the elastic net and LASSO methods, we further compare MSLRL with another two sparsity-based methods. One is multi-modal multi-task (M3T) [11] and the other is joint sparse learning [12]. Furthermore, we additionally compare MSLRL with low-rank learning and sparse learning and sparse low-rank learning (SLRL). The classification performance results are summarized in Table 1. It is clear that, the MSLRL method achieves higher accuracy than classical

Table 1. Classification performance of all competing methods with different classifiers.

Method	Classifier	ACC	SEN	SPEC	AUC
Elastic net	SVM	67.84	73.17	84.11	86.23
	Capped SVM	68.66	74.31	84.66	86.93
LASSO	SVM	65.27	73.45	85.23	84.65
	Capped SVM	65.68	74.92	86.30	85.17
M3T	SVM	74.55	80.05	94.05	88.23
	Capped SVM	75.81	81.55	97.45	89.45
Joint sparse learning	SVM	72.10	75.24	85.38	87.54
	Capped SVM	73.46	78.20	87.79	89.07
Low-rank learning	SVM	72.32	73.01	88.68	88.78
	Capped SVM	73.06	78.52	90.03	89.92
Sparse learning	SVM	70.63	77.19	87.07	87.45
	Capped SVM	71.88	77.85	87.93	88.97
SLRL	SVM	75.23	84.21	93.86	90.24
	Capped SVM	77.87	85.98	95.47	92.77
MSLRL	SVM	78.76	84.62	98.32	92.21
	Capped SVM	**79.49**	**87.24**	**99.21**	**94.31**

Elastic net and LASSO as well as sparse-based M3T and joint sparse learning using both SVM classifiers. SLRL turns out to be more effective than low-rank learning and sparse learning, which validates the strategy of combining l_1-norm $\|\mathbf{W}\|_1$ and trace norm $\|\mathbf{W}\|_*$ using sparsity and low-rank structure. MSLRL outperforming SLRL in both classifiers, which proves that multi-task learning successfully explores the intrinsic relation within multi-modal features. Receiver operating characteristic curves (ROC) for algorithm comparison are shown in Fig. 2. MSLRL obtains the best performance in all competing methods in each classifier, which shows the advantage and potential for early PD diagnosis.

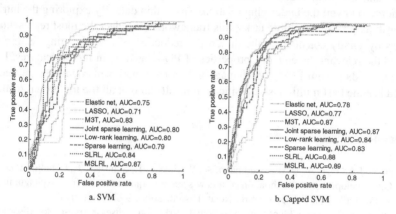

a. SVM   b. Capped SVM

Fig. 2. ROC plots of the competing methods using two classifiers (SVM and Capped SVM).

3.4 Most Distinctive Brain Regions

The identification of PD-related features and the monitoring of progression are of great significance in early diagnosis. We utilize the weight coefficient matrix generated in feature selection to study the discriminative brain regions most related to PD. The regions most related with PD are visualized in Fig. 3. The selected brain regions are

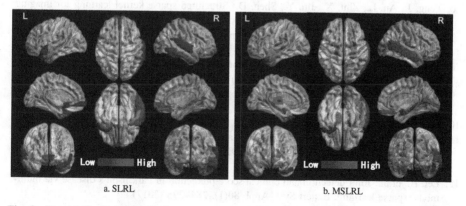

a. SLRL   b. MSLRL

Fig. 3. Top 10 discriminative brain regions obtained from SLRL and MSLRL. Brain regions are color-coded. High means high relevance with PD. Low means relatively low relevance with PD. (Color figure online)

slightly different in two methods. The higher relevance of MSLRL than SLRL reveals that MSLRL is more effective than SLRI for PD diagnosis. These distinctive brain regions can be further investigated for clinical practice.

4   Conclusion

In this paper, we introduce a multi-task sparse low-rank learning framework for early PD diagnosis between four progression stages. Specifically, for each task we add the sparsity and low-rank regularization to the weight coefficients with a l_1-norm and a trace norm to unveil the underlying relationships within data. By exploring the intrinsic relationships between multiple tasks, this framework can select the most representative features by jointly considering the dimension reduction of neuroimaging feature vectors and the relevant dependency properties of PD-related brain region features. Using multi-modal data from PPMI neuroimaging dataset, experiments demonstrate that our method has the best multi-class classification results among all the traditional methods.

References

1. Simons, J.A., Fietzek, U.M., Waldmann, A., Warnecke, T., Schuster, T., Ceballos-Baumann, A.O.: Development and validation of a new screening questionnaire for dysphagia in early stages of Parkinson's disease. Park. Relat. Disord. **20**(9), 992–998 (2014)
2. Postuma, R.B., et al.: Identifying prodromal Parkinson's disease: pre-motor disorders in Parkinson's disease. Mov. Disord. Off. J. Mov. Disord. Soc. **27**(5), 617–626 (2012)
3. Gaenslen, A., Swid, I., Liepelt-Scarfone, I., Godau, J., Berg, D.: The patients' perception of prodromal symptoms before the initial diagnosis of Parkinson's disease. Mov. Disord. Off. J. Mov. Disord. Soc. **26**(4), 653–658 (2011)
4. Erro, R., Schneider, S.A., Quinn, N.P., Bhatia, K.P.: What do patients with scans without evidence of dopaminergic deficit (SWEDD) have? New evidence and continuing controversies. J. Neurol. Neurosurg. Psychiatry (2015)
5. Adeli, E., et al.: Joint feature-sample selection and robust diagnosis of Parkinson's disease from MRI data. NeuroImage **141**, 206–219 (2016)
6. Peng, J., An, L., Zhu, X., Jin, Y., Shen, D.: Structured sparse kernel learning for imaging genetics based alzheimer's disease diagnosis. In: MICCAI, pp. 70–78 (2016)
7. Zhou, J., Chen, J., Ye, J.: Multi-task learning: theory, algorithms, and applications. SDM Tutor. (2012)
8. Chang, C.-C., Lin, C.-J.: LIBSVM: a library for support vector machines. ACM Trans. Intell. Syst. Technol. (TIST) **2**(3), 27 (2011)
9. Nie, F., Wang, X., Huang, H.: Multiclass capped p-Norm SVM for robust classifications. In: AAAI, pp. 2415–2417 (2017)
10. Friston, K.J.: Statistical parametric mapping (1994)
11. Zhang, D., Shen, D.: Multi-modal multi-task learning for joint prediction of multiple regression and classification variables in Alzheimer's disease. Neuroimage **59**(2), 895–907 (2012)
12. Lei, H., et al.: Joint detection and clinical score prediction in Parkinson's disease via multi-modal sparse learning. Expert Syst. Appl. **80**(1), 284–296 (2017)

Optic Disc Segmentation in Retinal Fundus Images Using Fully Convolutional Network and Removal of False-Positives Based on Shape Features

Sandip Sadhukhan[1]([✉]), Goutam Kumar Ghorai[1], Souvik Maiti[1], Vikrant Anilrao Karale[2], Gautam Sarkar[1], and Ashis Kumar Dhara[3]

[1] Jadavpur University, Kolkata 700032, WB, India
sansad@gmail.com
[2] Computer Vision Lab, IIT Kharagpur, Kharagpur 721302, India
[3] Dr. S P Mukherjee International Institute of Information Technology (IIIT Naya Raipur), Raipur 493661, Chattisgarh, India

Abstract. In today's world blindness is a major concern in working population and diseases like glaucoma, diabetic retinopathy are main causes for this. Early and fast detection using automated software system can be a great help in this area. For that one major step is to detect and segment the optic disc (OD) in retinal fundus image. In this paper we have used U-Net based fully convolutional network to segment OD. U-Net is a very efficient architecture in image segmentation particularly in the area where availability of input images are very less. We have first trained U-Net from scratch on the extended Messidor dataset. It is then evaluated using three-fold cross validation on MESSIDOR image dataset. During the process we have removed false positives based on morphological operation and shape features. We have seen this method has outperformed existing techniques in OD segmentation on the images affected by diabetic retinopathy.

Keywords: Retinal fundus image
Optic disc detection and segmentation · Fully convolutional network

1 Introduction

Throughout the world around 314 million people are suffering from Diabetic retinopathy, hypertensive retinopathy, glaucoma. These diseases gradually leads to vision loss of the patient which is a major area of concern in the developing counties [3]. Early identification and treatment can cure more than 85% visual impairments cases. In this field computer aided diagnosis system can make the process faster and assist ophthalmologists to cater more patients in less time.

Supported by organization x.

D. Stoyanov et al. (Eds.): DLMIA 2018/ML-CDS 2018, LNCS 11045, pp. 369–376, 2018.
https://doi.org/10.1007/978-3-030-00889-5_42

There are different approaches followed in identification and segmentation of Optic Disc (OD). Welfer *et al.* [21] identified the OD boundary using morphological operations and watershed transformation technique. Aquino *et al.* [2] segmented the OD using morphological operations, edge detection method and circular Hough transformation technique. Morales *et al.* [17] applied inpainting as preprocessing for removing blood vessels and stochastic watershed transformation for determining the OD boundary. Xu *et al.* [22] applied active contour model (ACM) and proved better segmentation. Lowell *et al.* [13] applied a direction sensitive gradient-based technique to remove the vessel obstructions and deformable ACM for finding the OD boundary in low resulotion images. Chrastek *et al.* [6] applied distance map algorithm to remove the blood vessels and then segmented the OD by using sequence of methods like morphological operation, Hough transformation and ACM. The method presented by Joshi *et al.* [11] improved the robustness of ACM proposed by Chan and Vese [4] by taking care of the variations in the OD region. Morales *et al.* [17] detected the boundary of optic disc by the principal component analysis.

To overcome all these types of shortcomings deep learning based algorithms are playing an important role because of its ability to learn features during training time. The success of convolutional neural network in object segmentation [5,7,18] has motivated us to investigate the performance of fully convolutioal network for optic disc detection and segmentation. The major contributions of the present work are (i) initial segmentation of optic disc using U-Net based fully convolutional network and (ii) removal of false-positives based on anatomy-aware features.

In this paper, Sect. 1 has covered the existing works in this area. Then we have described the proposed segmentation framework in Sect. 2. Experimental results and comparison of the proposed method with the state-of-the-art techniques is provided in Sect. 3. Conclusion and future scope of work is stated in Sect. 4.

2   Segmentation Framework

In our proposed method (Fig. 1) U-net [19] based fully convolutional network has been used for initial segmentation after preprocessing of the input images. Then false positives have been reduced using anatomy-aware features. The U-Net architecture is used for initial segmentation as it provides better segmentation using few number of training images.

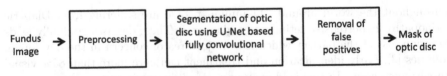

Fig. 1. Block diagram of the proposed segmentation framework

2.1 Preprocessing

First all the images are resized to 512 × 512 pixels. Then red channel image is threshold. Morphological opening, closing and erosion operations [8] with square structuring element are used to create a mask of circular retinal fundus region-of-interest, which allows focusing only on the foreground of retinal images.

2.2 Segmentation Using U-Net

Architecture of U-Net. The U-net [19] is a fully convolutional network which consists of convolution operation for down-sampling, max pooling, ReLU operation, concatenation and de-Convolution operation for up-sampling. The down-sampling path has 5 convolutional blocks and each block has two convolutional layers with a filter size of 3 × 3 and stride of 1. Max pooling with stride 2 is applied to the end of every blocks except the last block. The data is propagated through the network along all possible paths and generates the segmentation map at the end of the network. At the end input images of 512 × 512 size reduces to 32 × 32. The second part of the U-Net is the expansion layer which basically create the high resolution segmentation map. This part consists of a sequence of up-convolutions and concatenation with high-resolution features from contraction path. Therefore, the size of feature maps increases from 32 × 32 to 512 × 512. High-level information is represented at up-sampling blocks, and low-level features are transferred through skip connection.

Training of U-Net. First data augmentation techniques have been applied on the images of extended MESSIDOR database (MESSIDOR-II) [16] which is then used for training of U-Net from scratch. A stochastic gradient-based optimization [12] (*ADAM*) is applied to minimize the cross-entropy based cost function. The learning rate for the ADAM optimizer is set to 0.0001 and over-fitting is reduced by using dropout [10]. The weights of background and foreground are maintained as 1:10 and training were performed upto 60,000 iterations.

False Positive Removal. Morphological opening is applied to separate false positives from Optic disc. E.g., for Fig. 2(a), after initial segmentation Fig. 2(b) is showing some false positives caused by exudates. Compactness feature is used to eliminate false positive candidates from initial segmentation results which will create two objects. The object having bigger size is considered as optic disc Fig. 2(c).

3 Experimental Results and Discussions

3.1 Database Used for Evaluation of Segmentation Result

MESSIDOR. MESSIDOR [15] database contains 1200 colour retinal images, acquired using non-mydriatic camera, Topcon TRC NW6 with field-of-view set to 45°. Binary mask of the optic disc of MESSIDOR dataset was provided by the experts of the University of Huelva [1].

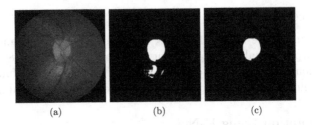

Fig. 2. (a) Original image (b) false positives caused by exudates (c) optic disc candidate.

3.2   Evaluation

The performance of optic disc detection is evaluated using Success Rate (SR) which represents the percentage of retinal images in a dataset where the centroid of optic disc is successfully localized within the boundary of the ground truth mask of optic disc. The performance of optic disc segmentation is evaluated in terms of Overlap Measure (OM) and Mean Absolute Distance (MAD) [20]. The OM represents the ratio of the intersecting area between the actual optic disc and segmented optic disc. MAD represents the mean of the shortest distances from the boundary of the actual optic disc to the boundary of the segmented optic disc.

3.3   Experimental Results

Quantitative Analysis. The evaluation of the proposed segmentation algorithm is performed on MESSIDOR datasets. During testing, we divided the images into three subsets. Out of three subsets, two are used for fine tuning of pre-trained network and remaining set is used for testing. Thus U-Net learns database specific features through transfer learning. The average value of SR, OM and MAD of the proposed framework and competing techniques are provided in Table 1. The OM of the proposed method is larger as compared to the competing techniques. Such improvement of OM is due to the application of fully convolutional network in initial segmentation.

There is only one failure case for optic disc detection for the MESSIDOR dataset. The MAD value of the proposed method is slightly better or comparable with the competing techniques. The high value of OM depict that the segmented mask of optic disc matches accurately with the ground truth mask. A comparison of segmentation performance in terms of percentage of test images included in various OM distributions, is provided in Table 2. The proposed method outperforms the competing techniques at all the four different OM levels such as $\geq$ 0.7, 0.75, 0.85 and 0.9.

Table 1. Comparative result of optic disc segmentation

Method	Author	OM	MAD	SR
MESSIDOR	Roychowdhury et al. [20]	0.84	3.9	100
	Marin et al. [14]	0.87	6.17	99.75
	Giachetti et al. [9]	0.88	-	99.83
	Aquino et al. [2]	0.86	-	98.83
	Yu et al. [23]	0.83	7.7	99.08
	Proposed	**0.91**	**1.97**	**99.92**

Table 2. Percentage of images in various OM levels

Method	Author	OM $\geq$ 0.7	OM $\geq$ 0.75	OM $\geq$ 0.85	OM $\geq$ 0.9
MESSIDOR	Roychowdhury et al. [20]	96.72	82.85	47.56	20
	Marin et al. [14]	95	-	83.75	48.92
	Giachetti et al. [9]	92–94	89–92	78–82	59–62
	Yu et al. [23]	77	77	45	25
	Aquino et al. [2]	93	90	73	46
	Proposed	**98.00**	**97.08**	**90.91**	**76.98**

Qualitative Results. We have analysed the proposed framework for images of healthy subjects [Fig. 3(a)–(c)], the images with the presence of pathologies [Fig. 4(a)–(c)], and low contrast [Fig. 4(b)]. These qualitative results reveal that the proposed algorithm is capable of identifying and segmenting the optic disc in bad quality retinal images. Few images with poor segmentation results is shown in Fig. 5(a)–(c). The poor segmentation is due to non-uniform illumination during image acquisition.

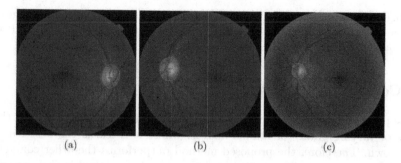

(a)   (b)   (c)

Fig. 3. Segmentation evaluation examples for normal fundus images. The contour of ground truth and segmented optic disc is shown in blue and green color respectively. (Color figure online)

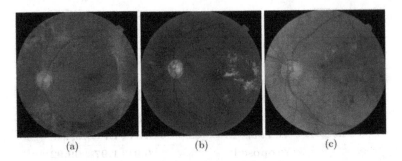

(a)   (b)   (c)

Fig. 4. Segmentation evaluation examples for images having pathologies,haemorrhage and low contrast. The contour of ground truth and segmented optic disc is shown in blue and green color respectively. (Color figure online)

3.4   Implementation

The U-Net architecture is implemented in Python using the PyTorch library in Linux environment using a 8 GB GPU (NVIDIA GeForce GTX 1070 with 8GB GDDR5 memory) on a system with Core-i7 processor and 32 GB RAM.

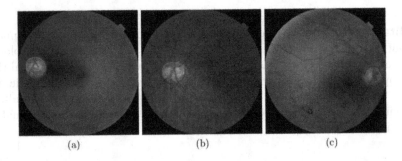

(a)   (b)   (c)

Fig. 5. Segmentation evaluation examples for some typical cases. The contour of ground truth and segmented optic disc is shown in blue and green color respectively. (Color figure online)

4   Conclusion

In the proposed method, fully convolutional network is trained by feeding thousands of varying grades of fundus images, where it is learns the best features on its own. Therefore, the proposed method outperforms the other competing techniques in most of the metrics measurements. The method is also successful in optic disc localization and segmentation, when tested on both dilated and non-dilated types of fundus images. The performance of this algorithm does not degrade while handling images containing strong distractors like yellowish exudates which prove the effectiveness and robustness of the proposed process. In future more research needs to be accomplished by testing on other independent datasets.

References

1. Expert system for early automated detection of DR by analysis of digital retinal images. http://www.uhu.es/retinopathy/muestr2as2.php
2. Aquino, A., Gegúndez-Arias, M.E., Marín, D.: Detecting the optic disc boundary in digital fundus images using morphological, edge detection, and feature extraction techniques. IEEE Trans. Med. Imaging 29(11), 1860–1869 (2010)
3. Bourne, R.R., et al.: Magnitude, temporal trends, and projections of the global prevalence of blindness and distance and near vision impairment: a systematic review and meta-analysis. Lancet Glob. Health 5(9), e888–e897 (2017)
4. Chan, T.F., Vese, L.A.: Active contours without edges. IEEE Trans. Image Process. 10(2), 266–277 (2001)
5. Chen, L.C., Papandreou, G., Kokkinos, I., Murphy, K., Yuille, A.L.: Deeplab: semantic image segmentation with deep convolutional nets, atrous convolution, and fully connected CRFS. arXiv preprint arXiv:1606.00915 (2016)
6. Chrstek, R., et al.: Med. Image Anal. Automated segmentation of the optic nerve head for diagnosis of glaucoma. 9(4), 297–314 (2005)
7. Cordts, M., et al.: The cityscapes dataset for semantic urban scene understanding. In: Proceedings of the IEEE Conference on Computer Vision and Pattern Recognition, pp. 3213–3223 (2016)
8. Gagnon, L., Lalonde, M., Beaulieu, M., Boucher, M.C.: Procedure to detect anatomical structures in optical fundus images. In: Medical Imaging 2001: Image Processing, vol. 4322, pp. 1218–1226. International Society for Optics and Photonics (2001)
9. Giachetti, A., Ballerini, L., Trucco, E.: Accurate and reliable segmentation of the optic disc in digital fundus images. J. Med. Imaging 1(2), 024001–024001 (2014)
10. Hinton, G.E., Srivastava, N., Krizhevsky, A., Sutskever, I., Salakhutdinov, R.R.: Improving neural networks by preventing co-adaptation of feature detectors. arXiv preprint arXiv:1207.0580 (2012)
11. Joshi, G.D., Sivaswamy, J., Krishnadas, S.: Optic disk and cup segmentation from monocular color retinal images for glaucoma assessment. IEEE Trans. Med. imaging 30(6), 1192–1205 (2011)
12. Kingma, D., Ba, J.: Adam: a method for stochastic optimization. arXiv preprint arXiv:1412.6980 (2014)
13. Lowell, J., et al.: Optic nerve head segmentation. IEEE Trans. Med. Imaging 23(2), 256–264 (2004)
14. Marin, D., Gegundez-Arias, M.E., Suero, A., Bravo, J.M.: Obtaining optic disc center and pixel region by automatic thresholding methods on morphologically processed fundus images. Comput. Methods Programs Biomed. 118(2), 173–185 (2015)
15. MESSIDOR: Messidor. digital retinal images, messidor techno-vision project, France. http://messidor.crihan.fr/download-en.php (download images section), May 2014
16. MESSIDOR-2: Messidor-2. digital retinal images, latim laboratory and the messidor program partners (2010). http://latim.univ-brest.fr/, http://messidor.crihan. fr/
17. Morales, S., Naranjo, V., Angulo, J., Alcañiz, M.: Automatic detection of optic disc based on pca and mathematical morphology. IEEE Trans. Med. Imaging 32(4), 786–796 (2013)

18. Papandreou, G., Kokkinos, I., Savalle, P.A.: Modeling local and global deformations in deep learning: epitomic convolution, multiple instance learning, and sliding window detection. In: 2015 IEEE Conference on Computer Vision and Pattern Recognition (CVPR), pp. 390–399. IEEE (2015)

19. Ronneberger, O., Fischer, P., Brox, T.: U-Net: convolutional networks for biomedical image segmentation. In: Navab, N., Hornegger, J., Wells, W.M., Frangi, A.F. (eds.) MICCAI 2015. LNCS, vol. 9351, pp. 234–241. Springer, Cham (2015). https://doi.org/10.1007/978-3-319-24574-4_28

20. Roychowdhury, S., Koozekanani, D.D., Kuchinka, S.N., Parhi, K.K.: Optic disc boundary and vessel origin segmentation of fundus images. IEEE J. Biomed. Health Inform. 20(6), 1562–1574 (2016)

21. Welfer, D., Scharcanski, J., Kitamura, C.M., Dal Pizzol, M.M., Ludwig, L.W., Marinho, D.R.: Segmentation of the optic disk in color eye fundus images using an adaptive morphological approach. Comput. Biol. Med. 40(2), 124–137 (2010)

22. Xu, C., Prince, J.L.: Snakes, shapes, and gradient vector flow. IEEE Trans. Image Process. 7(3), 359–369 (1998)

23. Yu, H., et al.: Fast localization and segmentation of optic disk in retinal images using directional matched filtering and level sets. IEEE Trans. Inf. Technol. Biomed. 16(4), 644–657 (2012)

Integrating Deformable Modeling with 3D Deep Neural Network Segmentation

Hui Tang, Mehdi Moradi[✉], Ken C. L. Wong, Hongzhi Wang,
Ahmed El Harouni, and Tanveer Syeda-Mahmood

IBM Research - Almaden Research Center, San Jose, USA
mmoradi@us.ibm.com

Abstract. Convolutional neural networks have advanced the state of
the art in medical image segmentation. However, there are two challenges in 3D deep learning segmentation networks. First, the segmentation masks from deep learning networks lack shape constraints, often
resulting in the need for post-processing. Second, the training and deployment of 3D networks require substantial memory resources. The memory
requirement becomes an issue especially when the target organs cover a
large footprint. Commonly down-sampling and up-sampling operations
are needed before and after the network. To address the post-processing
requirement, we present a new loss function that incorporates the level
set based smoothing loss together with multi Dice loss to avoid an additional post processing step. The formulation is general and can accommodate other deformable shape models. Further, we propose a way to
integrate the down- and up-sampling in the network such that the input
of the deep learning network can work directly on the original image
without a significant increase in the memory usage. The 3D segmentation
network with the proposed loss and sampling approach shows promising
results on a dataset of 48 chest CT angiography images with 16 target
anatomies. We obtained average Dice of 79.5% in 4 fold cross validation.

1 Introduction

Advances in deep learning segmentation methods have enabled faster 2D and
3D segmentation [1–3]. In these networks, compared to traditional methods,
high-level deeply learned features from a receptive field are used. Compared to
stacked 2D slice segmentation, 3D segmentation has a better chance of producing consistent and continuous object shapes. However, learning a 3D volume
neural network segmentation faces two challenges. First, each voxel is classified
using content from a receptive field with certain size but the overall shape of
the object is not taken into account. Therefore, a post processing step to further
refine the segmentation is usually needed. To address this problem, Kamnitasas
et al. [3] used fully connected conditional random fields (CRF) to refine brain
lesion segmentation in a post processing step. Lu et al. [4] used graph cut in the
post processing. Level set is also often used as a post processing step to refine

D. Stoyanov et al. (Eds.): DLMIA 2018/ML-CDS 2018, LNCS 11045, pp. 377–384, 2018.
https://doi.org/10.1007/978-3-030-00889-5_43

the segmentation output from deep learning networks [2,5,6]. In the deployment stage, the deep learning step takes milliseconds while the post processing step usually takes longer. Thus integrating the post processing step in the learning of the deep learning weights can further speed up and simplify the segmentation process in the deployment stage. Tang et al. [7] proposed a deep level set method for liver CT and left ventricle MRI segmentation. They use level set to refine an initial segmentation from a network trained with limited data, and then backpropagate the loss between the refined segmentation and the deep learning output. However, their method does not have an explicit mathematical formulation of the integration. Hu et al. [8] proposed a framework to let the network learn a levelset function for objects instead of a probability map. However, their levelset function is obtained by directly substracting 0.5 from the probability map, which is different from the commonly used signed distance transform method.

Second, 3D volume segmentation requires significant memory becuase of the huge number of weights learned. Constrained by the memory limit, usually small volumes, either from downsampling of the original image or smaller cropped regions are fed into a deep learning network. Milletari et al. [1] and Çiçek, et al. [9] downsampled the original image before feeding into the network and upsampled it back. However, this downsampling method results in lost information. Besides downsampling, Gibson et al. [2] also used batch-wise spatial dropout and Monte Carlo inference to reduce memory costs without affecting performance. Memory usage can also be reduced if fewer kernels in each layer or fewer layers are used in the network. However, reducing the number of kernels will reduce the number of learned latent features and increase the risk of getting a biased network. Reducing the number of layers will shorten the network depth and thus result in a smaller receptive field and lose part of the neighborhood information.

In this paper, our contribution focuses on addressing these two challenges. For the first challenge, we propose a novel way to integrate a level set energy function into Dice based loss. We show that the new proposed loss can drive the learning of the network weights such that the segmentation output of the network has the smooth property defined by a level set energy function. This smoothing energy is propagated back into the network to train a set of weights that can output a smoother segmentation. For the second challenge, our strategy of processing large volumes is integrating downsampling and upsampling into the network to process a larger volume. We evaluate the proposed method in 48 chest CTA datasets where 16 anatomies are manually segmented. We demonstrate the efficiency of integrating post processing into deep learning network while reducing the processing time for a volume to millisecond.

2   Method

We first propose the framework of integrating the surface smoothing into deep learning training, followed by a modified segmentation network that handles large volumes by adding very few parameters to the network.

2.1 Integrating Level Set Energy into Network Loss Function

The softmax output of a segmentation network is bounded between 0 and 1. As such, the n_{th} output can be treated as a Heaviside function $H^n(\mathbf{x})$ of a latent surface S and its corresponding level set embedding function $\phi^n(\mathbf{x})$ can be obtained using signed distance transform. From a given $\phi^n(\mathbf{x})$, the corresponding Heaviside function is approximated as $H^n(\mathbf{x}) = \frac{1}{2}(1 + \frac{2}{\pi} arctan(\frac{\phi^n(\mathbf{x})}{\epsilon}))$.

In level set representation, smoothing a surface is equal to evolving its corresponding embedding function. Thus the level set loss used for smoothing a surface is defined as:

$$E(\phi^n(\mathbf{x})) = \int_\Omega \delta(\phi^n(\mathbf{x})) \times |\nabla\phi^n(\mathbf{x})|d\mathbf{x} \tag{1}$$

where Ω is the volume inside the surface S. $\mathbf{x}$ is the voxel index. $\delta^n(\mathbf{x})$ is the gradient of $H^n(\mathbf{x})$ with regard to $\mathbf{x}$, and is equal to $\frac{\epsilon}{\pi(\epsilon^2 + \phi^n(\mathbf{x})^2)}$.

Different types of loss, such as cross entropy loss, Dice based loss for binary segmentation [1], or probabilistic Dice scores [2] were proposed to train a segmentation network. We took multi Dice, which is the sum of Dice for different organs as an example in this paper to integrate with level set based surface energy.

Using $H(\mathbf{x})$ to denote the group of $H^n(\mathbf{x})$ for all anatomies, the overall loss to minimize can be written as:

$$E(H(\mathbf{x})) = E_1(H(\mathbf{x})) + E_2(H(\mathbf{x})) \tag{2}$$

$$= -\sum_{n=0}^{N} Dice(H^n(\mathbf{x}), g^n(\mathbf{x})) + \sum_{n=0}^{N} w_n \times \int_\Omega \delta(\phi^n(\mathbf{x})) \times |\nabla\phi^n(\mathbf{x})|d\mathbf{x}$$

where E_1 is the multi Dice based loss and E_2 is the level set based loss. The level set based loss is defined to be the overall area of the segmentation surface for the n_{th} anatomy. $g^n(\mathbf{x})$ is the ground truth binary mask of the n_{th} anatomy, w_n is the weight used for different anatomies. N is the number of anatomies.

For back propagation, we need to compute the gradient of the loss with respect to the network prediction $H^n(\mathbf{x})$:

$$\frac{\partial E(H(\mathbf{x}))}{\partial H^n(\mathbf{x})} = \frac{\partial E_1(H(\mathbf{x}))}{\partial H^n(\mathbf{x})} + w_n \times \frac{\partial E_2(H(\mathbf{x}))}{\partial H^n(\mathbf{x})} \tag{3}$$

in which the first part can be calculated as:

$$\frac{\partial E_1(H(\mathbf{x}))}{\partial H^n(\mathbf{x})} = 2\left(\frac{g_j^n(\mathbf{x})(\sum_i^I H_i^n(\mathbf{x})^2 + \sum_i^I g_i^n(\mathbf{x})^2) - 2H_j^n(x)\sum_i^I H_i^n(\mathbf{x})g_i^n(\mathbf{x})}{(\sum_i^I H_i^n(\mathbf{x})^2 + \sum_i^I g_i^n(\mathbf{x})^2)^2}\right) \tag{4}$$

where i and j are voxel indices. The second term can be calculated as:

$$\frac{\partial E_2(H(\mathbf{x}))}{\partial H^n(\mathbf{x})} = \frac{\partial E_2(H(\mathbf{x}))}{\partial \phi^n(\mathbf{x})} \times \frac{\partial \phi^n(\mathbf{x})}{\partial H^n(\mathbf{x})} \tag{5}$$

where $\frac{\partial\phi^n(\mathbf{x})}{\partial H^n(\mathbf{x})}$ is difficult to be solved analytically, so we approximate it as $\frac{\triangle\phi^n(\mathbf{x})}{H^n(\phi^n(\mathbf{x})+\triangle\phi^n(\mathbf{x}))-H^n(\phi^n(\mathbf{x}))}$. The gradient of $E_2(H(\mathbf{x}))$ with respect to $\phi^n(\mathbf{x})$ is given as [10]:

$$\frac{\partial E_2(H(\mathbf{x}))}{\partial\phi^n(\mathbf{x})} = \delta(\phi^n(\mathbf{x}) \times div(\frac{\nabla\phi^n(\mathbf{x})}{|\nabla\phi^n(\mathbf{x})|}) \tag{6}$$

$div(\frac{\nabla\phi^n(\mathbf{x})}{|\nabla\phi^n(\mathbf{x})|})$ is the mean curvature of a surface. Equation 6 evolves $\phi^n(\mathbf{x})$ by the surface curvature in the direction of the surface norm, which will result in a smoother surface. The sign of the curvature determines whether a point on the surface should move inward or forward in the direction of surface normal.

2.2 Segmentation Network Architecture

Inspired by image guided filtering [11], which uses an additional image to guide the filtering of a target image, we propose the architecture in Fig. 1 to use the raw image to guide the upsampling of the low resolution segmentation maps.

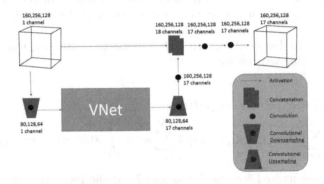

Fig. 1. The network architecture modifies VNet to integrate downsampling and upsampling procedures with additional layers with few parameters.

The raw image is first downsampled with ONE kernal downsampling convolution (this can be replaced by average pooling), and the downsampled image is fed to VNet [1]. We replace the last softmax layer in standard VNet with PRelu layer. The raw image is then upsampled by a deconvolution layer with the number of channels preserved, which is equivalent to the number of anatomies + background. The deconvolution layer can be replaced by a bilinear resampling layer and a convolution layer. The deconvolution output is then concatenated with the raw image in the channel dimension, followed by two convolution and activation layers. The downsampling and upsampling added only 31698 weights when the number of anatomies n equals 16 ($3 \times 3 \times 3$ for the downsampling convolution layer, $(n+1) \times 3 \times 3 \times 2 \times (n+1)$ for the deconvolution layer and the followed convolution layer, as well as

$(n+2) \times 3 \times 3 \times 3 \times (n+1) + (n+1) \times 3 \times 3 \times 3 \times (n+1)$ for the last two convolution layers), this number can be reduced to 513 for a binary segmentation. Thus, most of the computation stays inside the VNet architecture whose input size is half the original input size in each dimension. This allows the processing of a large image without adding much to memory cost.

2.3 Implementation Details

This method is implemented in Caffe and runs on one TITAN X GPU with 12 GB of memory. The proposed architecture is first trained using multi Dice loss for 300 epochs until it converges. And then we continue training using the proposed loss which integrates the level set smoothing energy for 15 epochs. Since we have anatomies with naturally different surface curvature, we also set different smoothing weights for different anatomies. For the vertebrae, the myocardium and the left ventricle, we set the weights to be 1e–5, while for others we use weight of 1e–4.

3 Experiments and Results

3.1 Data

We collect 48 cardiac CTA images annotated for 16 anatomical structures by one annotator. The 16 anatomies are: sternum, ascending aorta, descending aorta, aortic arch, aortic root, left pulmonary artery, right pulmonary artery, trunk pulmonary artery, vertebrae, left atrium, right atrium, left ventricle, right ventricle, left ventricular myocardium, superior vena cava, and inferior vena cava similar to [12]. The cardiac CT studies used here were acquired by a Siemens CT scanner. All images have voxel size of 1.5 mm in all directions.

3.2 Results

For the first stage of training which does not have the level set integrated loss, we obtain average Dice of 79.3% for 4-fold cross validation. After continued training with level set based smoothing energy, we obtain Dice of 79.5%. We must specify that the sole expert that provided the ground truth segmentation was not asked to target smoothness, thus adding the smoothing term does not necessarily improve Dice coefficient. But we can visually observe a smoother segmentation. Figure 2 shows two superior vena cava segmentation outputs generated from two trained models with and without level set smoothing energy. We see that some false positives due to image noise and lack of shape information are removed because of their high curvature property.

As a qualitative way of understating the effects of the new loss function on smoothing the structures, consider the case of spine as illustrated in Fig. 3. The progressively smooth volume after epochs 8 and 15 are visible. To better visualize the smoothing effect, we use a large weight (1e–4) in this example only for demonstration. When applying this method to other applications, the number of training epochs and the weight w_n should be tuned as hyper parameters.

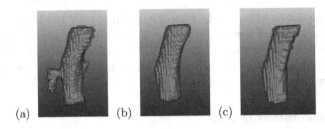

Fig. 2. Effect of adding a level set smoothing term in the loss for smoothing surfaces: (a) trained with multi Dice loss, (b) trained with the proposed loss which integrates level set smoothing energy, (c) ground truth segmentation

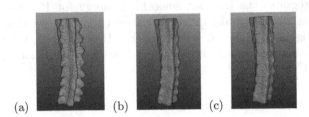

Fig. 3. Effect of adding a level set smoothing term in the loss for smoothing surfaces, (a) without smoothing, (b) smoothing effect after 8 epochs, (c) smoothing effect after 15 epochs.

3.3   Performance Comparison

We compared our results with the state of the art multi atlas based segmentation method followed by corrective learning as post processing [12]. Figure 4 shows the bar plot comparing Dice per anatomy for five different methods: the multi atlas based method, the standard VNet which takes resampled volumes, the standard VNet followed by a level set smoothing step as post processing, the proposed modified VNet architecture trained by multi Dice loss, and the proposed modified VNet architecture trained by our proposed loss. For the standard VNet, due to the memory limit, the input was downsample with voxel size of 2 mm × 2 mm × 3.5 mm and volume size of 128 × 192 × 64.

From Fig. 4, we can see that the deep learning method is comparable to the state of the art multi atlas based segmentation. The proposed modified VNet architecture trained with the proposed loss performs the best among the deep learning methods. For small anatomies such as aortic root, left pulmonary artery and superior vena cava, we get a larger boost in the performance than large anatomies. We show the summary of the comparisons in Table 1. An example of the segmented volume compared to the ground truth is shown in Fig. 5.

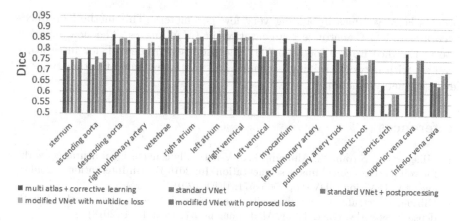

Fig. 4. Results compared to using original VNet and state of the art multi atlas based segmentation from [12]

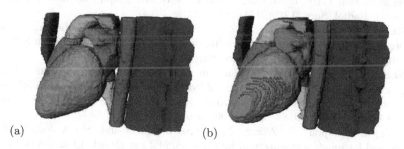

Fig. 5. Example of segmented anatomies (a) results from weights trained with 10 epochs using the proposed loss, (b) ground truth.

Table 1. Summary of performance of different methods. Method 1: multi atlas method followed by corrective learning. Method 2: standard VNet. Method 3: standard VNet + post processing. Method 4: modified VNet trained with multi dice loss. Method 5: modified VNet trained with proposed loss which integrates the level set smoothing energy.

	Method 1	Method 2	Method 3	Method 4	Method 5
Mean	0.816	0.744	0.766	0.793	0.795
Std	0.076	0.088	0.090	0.081	0.073

4   Conclusion

In this paper, we propose a new loss function to integrate the level set smoothing energy into multi Dice loss to eliminate an additional post processing step. We also propose a new strategy for designing segmentation architectures that can process large volumes by adding very few parameters. This method produces accurate and fast anatomic segmentation in CTA images. The new network boosts the dice from 0.766 to 0.795. The proposed framework for integrating level set with network training is general and can be extended to other types of level set energy functions.

References

1. Milletari, F., Navab, N., Ahmadi, S.A.: V-net: fully convolutional neural networks for volumetric medical image segmentation. In: 2016 Fourth International Conference on 3D Vision (3DV), pp. 565–571. IEEE (2016)
2. Gibson, E., et al.: Automatic multi-organ segmentation on abdominal CT with dense v-networks. IEEE Trans. Med. Imaging **37**, 1822–1834 (2018)
3. Kamnitsas, K., et al.: Efficient multi-scale 3D CNN with fully connected CRF for accurate brain lesion segmentation. Med. Image Anal. **36**, 61–78 (2017)
4. Lu, F., Wu, F., Hu, P., Peng, Z., Kong, D.: Automatic 3D liver location and segmentation via convolutional neural network and graph cut. Int. J. Comput. Assist. Radiol. Surg. **12**(2), 171–182 (2017)
5. Hu, P., Wu, F., Peng, J., Bao, Y., Chen, F., Kong, D.: Automatic abdominal multi-organ segmentation using deep convolutional neural network and time-implicit level sets. Int. J. Comput. Assist. Radiol. Surg. **12**(3), 399–411 (2017)
6. Veni, G., Moradi, M., Bulu, H., Narayan, G., Syeda-Mahmood, T.: Echocardiography segmentation based on a shape-guided deformable model driven by a fully convolutional network prior. In: 2018 IEEE 15th International Symposium on Biomedical Imaging (ISBI 2018), pp. 898–902, April 2018
7. Tang, M., Valipour, S., Zhang, Z., Cobzas, D., Jagersand, M.: A deep level set method for image segmentation. In: Cardoso, M.J., et al. (eds.) DLMIA/ML-CDS -2017. LNCS, vol. 10553, pp. 126–134. Springer, Cham (2017). https://doi.org/10. 1007/978-3-319-67558-9_15
8. Hu, P., Shuai, B., Liu, J., Wang, G.: Deep level sets for salient object detection. In: IEEE CVPR (2017)
9. Çiçek, Ö., Abdulkadir, A., Lienkamp, S.S., Brox, T., Ronneberger, O.: 3D U-Net: learning dense volumetric segmentation from sparse annotation. In: Ourselin, S., Joskowicz, L., Sabuncu, M.R., Unal, G., Wells, W. (eds.) MICCAI 2016. LNCS, vol. 9901, pp. 424–432. Springer, Cham (2016). https://doi.org/10.1007/978-3-319-46723-8_49
10. Osher, S., Sethian, J.A.: Fronts propagating with curvature-dependent speed: algorithms based on Hamilton-Jacobi formulations. J. Comput. Phy. **79**(1), 12–49 (1988)
11. He, K., Sun, J., Tang, X.: Guided image filtering. In: Daniilidis, K., Maragos, P., Paragios, N. (eds.) ECCV 2010. LNCS, vol. 6311, pp. 1–14. Springer, Heidelberg (2010). https://doi.org/10.1007/978-3-642-15549-9_1
12. Wang, H., Prasanna, P., Syeda-Mahmood, T.: Fast anatomy segmentation by combining low resolution multi-atlas label fusion with high resolution corrective learning: an experimental study. In: 2017 IEEE 14th International Symposium on Biomedical Imaging (ISBI 2017), pp. 223–226. IEEE (2017)

Correction to: Unpaired Deep Cross-Modality Synthesis with Fast Training

Lei Xiang, Yang Li, Weili Lin, Qian Wang, and Dinggang Shen

Correction to:
Chapter "Unpaired Deep Cross-Modality Synthesis with Fast Training" in: D. Stoyanov et al. (Eds.): *Deep Learning in Medical Image Analysis and Multimodal Learning for Clinical Decision Support*, **LNCS 11045, https://doi.org/10.1007/978-3-030-00889-5_18**

In the originally published version of this chapter, the Acknowledgements section was missing. This has been corrected and an Acknowledgements section has been added.

The updated version of this chapter can be found at
https://doi.org/10.1007/978-3-030-00889-5_18

Author Index

Printed in the United States
By Bookmasters